Clinical Anesthesia

Clinical Anesthesia

Edited by Mercy Rogers

STATES
ACADEMIC PRESS
www.statesacademicpress.com

States Academic Press,
109 South 5th Street,
Brooklyn, NY 11249, USA

Visit us on the World Wide Web at:
www.statesacademicpress.com

ISBN: 978-1-63989-782-7

Cataloging-in-Publication Data

Clinical anesthesia / edited by Mercy Rogers.
p. cm.
Includes bibliographical references and index.
ISBN 978-1-63989-782-7
1. Anesthesiology. 2. Anesthesia. I. Rogers, Mercy.
RD81 .H36 2023
617.96--dc23

Table of Contents

Preface

This book has been a concerted effort by a group of academicians, researchers and scientists, who have contributed their research works for the realization of the book. This book has materialized in the wake of emerging advancements and innovations in this field. Therefore, the need of the hour was to compile all the required researches and disseminate the knowledge to a broad spectrum of people comprising of students, researchers and specialists of the field.

Anesthesia is a state of temporarily induced loss of awareness or sensation to primarily achieve hypnosis, analgesia and muscle relaxation. There are varied drugs used for anesthesia such as general anesthetics, analgesics, neuromuscular-blocking drugs, etc. These drugs affect interconnected parts of the nervous system. Anesthesia is not a treatment on its own, but it facilitates other types of treatments, which would be too painful for the patient otherwise. An important stage of anesthesia is risk assessment, which is crucial for reducing anesthetic risks. It is a pre-operative procedure that covers the medical history, physical examination and lab tests, and obtains information about any medical conditions or genetic disorders that might afflict the patient. The various advancements in clinical anesthesia are glanced at in this book and their applications as well as ramifications are looked at in detail. It includes contributions of experts and scientists, which will provide innovative insights into the study of anesthesia. Researchers and students engaged in the study of anesthesia will be assisted by this book.

At the end of the preface, I would like to thank the authors for their brilliant chapters and the publisher for guiding us all-through the making of the book till its final stage. Also, I would like to thank my family for providing the support and encouragement throughout my academic career and research projects.

Editor

1

Regional anaesthesia is associated with less patient satisfaction compared to general anaesthesia following distal upper extremity surgery

Wouter Droog[1*], Sanne E. Hoeks[1], G. Peter van Aggelen[2], D-Yin Lin[1], J. Henk Coert[3], Robert Jan Stolker[1] and Eilish M. Galvin[1]

Abstract

Background: Patient satisfaction is a well-established indicator to evaluate the quality of medical care and there is an increasing support for the use of patient-reported experience measures (PREMs) to evaluate satisfaction. To anesthetize the upper limb for surgery, both general and regional plexus anaesthesia are appropriate techniques. However, the best technique in the anaesthesiologist's perspective might not necessarily result in the highest patient satisfaction. The aim of this study is to investigate patient satisfaction following general and regional anaesthesia, and to identify areas where anaesthesiologists can focus on improving patient care.

Methods: Patients scheduled for elective distal upper extremity surgery under either general or regional plexus anaesthesia were prospectively included. On the first postoperative day, patient satisfaction and main reason for dissatisfaction with the anaesthesia technique were investigated during a telephone interview.

Results: Of the 243 patients included in the current study, 79.8% report being "fully satisfied" with their anaesthesia technique. 32.1% of the patients who received regional anaesthesia reported not feeling "fully satisfied". This figure is 5.5% following general anaesthesia. Main reason for dissatisfaction following regional anaesthesia are reported as "insufficient anaesthesia prior to surgery", and "the discomfort of having a long-lasting insensate extremity postoperatively".

Conclusions: Following regional plexus anaesthesia, a third of the patients are not "fully satisfied". To optimize patient satisfaction following regional anaesthesia techniques, we advocate stronger focus on patient counselling preoperatively, addressing the issues of block failure and prolonged postoperative sensory and motor block.

Keywords: Patient satisfaction, Anaesthesia, conduction, Anaesthesia, general, Patient care

* Correspondence: w.droog@erasmusmc.nl
[1]Department of Anaesthesia, Erasmus University Medical Centre Rotterdam, P.O. Box 2040, 3000, CA, Rotterdam, The Netherlands

Background

Patient satisfaction is a well-established indicator to evaluate the quality of medical care and it is an important tool for prompting improvements in clinical care [1–3]. There is increasing support for the use of patient-reported experience measures (PREMs) and The American Society of Anesthesiologists (ASA) recognizes the importance of assessing patient satisfaction and experience [4]. In general, patient satisfaction with anaesthesia care is reported as very high [3, 5], but during times of rising patient expectations, areas for potential improvement are worthy of investigation.

For distal upper extremity surgery a variety of anaesthetic techniques are available to anesthetize the upper limb; general anaesthesia and regional (plexus) blocks are commonly applied techniques. Both techniques have their advantages and disadvantages, and the choice of technique largely depends on the planned surgery and patient's overall health status and preferences. The anaesthesiologist is faced with the task of choosing the "best" anaesthesia technique for an individual patient. In clinical practice however, the best technique in anaesthesiologist's perspective, might not necessarily result in the highest patient satisfaction. Therefore, the aim of the current study is to investigate patient satisfaction following both general and regional plexus anaesthesia. The secondary aim of this study is to identify areas for clinical practice improvement.

Methods

This study was carried out by the Departments of Anaesthesia and Plastic Surgery of two hospitals; a large university hospital and a smaller teaching hospital. The study formed part of a prospective study on nerve injury following distal upper extremity surgery including a total of 335 patients. For this analysis on patient satisfaction following general and regional plexus anaesthesia, we only included those patients scheduled for elective upper extremity surgery under these two anaesthesia techniques. We excluded patients operated under other forms of anaesthesia techniques, such as Bier block or distal individual nerve blocks, and those with a planned combination of general and regional anaesthesia. All patients included gave written informed consent and were 18 years and older. The local Medical Ethics Committee of both hospitals reviewed and approved this study (October 11, 2012, number 2012–327).

Preoperatively

All patients scheduled for elective upper extremity surgery were referred to the anaesthesia outpatient clinic by the treating plastic hand surgeon. Structured history-taking and clinical examination was used to evaluate overall health status. The choice between general or regional anaesthesia for the planned surgery was made on the basis of patient factors, patient preferences, and the planned procedure. Patients were verbally informed about the planned anaesthetic technique and possible complications. If patients were medically suitable candidates for both regional and general anaesthesia, they were informed on both techniques and in shared discussion the actual technique was chosen. All patients agreed on the proposed anaesthesia technique.

Intraoperatively

Data on the anaesthetic technique and medication used were collected using the computerized Hospital Information System. The technical performance of the anaesthesia technique and medication used was at the discretion of the treating anaesthesiologist. The same applies for the use of ultrasound, nerve stimulator, needle type and diameter, and other equipment necessary for the regional block performance. Regional plexus blocks were performed using ropivacaine 7.5 mg/mL, mepivacaine 2 mg/mL, lidocaine 10 mg/mL, prilocaine 10 mg/mL or a combination of these agents. Dose (mg/kg) and volume (mL) of local anaesthetic used, was determined by the treating physician. Analgesia and sedation used during performance of regional anaesthesia or during surgery, consisted of one or a combination of alfentanil, sufentanil, propofol, and midazolam. Targeted sedation level during block performance was Ramsay sedation scale level 2, which means that patients are cooperative, orientated and tranquil [6].

All patients were scheduled for day-care surgery and all patients were expected to be discharged on the day of surgery. Before discharge home, patients had to meet local post-operative discharge criteria for day-care surgery. These criteria include: stable vital signs, proper orientation, able to drink/eat/void/dress/walk (without assistance), minimal nausea/vomiting/pain, and the presence of an adult escort home. In all patients, postoperative medication included acetaminophen plus a nonsteroidal anti-inflammatory drugs and/or opioids (tramadol or oxycodone).

Postoperatively

On the first postoperative day, all patients received a telephone call from a nurse from the hospital ward, assessing postoperative pain scores, patient satisfaction, and main reason for dissatisfaction. The day-one postoperative questionnaire used in this study was developed by the research team (Appendix). Before analysis of the data, main reasons for dissatisfaction were clustered. The nurse was not affiliated with the anaesthesia department and was not aware of the anaesthesia technique.

Outcome

Satisfaction was measured on a three-point Likert rating scale, by asking patients to rate if they were "fully satisfied", "partly satisfied", or "dissatisfied" with their anaesthesia technique. A three-point scale was used to simplify identification of patients who were dissatisfied and those who were not. Comparable reasons for patient dissatisfaction were clustered into groups. Postoperative pain was measured using the Numeric Rating Scale (NRS). The NRS is a verbally administered 11-point numeric rating scale, on which a patient can report pain intensity ranging from 0 ("no pain") to 10 ("worst pain imaginable") [7]. All scores of four or higher were considered abnormal. All scores under four were labelled as "pain level acceptable to the patient".

Statistical analysis

Statistical analysis was performed using SPSS 25.0 (IBM Corporation, Armonk, NY, USA). Continuous variables were tested for normality of the distribution and were presented as mean (± SD) or median (+ IQR). Kruskal-Wallis and Mann-Whitney U tests were used for continuous variables. For categorical variables the Fisher's exact test was used. A *P*-value of 0.05 or less was considered to be statistically significant.

Results

A total of 335 patients scheduled for elective upper extremity surgery were consecutively screened and asked to participate in the study. After excluding the patients that did not meet the inclusion criteria for the current analysis ($n = 77$), and patients who were not contactable day 1 post surgery ($n = 15$), a total of 243 patents were investigated. Of these 243 patients 134 received regional and 109 general anaesthesia prior to surgery.

Patient and surgical characteristics, pain-scores (NRS), and patient satisfaction scores are summarized in Table 1. Details on anaesthesia technique and patient satisfaction are shown in Table 2.

One hundred ninety-four patients of a total of 243 patients (79.8%) reported being "fully satisfied" with their anaesthesia technique (Table 1). 36 patients are "partly satisfied" (14.8%), and 13 patients (5.3%) are "dissatisfied" with their anaesthesia technique (Table 1). There is no difference in satisfaction scores comparing for gender, age, BMI, or ASA-classification (Table 1). Median pain scores are statistically significantly higher in patients who are "dissatisfied" in comparison to patients who are "partly satisfied" or "fully satisfied" in both groups (Table 1). Median preoperative pain scores are 3 (0 – 6) and 4 (0 – 7) in the general and regional anaesthesia group respectively (Table 3). Median postoperative pain scores are 3 (1–5) and 4 (1–7) following general or regional anaesthesia respectively (Table 3). There is no statistically significant difference in median pre- and postoperative pain scores between the general and regional anaesthesia group (Table 3).

Patients following regional anaesthesia have lower levels of being "fully satisfied" with their anaesthesia technique than those following general anaesthesia (Table 2). Of the total of 134 patients who received regional anaesthesia as the primary anaesthesia technique, 43 patients (32.1%) are not "fully satisfied" versus 6 patients of a total of 109 (5.5%) general anaesthesia patients (Table 2). Due to insufficient anaesthesia prior to surgery, conversion from regional to general anaesthesia occurred in 17 of the 134 patients (13%) and additional or rescue blocks were performed in 12 of the 134 patients (9%).

Main reasons for dissatisfaction with regional anaesthesia in this study are: insufficient anaesthesia prior to surgery, and patient's discomfort with their insensate and uncontrollable extremity postoperatively (Table 4). 14 patients do not reveal details on their reason for dissatisfaction (Table 4). In the 134 patients who received regional plexus anaesthesia, medication (sedatives/analgesics) administered during block placement procedure did not result in more patients being "fully satisfied" (Table 2).

Discussion

In the current study, 79.8% of the 243 participants report being "fully satisfied" with the anaesthetic technique used during their surgery. Previous research shows that satisfaction with all aspects of health care is high (> 85%), and satisfaction with the anaesthetic care provided is often even higher (up to 96.8%) [3, 5]. Compared to these findings, patients in the current study are less frequently "fully satisfied". This can partly be explained by the fact that the current study focuses specifically on anaesthesia technique used, as supposed to others who have focussed on quality of recovery after anaesthesia [3, 5]. Patient characteristics commonly associated with high satisfaction scores are: older age, male gender, and co-existing medical conditions (or ASA-class ≥ 3) [3, 5, 8, 9]. These patient characteristics are of no influence on satisfaction scores in the current study.

Patients following regional anaesthesia have significantly lower levels of being "fully satisfied" in comparison to those following general anaesthesia. Following regional anaesthesia, 32.1% of the patients are not "fully satisfied" versus only 5.5% following general anaesthesia. Further evaluation of those patients who are not "fully satisfied" with their anaesthesia technique reveals two frequently reported complaints. Firstly, a feeling of insufficient anaesthesia prior to surgery. Obviously this is a reason for dissatisfaction; patients assume a fully working regional block, as this was communicated during the outpatient visit. Unfortunately, in 28 patients receiving regional anaesthesia,

Table 1 Patient and Surgical Characteristics and Satisfaction Scores

	Total	Fully Satisfied	Partly Satisfied	Dissatisfied	*P*-value
Total	243	194 (79.8%)	36 (14.8%)	13 (5.3%)	
Gender					0.425
Female (*n*)	131	101	23	7	
Male (*n*)	112	93	13	6	
Age (yrs.)[a]					0.482
median	52.0	52.5	49.5	47.9	
(IQR)	(36.6–61.8)	(37.8–62.9)	(32.5–58.0)	(41.9–57.8)	
BMI (kg/m^2)[a]					0.693
median	24.9	24.9	24.9	22.9	
(IQR)	(23.0–27.4)	(23.4–27.5)	(22.9–26.9)	(21.5–29.8)	
ASA-classification[b]					0.902
ASA 1 (*n*)	116	92	17	7	
ASA 2 (*n*)	118	95	18	5	
ASA 3 (*n*)	9	7	1	1	
NRS-Score[a]					
median	3	3	5	7	0.011
(IQR)	(1–6)	(1–6)	(1.25–7)	(2–8.5)	
NRS $\geq$ 4	118	88	22	8	0.139
NRS < 4	125	106	14	5	
Type of Surgery[c]					
Arthrodesis/arthroplasty (*n*)	37	27	4	6	
Carpal Tunnel Syndrome (*n*)	8	8	0	0	
Cubital Tunnel Syndrome (*n*)	2	1	0	1	
Dupuytren's contracture (*n*)	57	48	7	2	
Finger-joint replacement (*n*)	1	1	0	0	
Ganglion cyst removal (*n*)	5	3	2	0	
Ligament repair surgery (*n*)	8	7	1	0	
Neuroma excision (*n*)	3	3	0	0	
Placement of osteosynthesis material (*n*)	4	4	0	0	
Proximal row carpectomy (*n*)	3	1	2	0	
Quervain's release surgery (*n*)	3	2	1	0	
Removal of osteosynthesis material (*n*)	7	5	2	0	
Tendon repair surgery (*n*)	13	11	2	0	
Tenolysis (*n*)	5	4	1	0	
Trigger finger release (n)	2	2	0	0	
Ulnar nerve transposition (*n*)	9	8	1	0	
Wrist arthroscopy (*n*)	21	12	8	1	
Miscellaneous (*n*)	55	47	5	3	
Tourniquet use[c]					
Yes (*n*)	235	186	36	13	
No (*n*)	8	8	0	0	
Duration of Tourniquet use (minutes)					
median	46.5	45	50	46	0.875
(IQR)	(30–65)	(30–65)	(31–61)	(37.5–64.5)	

[a]*Age, BMI and NRS-Score are not normally distributed and therefore presented as 'median (IQR)'*
[b]*ASA-classification (class 1–6), according to The American Society of Anesthesiologists (ASA) physical status classification system*
[c]*Due to the small numbers in some cells, no statistical analyses was performed on type of surgery details*

Table 2 Anaesthesia Characteristics and Satisfaction Scores

	Total	Fully Satisfied	Partly Satisfied	Dissatisfied	*P*-value
Total	243	194 (79.8%)	36 (14.8%)	13 (5.3%)	
Type of Anaesthesia					< 0.001
General Anaesthesia	109	103	5	1	
Regional Anaesthesia[a]	134	91	31	12	
Adjuvants used during regional anaesthesia procedure[b]	134	91	31	12	
Nerve Stimulator	12	7	4	1	
Ultrasound	29	20	5	4	
Nerve Stimulator & Ultrasound	93	64	22	7	
Local anaesthetic used during regional anaesthesia procedure[b]	134	91	31	12	
Ropivacaine (7.5 mg/mL)	116	78	29	9	
Mepivacaine (2 mg/mL)	7	5	1	1	
Mix of Ropivacaine and Mepivacaine	6	6	0	0	
Other[c]	5	2	1	2	
Medication during regional anaesthesia procedure	134	91	31	12	0.392
Yes	81	52	22	7	
No	53	39	9	5	
Medication administered during surgical procedure [d]	117	84	26	7	0.018
Yes	33	19	13	1	
No	84	65	13	6	

[a]Regional Anaesthesia Details (n = 134): Pippa Block 1, Interscalene Brachial Plexus Block 3, Supraclavicular Brachial Plexus Block 18, Axillary Block 112
[b]Due to the small numbers in some cells, no statistical analyses was performed on these regional anaesthesia details
[c]Other local anaesthetics used were: Prilocaine (10 mg/mL), Lidocaine (10 mg/ml) or a mix of Lidocaine and Ropivacaine
[d]Medication during procedure was only administered in the 117 patients receiving regional anaesthesia alone, without the 17 patients who received general anaesthesia due to insufficient regional anaesthesia

additional (rescue) blocks or conversion to general anaesthesia was needed.

The second most common reason given for lower satisfaction is patient's discomfort with their insensate and uncontrollable extremity postoperatively. Prolonged postoperative analgesia is a frequently referenced as a major advantage of regional anaesthesia over general anaesthesia [10]. However, in the current study, the prolonged postoperative anaesthesia is a reason for not being "fully satisfied". This finding highlights a mismatch between doctor's opinion of a successful outcome and that of the patient. PREMs are therefore of utmost importance to evaluate outcome and improve quality of care.

Table 3 NRS-Score and Anaesthesia Technique

	Total	General Anaesthesia	Regional Anaesthesia	*P*-value
Number	243	109	134	
Preoperative NRS-Score				
median	4	3	4	0.201
(IQR)	(0–7)	(0–6)	(0–7)	
NRS ≥ 4	124	50	74	0.147
NRS < 4	119	59	60	
Postoperative NRS-Score				
median	3	3	4	0.139
(IQR)	(1–6)	(1–5)	(1–7)	
NRS ≥ 4	118	50	68	0.450
NRS < 4	125	59	66	

Data is presented as number and 'valid percentage'

Table 4 Patient Comments for not being "fully satisfied" with their Anaesthesia Technique

Comment	Number
Insufficient regional anaesthesia (resulting in additional blocks, or conversion to general anaesthesia)	18
Patient discomfort with the insensate and uncontrollable extremity postoperatively	6
Symptoms of local anaesthetic toxicity	1
Pain during regional anaesthesia procedure	2
Pain following regional anaesthesia wear-off	3
Uncomfortable sensations during wear-off of regional anaesthesia (e.g. tingling)	2
Horner's syndrome	1
Nausea following general anaesthesia	2
No specific reason given	14
Total	49

In the current study, median pain scores are significantly higher in patients who are "dissatisfied" in comparison to patients who are or "partly satisfied" or "fully satisfied" following both general and regional anaesthesia. A correlation between higher pain scores and dissatisfaction would seem intuitive, but our findings indicate that this relationship is more complex. Of the 118 patients with high intensity pain scores (NRS $\geq$ 4) a total of 88 patients (74.6%) are still "fully satisfied" with their anaesthesia technique. Thus, for some patients a certain level of postoperative pain is self-evident following surgery and lowering pain scores will not necessarily result in higher satisfaction scores.

How can we improve patient satisfaction in our daily clinical practice? In this particular study group, taking the limitations into account, regional anaesthesia results in less patients being fully satisfied compared to general anaesthesia. This finding suggests there is room for clinical practice improvement. In patients receiving regional anaesthesia, main reasons for dissatisfaction are: a feeling of insufficient anaesthesia prior to surgery, and patient's discomfort with their insensate and uncontrollable extremity postoperatively. We therefore advocate that both these items are addressed in detail during pre- and postoperative counselling in those patients receiving regional anaesthesia. Of course, patients should be made aware of the risk of an insufficient regional block prior to surgery and the need for additional blocks, or sometimes conversion to general anaesthesia. Unfortunately, failure of regional anaesthesia techniques cannot always be prevented. Secondly, all regional anaesthesia patients should be counselled on prolonged postoperative sensory and motor block; because for some patients, this results in discomfort and a feeling of uncertainty. Duration of the motor/sensory block is highly variable and is difficult to predict with accuracy in individual patients [11]. We therefore strongly suggest that all patients are made aware of such variability in duration prior to block placement and before discharge home. Additionally, pain management should not end at discharge home, but an individual and intensive multi-modal analgesic plan should be in place for all patients.

A limitation of the current study, and many other studies on patient satisfaction, is the use of a simplistic three-point Likert rating scale to assess the highly complex and multidimensional concept of patient satisfaction [12]. Patient satisfaction is determined by many different variables, such as the quality of provided medical care, perceived outcomes, and preoperative expectations [2]. Proper assessment of satisfaction is therefore a complex task, and high satisfaction scores not necessarily reflect high quality of medical care [1, 3, 13]. To simplify this complex assessment, we entirely centred our attention on a single part of the total anaesthetic care given to a patient, and primarily focus on anaesthesia technique provided. Also, satisfaction scores in this current study are primarily used as an instrument to identify potentially modifiable factors associated with dissatisfaction, to provide an opportunity for clinical practice improvement.

Another limitation of the current study is the lack of randomization of patients between regional and general anaesthesia. This may introduces several biases, such as anaesthesiologists' preference, patients' preference, and bias through inclusion of patients who were medically not eligible for a specific anaesthesia technique. For example, if an anaesthesiologist prefers general anaesthesia, his exposure (and subsequently his success-rate) might be lower than in those who prefer regional anaesthesia. Also, satisfaction scores can be influenced in patient who prefer a specific anaesthesia technique, but find out this technique is (medically) not advisable.

A final limitation of the current study is the small sample size, with a wide variability in the types of surgical procedures, types of regional anaesthesia techniques, and low overall ASA-score. We chose to study a pragmatic cohort of patients undergoing elective distal upper extremity surgery, and therefore the present conclusions should be interpreted accordingly.

Conclusions

For distal upper extremity surgery a variety of anaesthetic techniques are available to anesthetize the upper limb. The results of the current study suggest that one third of the patients are not "fully satisfied" following regional (plexus) anaesthesia techniques. To optimize patient satisfaction following regional anaesthesia techniques, we advocate focusing on patient counselling and more expansively addressing the issues of block failure and prolonged postoperative sensory and motor block.

Appendix

Table 5 Day-one postoperative Questionnaire (Translated from Dutch)

Question	Answer
Pain at the current moment (NRS)	0 / 1 / ... / 10 *
Are you satisfied with the Anaesthesia Technique performed?	"fully satisfied" / "partly satisfied" / "dissatisfied"
What is your main reason for dissatisfaction?	… (open question)
Additional Comments	… (open question)

** NRS 0–10: 0 stands for "no pain" and 10 for "worst pain imaginable"*

Abbreviations
ASA: American Society of Anesthesiologists; NRS: numeric rating scale; PREMs: patient-reported experience measures

Acknowledgments
Not applicable.

Author's contributions
WD helped design and conduct the study, analyse the data, and write the manuscript. SH helped analyse the data, write and edit the manuscript. PA helped conduct the study, and reviewed the manuscript. DL helped conduct the study, and reviewed the manuscript. HC helped design and conduct the study, and reviewed the manuscript. RS helped design and conduct the study, and reviewed the manuscript. EG helped design and conduct the study, write and edit the manuscript. All authors read and approved the final manuscript.

Author details
[1]Department of Anaesthesia, Erasmus University Medical Centre Rotterdam, P.O. Box 2040, 3000, CA, Rotterdam, The Netherlands. [2]Department of Anaesthesia, Franciscus Gasthuis & Vlietland, P.O. Box 10900, 3004, BA, Rotterdam, The Netherlands. [3]Department of Plastic Surgery, University Medical Centre Utrecht, P.O. Box 85500, 3508, GA, Utrecht, The Netherlands.

References
1. Wu CL, Naqibuddin M, Fleisher LA. Measurement of patient satisfaction as an outcome of regional anesthesia and analgesia: a systematic review. Reg Anesth Pain Med. 2001;26:196–208.
2. Teunkens A, Vanhaecht K, Vermeulen K, Fieuws S, Van de Velde M, Rex S, Bruyneel L. Measuring satisfaction and anesthesia related outcomes in a surgical day care center: a three-year single-center observational study. J Clin Anesth. 2017;43:15–23.
3. Royse CF, Chung F, Newman S, Stygall J, Wilkinson DJ. Predictors of patient satisfaction with anesthesia and surgery care: a cohort study using the postoperative quality of recovery scale. Eur J Anaesthesiol. 2013;30:106–10.
4. Kingsley C, Patel S. Patient-reported outcome measures and patient-reported experience measures. BJA Education. 2017;17:137–44.
5. Myles PS, Williams DL, Hendrata M, Anderson H, Weeks AM. Patient satisfaction after anesthesia and surgery: results of a prospective survey of 10,811 patients. Br J Anaesth. 2000;84:6–10.
6. Ramsay MA, Savege TM, Simpson BR, Goodwin R. Controlled sedation with alphaxalone-alphadolone. BMJ. 1974;2:656–9.
7. Hawker GA, Mian S, Kendzerska T, French M. Measures of adult pain: visual analog scale for pain (VAS pain), numeric rating scale for pain (NRS pain), McGill pain questionnaire (MPQ), short-form McGill pain questionnaire (SF-MPQ), chronic pain grade scale (CPGS), short Form-36 bodily pain scale (SF-36 BPS), and measure of intermittent and constant osteoarthritis pain (ICOAP). Arthritis Care Res (Hoboken). 2011;63(Suppl 11):S240–52.
8. Coyle TT, Helfrick JF, Gonzalez ML, Andresen RV, Perrott DH. Office-based ambulatory anesthesia: factors that influence patient satisfaction or dissatisfaction with deep sedation/general anesthesia. J Oral Maxillofac Surg. 2005;63:163–72.
9. Cooper K, Kelley H, Carrithers J. Perceptions of side effects following axillary block used for outpatient surgery. Reg Anesth. 1995;20:212–6.
10. Klein SM, Buckenmaier CC 3rd. Ambulatory surgery with long acting regional anesthesia. Minerva Anestesiol. 2002;68(833–41):841–7.
11. Droog W, Lin DY, Huisman JS, Franssen FA, van Aggelen GP, Coert JH, Galvin EM. Individual duration of axillary brachial plexus block is unpredictable: a prospective double centered observational study. Minerva Anestesiol. 2017;83:1146–51.
12. Barnett SF, Alagar RK, Grocott MP, Giannaris S, Dick JR, Moonesinghe SR. Patient-satisfaction measures in anesthesia: qualitative systematic review. Anesthesiology. 2013;119:452–78.
13. Capuzzo M, Gilli G, Paparella L, Gritti G, Gambi D, Bianconi M, Giunta F, Buccoliero C, Alvisi R. Factors predictive of patient satisfaction with anesthesia. Anesth Analg. 2007;105:435–42.

2

A novel approach to neuraxial anesthesia: Application of an automated ultrasound spinal landmark identification

Ting Ting Oh[1], Mohammad Ikhsan[2], Kok Kiong Tan[2], Sultana Rehena[3], Nian-Lin Reena Han[4], Alex Tiong Heng Sia[1,5] and Ban Leong Sng[1,5*]

Abstract

Background: Neuraxial procedures are commonly performed for therapeutic and diagnostic indications. Currently, they are typically performed via palpation-guided surface landmark. We devised a novel intelligent image processing system that identifies spinal landmarks using ultrasound images. Our primary aim was to evaluate the first attempt success rate of spinal anesthesia using landmarks obtained from the automated spinal landmark identification technique.

Methods: In this prospective cohort study, we recruited 100 patients who required spinal anesthesia for surgical procedures. The video from ultrasound scan image of the L3/4 interspinous space in the longitudinal view and the posterior complex in the transverse view were recorded. The demographic and clinical characteristics were collected and analyzed based on the success rates of the spinal insertion.

Results: Success rate (95%CI) for dural puncture at first attempt was 92.0% (85.0–95.9%). Median time to detection of posterior complex was 45.0 [IQR: 21.9, 77.3] secs. There is good correlation observed between the program-recorded depth and the clinician-measured depth to the posterior complex (r = 0.94).

Conclusions: The high success rate and short time taken to obtain the surface landmark with this novel automated ultrasound guided technique could be useful to clinicians to utilise ultrasound guided neuraxial techniques with confidence to identify the anatomical landmarks on the ultrasound scans. Future research would be to define the use in more complex patients during the administration of neuraxial blocks.

Keywords: Automated, Ultrasound, Spinal Anaesthetics: anatomy, Neuraxial anesthesia

Background

Neuraxial procedures are commonly performed for therapeutic and diagnostic indications. These procedures are employed for surgical anesthesia, postoperative pain control, epidural labour analgesia and chronic pain management. More than 1.4 million Caesarean deliveries are performed in the United States with a majority using neuraxial anesthesia [1]. and more than 700,000 epidural procedures performed in 2006 [2, 3]. Epidural labour analgesia is utilized by increasing number of women in labour [4]. ,Therefore, it is essential to make neuraxial procedures safe and reliable.

Lumbar neuraxial procedures are typically performed via a 'blind' surface landmark and palpation guidance. Unfortunately, surface landmark identification may be highly inaccurate in identifying the underlying spinal structures [5, 6]. The identification of this space demands good knowledge of the anatomy and some skills due to its complexity. The failure in palpation from patient factors such as obesity, abnormal spine or

* Correspondence: sng.ban.leong@singhealth.com.sg
[1]Department of Women's Anaesthesia, KK Women's and Children's Hospital, Singapore, Singapore
[5]Anesthesiology and Peroperative Sciences Academic Clinical Program, Duke-NUS Medical School, 8 College Road, Singapore, Singapore

previous spinal surgery results in difficult needle placement, leading to higher rate of complications. Permanent neurological injury may occur when spinal anesthesia is administered at a high spinal space [7]. Multiple attempts at neuraxial procedures could be associated with an increased risk of post-dural puncture headache, paraesthesia and spinal hematoma.

Neuraxial ultrasonography is a recent development in neuraxial anesthesia practice particularly in epidural space identification [8, 9]. It has been shown to be a safe and effective technique, with increasing use as an auxiliary tool to physical examination, enhancing the overall success rate of lumbar puncture and reducing the number of injection attempts. Even in normal surgical patients, the neuraxial anesthesia needle insertion first attempt success rate (success in achieving dural puncture on the first needle pass) is only about 50 to 60% when the palpation technique is used [10, 11].

However, despite its benefits and recommendations by international guidelines, ultrasound-guided neuraxial blocks are still not considered as routine clinical practice in many centres. A survey of 150 anesthesiologists in the United Kingdom showed that more than 90% of respondents have never used ultrasound for neuraxial blockade [12]. The reason is likely multifactorial, the most significant of which is that use of ultrasound for neuraxial blockade could be complex. Most of the clinical studies elucidating the benefits of ultrasound-guided neuraxial techniques originated from highly skilled operators, and learning and pattern recognition of spinal structures may be challenging especially in novice learners and even in those experienced operators when difficult spinal anatomy is present.

To fill this gap in current practice, we devised an intelligent image processing system with the ability to identify spinal landmarks in the ultrasound images [13–18]. In our preliminary studies done in a pilot proof of concept study in healthy volunteers, good accuracy in correct identification of L3/4 interspinous space in 93% of subjects (56 out of 60) was obtained. Primary inaccuracy was mainly due to the poor identification of the L5/S1 interspinous space. Hence, L2/3 instead of L3/4 interspinous space was identified. However, this had no implications on patient safety as spinal cord was above this level [16, 19]. We have further developed and refined the software to be used in a commercially available ultrasound machine (Sonosite M-Turbo Color Digital Ultrasound System).

We conducted a prospective cohort study with the primary aim of evaluating the first attempt success rate of spinal anesthesia using landmarks obtained from the novel automated spinal landmark identification technique. The primary hypothesis of the study was that automated spinal landmark identification algorithm using image processing system would achieve a mean 90% first attempt success rate of spinal anesthesia.

Methods

The study was conducted at KK Women's and Children's Hospital and ethics approval was obtained (Singhealth Centralised Institutional Review Board: CIRB 2016/2262). The trial was registered on clinicaltrials.gov registry (NCT 03535155). Patients who met the inclusion criteria including women with age between 21 and 75 years old who required spinal anesthesia for surgical procedure, weight of 40-90 kg and height of 140-180 cm. The exclusion criteria included history of scoliosis, history of spinal instrumentation, drug allergy to ultrasound transmission gel and visible wound or injury in the lumbar spine. The patients were given the patient information sheet, before informed written consent was obtained from every patient by the investigators.

The patient assumed a seated position with the lower back exposed. Ultrasound gel was applied to the lower back before the investigator placed an ultrasound curved array probe around the sacral region. The graphical interface of the software, integrated with the ultrasound machine, guided the investigator to first identify the sacrum as a hyperdense line which was reflected as a computer marked red line as shown in Fig. 1a at the sacral region [20]. The investigator then moved the ultrasound probe in a steady vertical upward longitudinal direction of the lumbar spine and identified the lamina that were reflected as triangular peaks. Subsequently the laminas were identified and marked as rectangular white box (Fig. 1a). Upon identification of the L3/4 interspinous space, the system marked with a horizontal line along the midline of the probe by a surgical skin marker (Fig. 1b, Fig. 2). After the longitudinal section of the scan was completed, the investigator turned the probe 90 degrees clockwise around the probe centred to the transverse view. The transverse scan consisted of horizontal movements of the ultrasound probe along the previously marked line at the level of L3/4 by the investigator with minimal rotational movements to obtain the best view. The software program assists the operator in finding the best view- the appearance of a green tick on the screen indicates the achievement of a good view. The green tick would not appear if no good view can be obtained. The software would signal when the correct identification of the posterior complex was visualized. (Fig. 3) This position was then marked with a vertical line at the midline of the probe using a surgical skin marker. The program will only give instructions when all the anatomical landmarks are identified. After this scan sequence was completed, the anaesthetist used the identified needle entry insertion point to attempt spinal anesthesia insertion without traditional palpation.

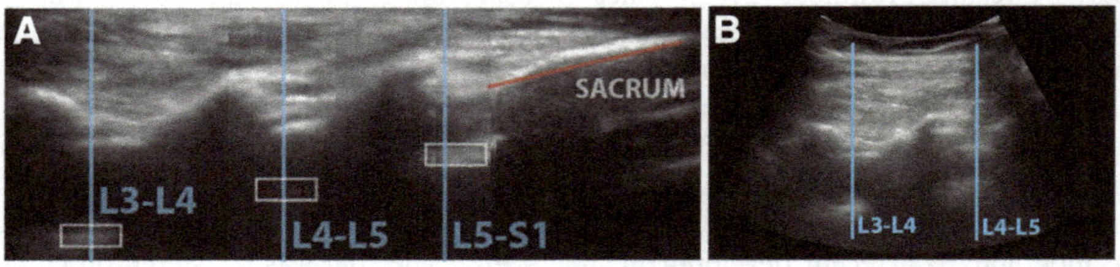

Fig. 1 The step by step process of automated ultrasound spinal landmark identification.Please refer to the Methods, second paragraph

If the required dural puncture was not obtained at first attempt at the marked site, subsequent attempts could include the use of traditional palpation led skin surface markings. The number of spinal attempts was recorded and defined as the number of spinal needle insertion points on the skin.

Images produced were longitudinal and transverse images and videos of the scans, including the image of the L3/4 interspinous space in the longitudinal view and the posterior complex in the transverse view. The parameters in the image processing systems have undergone the offline training based on anatomical landmark images from patient's database, hence less artefacts are less likely to affect the image processing system. All the identified images landmarks have been validated by the clinician investigators during the study.

Patient demographic data including age, weight, height and history of spine disorders were recorded. The number of spinal attempts and the time taken to identify the posterior complex in the transverse view were also recorded. The distance from skin to posterior complex was measured by the program. This was followed by the reading of the recorded scans by an experienced clinician investigator, blinded to the recorded images and videos by using study numbers, to determine the distance from skin to posterior complex from the scans.

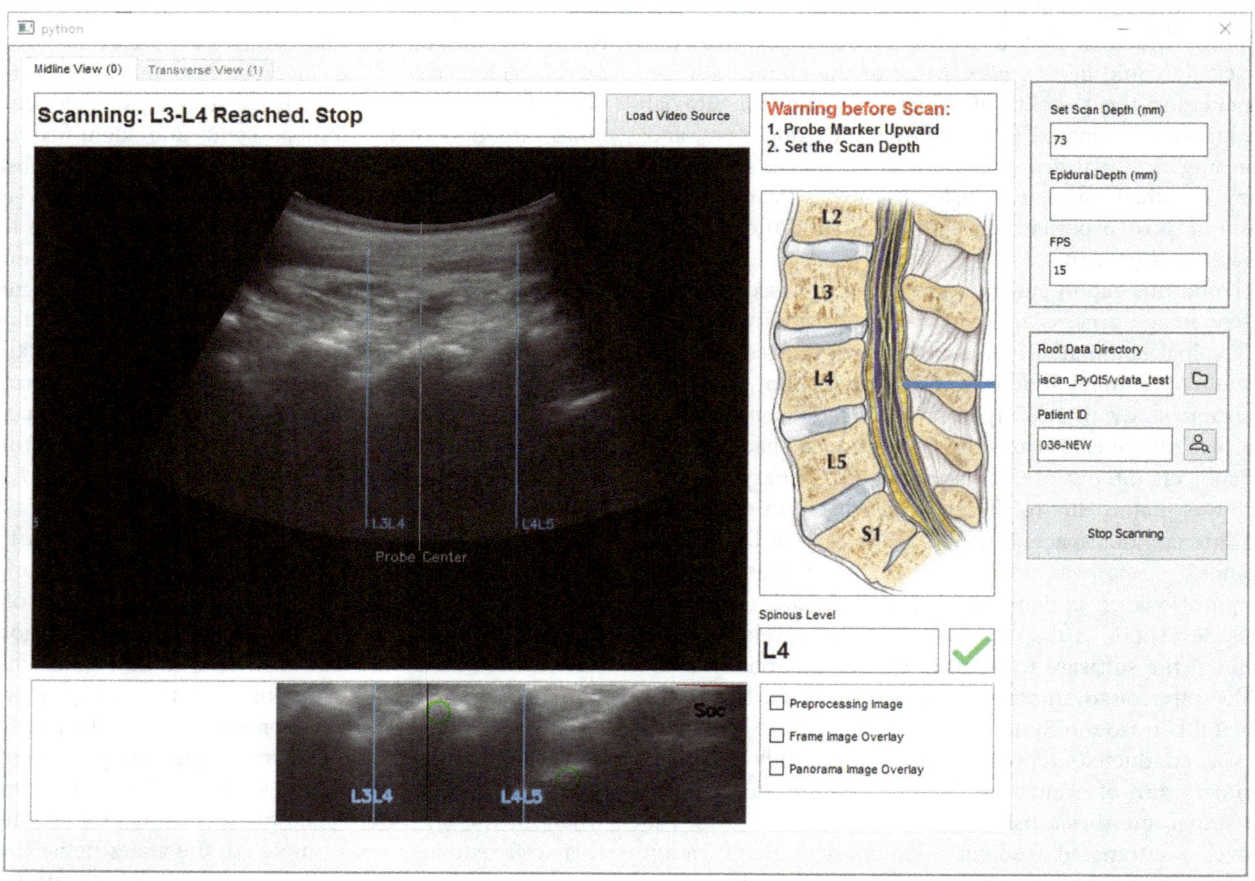

Fig. 2 Midline View

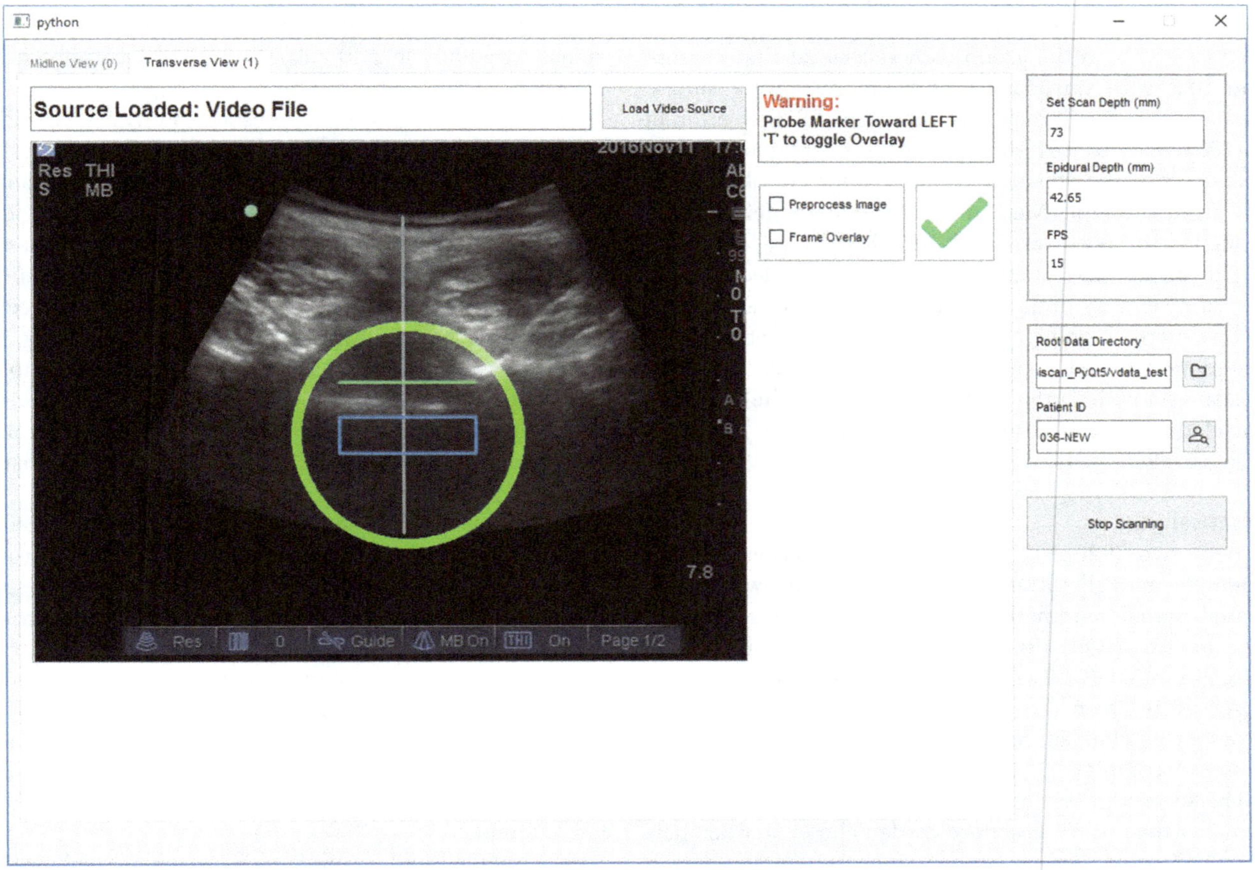

Fig. 3 Transverse view

Congruency between the distance measured by the program and by the clinician investigator was then determined. The scans were done by only the principal investigator and co-investigator who are anesthesiology specialists. However, the needle insertions were done mostly by anesthesiology trainees who were assigned to the operating theatre as our center is a teaching hospital in obstetric anesthesia.

The planned sample size for the primary aim of the study was 100 subjects and it was calculated based on the following assumptions: expected first attempt spinal needle success rate of 90% using the automated spinal landmark identification system, a margin of error as 6.25% i.e. first attempt success rate between 83.5 to 96.0% and 95% confidence interval (95% CI) [21, 22]. Our pilot data showed that the accuracy of our system was 93% (56 out of 60 subjects) and we adjusted for 10% failure rate to obtain successful ultrasound imaging. We wanted to investigate this newer image processing system during this study. The primary outcome analysis was done using incidence proportion; with its corresponding 95% CI estimated using the Wilson score interval method for binomial data.

Primary outcome, *success at first attempt* at spinal needle insertion, was treated as binary data with status as *"yes"* or *"no"*. Success rate was expressed as proportion with corresponding 95% confidence interval (95%CI). Demographic and ultrasound imaging data were summarized based on status of success at first attempt. Continuous variables were summarized using mean standard deviation (SD) and median [interquartile range (IQR)] values while categorical variables were summarized as frequency (proportions). Pearson's correlational and Cronbach's coefficient alpha analysis were performed to assess internal reliability of program-recorded depth and the experienced clinician-measured depth to the posterior complex. SAS version 9.4 software (SAS Institute, Cary, North Carolina) was used for the analysis.

Results

From May 2016 to May 2017, 100 patients who underwent spinal anesthesia for surgical procedure were recruited in the study. All the ultrasound imaging scans with automated spinal landmark identification were successfully performed. There were 99 patients who underwent Caesarean delivery and 1 patient underwent gynaecological procedure. Success rate for dural puncture at first attempt was 92% (95%CI 85–96%). Baseline characteristics in the group with success at first attempt and that with unsuccessful first attempt were similar (Table 1) In the group with unsuccessful first attempt (8/100 = 8%), 5 had dural punctures obtained at the second attempt, while 3 had dural punctures obtained at the third attempt. Median (IQR) time to detection of posterior complex was 45.0 [21.9, 77.3] secs.

The mean (SD) number of attempts needed to scan the lumbar area until obtaining the L3/4 level was 3.1 (3.0). There is good correlation observed between the program-recorded depth and the experienced clinician-measured depth to the posterior complex. The Pearson's correlation and Cronbach's alpha was 0.94 and 0.97 respectively (Fig. 4).

Discussion

Ninety two (92 of 100) patients had successful first attempts and all ultrasound imaging scans with automated spinal landmark identification were successful. The median (IQR) time to detection of posterior complex was 45.0 [21.9, 77.3] secs. Good correlation was observed between the program-recorded depth and the experienced clinician investigator-measured depth to the posterior complex.

The successful first attempt rate in neuraxial anesthesia is higher than 61.6% described by de Filho et al. when palpation directed surface landmarking was employed in a population that was similar in demographics of age and BMI [10]. In addition, 99% of our patients (99 of 100) recruited were obstetric cases that could pose a more challenging anatomy for neuraxial techniques. The high first attempt success rate could reduce complications associated with multiple attempts such as patient discomfort, increased incidence of post-dural puncture headache, paraesthesia and spinal hematoma. Patient safety could be improved as this automated ultrasound spinal landmark identification system allows for correct identification of spinal structures in particular the spinal level of needle insertion.

Ultrasound imaging may be especially useful for difficult patients with obesity, abnormal spinal anatomy and previous spinal surgery where palpation of spinal landmarks can be challenging [23]. In patients with abnormal spinal anatomy, ultrasound imaging has been shown to improve the neuraxial anesthesia needle insertion first attempt success rate from 32% using the palpation technique to 65% with the use of ultrasound imaging by Chin KJ et al [23]. Furthermore, lumbar ultrasonography has been recommended for clinical use when performing neuraxial anesthesia by the National Institute for Health and Care excellence (NICE) guidelines and systematic review [24, 25].

We are evaluating if identification of the site of needle insertion will improve successful needle insertion with the first attempt. Often, especially with junior trainees or in patients with more challenging anatomy, the wrong identification of site of needle insertion is a significant contribution to the inability to obtain a successful needle insertion with the first attempt. The utility of this automated spinal landmark identification is to circumvent errors in identifying site of needle insertion and henceforth, improve successful needle insertion with the first attempt.

Poor uptake to ultrasound guided neuraxial techniques could in part be due to the lack of technical skills in identifying the anatomical landmarks and the perceived belief that using an ultrasound to guide neuraxial techniques may be too time-consuming compared to the traditional palpation led surface landmarking technique. The automation in this novel system could allow operators to have confirmation of the sonographic images and structures. This allows for both novice trainees and

Table 1 Demographic and clinical characteristics based on the success rates of the epidural insertion

Variable	Success		Total $N = 100$
	First Attempt $N = 92$	Not First Attempt $N = 8$	
Race, n (%)			
Chinese	51 (55.4)	05 (62.5)	056 (56.0)
Indian	12 (13.0)	00	012 (12.0)
Malay	12 (13.0)	01 (12.5)	013 (13.0)
Others	17 (18.5)	02 (25.0)	019 (19.0)
Age (Years), mean (SD)	33.5 (5.79)	36.4 (12.9)	033.7 (6.57)
Weight (kg), mean (SD)	69.2 (9.43)	66.0 (6.34)	69.0 (9.24)
Height (m), mean (SD)	1.6 (0.06)	1.6 (0.03)	1.6 (0.06)
BMI (kg/m^2), mean (SD)	28.1 (3.16)	26.4 (2.34)	28.0 (3.13)
Level of scan operator Consultant, n (%)	92 (100)	8 (100)	100 (100)
Skin to posterior complex depth (mm), mean (SD)	44.7 (6.3)	39.6 (6.7)	44.3 (6.5)

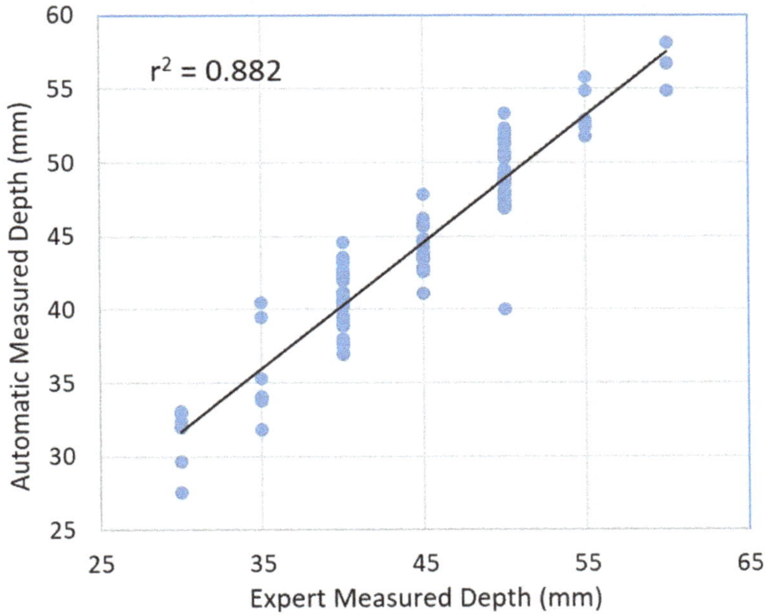

Fig. 4 Pearson's correlation between program-recorded depth and the experienced clinician- measured depth to the posterior complex

experienced clinicians who are unfamiliar with ultrasound techniques to be able to harness the benefits of ultrasound-guided neuraxial techniques. This study showed that using ultrasound would not compromise on procedural time as the time taken to obtain the surface landmark with the automated ultrasound-guided neuraxial technique was under a minute. Furthermore, the high rate of first attempt success rate could potentially reduce the complications caused by multiply entry attempts.

Limitations of this study

Limitations of this study would include a lack of a comparator arm. However, we were investigating a novel automated spinal landmark system and future studies with a randomized trial design would be planned. In addition, the limitation of the proposed image processing program is the high sensitivity required of quality of ultrasound images. However, it is crucial to achieve a high accuracy (less false positives) at the sacrifice of non-optimal recall rate. This may lead to possible additional attempts in scanning as the algorithm is highly specific to only accept given information when all landmarks are detected. The system is validated by our study population (young obstetric women with BMI below 30 kg/m^2) and it is not designed or validated by complex spinal anatomy, obesity patients, paediatric patients and geriatric patients. As the software program requires first identifying the sacrum and then counting the spinal level till L3/4. The abnormal anatomy such as fusion or reduced interspinous distance could increase the risk of misinterpretation.

We chose our primary aim to evaluate the clinical relevance of the automated ultrasound guided system as we had previously evaluated the correlation between spinal landmark identified by the automated machine and identified by an expert anesthesiologist skilled in spine imaging in our preliminary study, which had showed a 93% correlation [13]. We agree that the image processing system does not improve operator error in needle insertion technique, but we are evaluating how the automated ultrasound guided technique can improve first pass attempts despite variations in operator errors in needle insertion technique.

Future directions

We observed a good correlation was observed between the program-recorded depth and the experienced clinician-measured depth to the posterior complex. This would be useful in future applications of using the program to guide epidural insertion. Its clinical correlation and applicability can be investigated in subsequent studies where congruency between distance to epidural space measured by the program against that measured by the epidural needle during epidural insertion. Hence, future work would be to investigate the correlation between program-recorded depth to the posterior complex and the actual distance to epidural space during epidural catheter insertion.

We plan to further determine the accuracy of locating the spinal level and the success of needle insertion by anesthesia trainees, and investigate the use of this system in the obese population, where this automated ultrasound guided neuraxial technique would be more useful, as surface landmarks for neuraxial anesthesia could be more challenging.

Conclusions

This study found that the use of this novel automated ultrasound-guided surface landmark system is a promising option to assist clinicians in improving identification of spinal landmarks, which could contribute to the high first attempt success of spinal anesthesia with acceptable procedural scan time.

Abbreviations

BMI: Body mass index; CI: Confidence interval; CIRB: Centralised Institutional Review Board; IQR: Interquartile range; NICE: National Institute for Health and Care excellence; SD: Standard deviation

Acknowledgements

We would like to acknowledge our clinical research coordinators Ms. Charis Lim and Ms. Agnes Teo for their administrative support in this study.

Authors' contributions

TTO: data collection, data analysis, drafted the manuscript and revised the manuscript. MI: data collection, data analysis and revised the manuscript. KKT: study design, data analysis and revised the manuscript. RS: study design, data analysis and revised manuscript. NLRH: study design, data analysis and revised the manuscript. ATHS: study design, data analysis and revised the manuscript. BLS: study design, data analysis, revised the article and final approval of the version to be submitted. All authors read and approved the final manuscript.

Author details

[1]Department of Women's Anaesthesia, KK Women's and Children's Hospital, Singapore, Singapore. [2]Department of Electrical and Comupter Engineering, Faculty of Engineering, National University of Singapore, Singapore, Singapore. [3]Center for Quantitative Medicine, Duke-NUS Medical School, 8 College Road, Singapore, Singapore. [4]Division of Clinical Support Services, KK Women's amd Children's Hospital, Singapore, Singapore. [5]Anesthesiology and Peroperative Sciences Academic Clinical Program, Duke-NUS Medical School, 8 College Road, Singapore, Singapore.

References

1. Ortner CM, Granot M, Richebe P, Cardoso M, Bollag L, Landau R. Preoperative scar hyperalgesia is associated with post-operative pain in women undergoing a repeat caesarean delivery. Eur J Pain. 2013;17(1):111–23.
2. Friedly J, Chan L, Deyo R. Increases in lumbosacral injections in the Medicare population: 1994 to 2001. Spine (Phila Pa 1976). 2007;32(16):1754–60.
3. Manchikanti L, Pampati V, Boswell MV, Smith HS, Hirsch JA. Analysis of the growth of epidural injections and costs in the Medicare population: a comparative evaluation of 1997, 2002, and 2006 data. Pain Physician. 2010;13(3):199–212.
4. Alran S, Sibony O, Oury JF, Luton D, Blot P. Differences in management and results in term-delivery in nine European referral hospitals: descriptive study. Eur J Obstet Gynecol Reprod Biol. 2002;103(1):4–13.
5. Margarido CB, Mikhael R, Arzola C, Balki M, Carvalho JC. The intercristal line determined by palpation is not a reliable anatomical landmark for neuraxial anesthesia. Can J Anaesth. 2011;58(3):262–6.
6. Kim JT, Bahk JH, Sung J. Influence of age and sex on the position of the conus medullaris and Tuffier's line in adults. Anesthesiology. 2003;99(6):1359–63.
7. Reynolds F. Peripheral nerve injuries associated with anaesthesia. Anaesthesia. 2001;56(2):196.
8. Carvalho JC. Ultrasound-facilitated epidurals and spinals in obstetrics; Anesthesiol Clin 2008, 26(1):145–158, vii-viii.
9. Perlas A. Evidence for the use of ultrasound in neuraxial blocks. Reg Anesth Pain Med. 2010;35(2 Suppl):S43–6.
10. de Filho GR, Gomes HP, da Fonseca MH, Hoffman JC, Pederneiras SG, Garcia JH. Predictors of successful neuraxial block: a prospective study. Eur J Anaesthesiol. 2002;19(6):447–51.
11. Lim YC, Choo CY, Tan KT. A randomised controlled trial of ultrasound-assisted spinal anaesthesia; Anaesth Intensive Care 2014, 42(2):191–198.
12. Mathieu S, Dalgleish DJ. A survey of local opinion of NICE guidance on the use of ultrasound in the insertion of epidural catheters. Anaesthesia. 2008;63(10):1146–7.
13. Yu S, Tan KK, Sng BL, Li SJ, Sia A. Automatic identification of needle insertion site in epidural anesthesia with a cascading classified. Ultrasound Med Biol. 2014;40(9):1980–90.
14. Yu S, Tan KK, CY Shen, Sia A. Ultrasound guided automatic localization of needle insertion site for epidural anesthesia; 2013 IEEE International Conference on Mechatronics and Automation. 2013. p. 985–90.
15. Yu S, Tan KK, Sng BL, Li SJ, Sia A. Real-time automatic spinal level identification with ultrasound image processing; 2015 IEEE 12th International Symposium on Biomedical Imaging (ISBI). 2015. p. 243–6.
16. Yu S, Tan KK, Sng BL, Li S, Sia A. Lumbar ultrasound image feature extraction and classification with support vector machine. Ultrasound Med Biol. 2015;41(10):2677–89.
17. Leng YS, Yu S, Tan KK, Tildsley P, Sia A, Sng BL. Feature extraction and classification for ultrasound images of lumbar spine with support vector machine; 2014 36th Annual International Conference of the IEEE Engineering in Medicine and Biology Society. 2014. p. 4659–62.
18. Yu S, Tan KK. Classification of lumbar ultrasound images with machine learning; simulated evolution and learning SEAL 2014 lecture notes in computer science, vol. 8886; 2014. p. 287–98.
19. Leng YS, Yu S, Ta KK, Tildsley P, Sia A, Sng BL. Development of a real-time lumbar ultrasound image processing system for epidural needle entry site localization; 2016 38th Annual International Conference of the IEEE Engineering in Medicine and Biology Society (EMBC). 2016. p. 4093-6.
20. Ikhsan M, Tan KK, Oh TT, Lew JP, Sng BL. Gabor-based automatic spinal level identification in ultrasound; 2017 39th Annual International Conference of the IEEE Engineering in Medicine and Biology Society (EMBC). 2017. p. 3146-9.
21. EB W. Probable inference, the law of succession, and statistical inference. J Am Stat Assoc. 1927;22(158):209–12.
22. Brown LDCT, DasGupta A. Interval estimation for a binomial proportion. Stat Sci. 2001:101–17.
23. Chin KJ, Perlas A, Chan V, Brown-Shreves D, Koshkin A, Vaishnav V. Ultrasound imaging facilitates spinal anesthesia in adults with difficult surface anatomic landmarks. Anesthesiology. 2011;115(1):94–101.
24. Excellence NIoHaC. Ultrasound-guided catheterisation of the epidural space. In: NICE Guidelines; 2008.
25. Shaikh F, Brzezinski J, Alexander S, Arzola C, Carvalho JC, Beyene J, Sung L. Ultrasound imaging for lumbar punctures and epidural catheterisations: systematic review and meta-analysis. BMJ. 2013;346:f1720.

3

Changes of cerebral regional oxygen saturation during pneumoperitoneum and trendelenburg position under propofol anesthesia

Toru Matsuoka[1], Tadahiko Ishiyama[2*], Noriyuki Shintani[2], Masakazu Kotoda[1], Kazuha Mitsui[2] and Takashi Matsukawa[1]

Abstract

Background: We evaluated the change of cerebral regional tissue oxygen saturation (rSO_2) along with the pneumoperitoneum and the Trendelenburg position. We also assessed the relationship between the change of rSO_2 and the changes of mean arterial blood pressure (MAP), heart rate (HR), arterial carbon dioxide tension ($PaCO_2$), arterial oxygen tension (PaO_2), or arterial oxygen saturation (SaO_2).

Methods: Forty-one adult patients who underwent a robotic assisted endoscopic prostatic surgery under propofol and remifentanil anesthesia were involved in this study. During the surgery, a pneumoperitoneum was established using carbon dioxide. Measurements of rSO_2, MAP, HR, $PaCO_2$, PaO_2, and SaO_2 were performed before the pneumoperitoneum (baseline), every 5 min after the onset of pneumoperitoneum, before the Trendelenburg position. After the onset of the Trendelenburg position, rSO_2, MAP, HR were recorded at 5, 10, 20, 30, 45, and 60 min, and $PaCO_2$, PaO_2, and SaO_2 were measured at 10, 30, and 60 min.

Results: Before the pneumoperitoneum, left and right rSO_2 were $67.9 \pm 6.3\%$ and $68.5 \pm 7.0\%$. Ten minutes after the onset of pneumoperitoneum, significant increase in the rSO_2 was observed (left: $69.6 \pm 5.9\%$, right: $70.6 \pm 7.4\%$). During the Trendelenburg position, the rSO_2 increased initially and peaked at 5 min (left: $72.2 \pm 6.5\%$, right: $73.1 \pm 7.6\%$), then decreased. Multiple regression analysis showed that change of rSO_2 correlated with MAP and $PaCO_2$.

Conclusions: Pneumoperitoneum and the Trendelenburg position in robotic-assisted endoscopic prostatic surgery did not worsen cerebral oxygenation. Arterial blood pressure is the critical factor in cerebral oxygenation.

Keywords: Cerebral oxygenation, Endoscopic prostatic surgery, Pneumoperitoneum, Trendelenburg position

* Correspondence: ishiyama@yamanashi.ac.jp
[2]Surgical Center, University of Yamanashi Hospital, University of Yamanashi, 1110 Shimokato, Chuo, Yamanashi 409-3898, Japan

Background

In robotic-assisted endoscopic prostatic surgery, a carbon dioxide pneumoperitoneum and the Trendelenburg position are essential. In the pneumoperitoneum and the Trendelenburg position, intracranial pressure was reported to increase [1]. In addition, pneumoperitoneum increases intraperitoneal pressure that leads to increase in intrathoracic pressure. Furthermore, the Trendelenburg position increases intrathoracic pressure. Increase in intrathoracic pressure should result in increase in central venous pressure [2]. Both intracranial pressure and central venous pressure increase in the pneumoperitoneum and the Trendelenburg position. The cerebral perfusion pressure is regarded as the mean arterial blood pressure (MAP) minus the intracranial pressure (when intracranial pressure > central venous pressure) or the central venous pressure (when central venous pressure > intracranial pressure) [3]. Therefore, unless the MAP changes the cerebral perfusion pressure decreased and cerebral circulation might be impaired in the pneumoperitoneum combined with the Trendelenburg position. Nevertheless, cerebral blood flow is maintained constantly within a wide range of cerebral perfusion pressure that is known as cerebral autoregulation [4]. On the other hand, cerebral blood flow has been reported to fluctuate even within autoregulation [5]. Therefore, cerebral blood flow may be unchanged or reduced after the pneumoperitoneum and the Trendelenburg position.

Measurement of cerebral regional tissue oxygen saturation values (rSO_2) using near infrared spectroscopy can allow to assess cerebral circulation [6]. A previous study investigated that cerebral oxygenation during pneumoperitoneum in the Trendelenburg position [7]. However, the Trendelenburg position was firstly placed followed by pneumoperitoneum in that study. In robotic-assisted endoscopic prostatic surgery, pneumoperitoneum is performed before the Trendelenburg position.

We tested the following hypotheses. Firstly, rSO_2 does not change after the pneumoperitoneum. Secondary, the Trendelenburg position combined with pneumoperitoneum does not alter rSO_2. The primary outcome was the change of rSO_2 along with the pneumoperitoneum and postural change. The secondary outcome was the relationship between the change of rSO_2 and MAP, heart rate (HR), arterial carbon dioxide tension ($PaCO_2$), arterial oxygen tension (PaO_2), or arterial oxygen saturation (SaO_2).

Methods

This study was approved by the institutional review board of University of Yamanashi (study No. 488), and and was registered in the University Hospital Medical Information Network Clinical Trials Registry (UMIN-CTR) under study number UMIN000026227. Written informed consent was obtained from all patients.

Anesthesia

Fifty-six adult patients (ASA physical status I or II) who underwent robotic-assisted endoscopic prostatic surgery were recruited. Patients having history of cerebral diseases such as cerebral infarction, cerebral hemorrhage, transient ischemic attack, or subarachnoid hemorrhage were excluded. No premedication was given. In the operating room, two sensors of near infrared spectroscopy (SAFB-SM, Covidien, Dublin, Ireland) were attached on the patient's forehead to measure the left and right rSO_2. A pulse oximeter was used to monitor percutaneous arterial oxygen saturation (SpO_2). A bispectral index (BIS) sensor was also attached on the forehead (Model QUATRO, Covidien). An earphone-type infrared tympanic thermometer (CE Thermo, Nipro, Tokyo, Japan) was used to monitor body temperature. Non-invasive arterial blood pressure, HR, rSO_2, SpO_2, and body temperature were measured before induction of general anesthesia while the patient breathed room air (Pre values). Fluid was infused at 6 ml/kg/hr. Anesthesia was induced and maintained with propofol using target controlled infusion and remifentanil. Tracheal intubation was facilitated with rocuronium. After the induction of anesthesia, radial arterial catheter was placed to allow continuous monitoring of MAP and blood gas analysis (SaO_2, PaO_2, and $PaCO_2$). The patient's lungs were mechanically ventilated in a volume controlled mode (tidal volume: 6–8 ml/kg) with a positive end-expiratory pressure of 3 cm H_2O. Peak airway pressure was controlled below 22 cmH_2O. $PaCO_2$ was maintaind between 35 and 45 mmHg. Fraction of inspired oxygen was adjusted to maintain PaO_2 between 150 and 250 mmHg. Position of the blood pressure transducer was standardized to place at the level of the ear for every patient. Mean arterial blood pressure was controlled within 60–120 mmHg. If MAP fell below 60 mmHg, ephedrine or phenylephrine was given. If MAP went up over 120 mmHg, the infusion rate of remifentanil was increased. Bispectral index (BIS) was adjusted between 40 and 60 by controlling the target of propofol infusion. If rSO_2 went down below 50%, or by 20% of the preanesthetic value, inspired oxygen was increased.

Measurements

Before pneumoperitoneum, baseline measurements of rSO_2, MAP, HR, SpO_2, SaO_2, PaO_2, and $PaCO_2$ were made. Pneumoperitoneum with intra-abdominal pressure of 10–15 mmHg was established and measurements were repeated every 5 min. Approximately 15 min after the establishment of the pneumoperitoneum, the Trendelenburg position with 30° head-down tilt was started. Before the start of the Trendelenburg position, rSO_2, MAP, HR, SpO_2, SaO_2, PaO_2, and $PaCO_2$ were measured. Measurements of rSO_2, MAP, HR, and SpO_2 were made at 5, 10, 20, 30, 45, 60 min after the start of Trendelenburg position. After the onset of the Trendelenburg position, blood gas analysis was performed at 10, 30, 60 min. The measurements were not blinded to the anesthesiologists.

Statistical analysis

We used Stat Flex version 6.0 (Artec, Osaka, Japan) for statistical analysis. Power analysis revealed that the sample size of 41 patients was sufficient to provided 80% power with an α level of 0.05 to detect mean differences of 5% in rSO_2. Change in rSO_2, MAP, HR, SpO_2, SaO_2, PaO_2, and $PaCO_2$ were examined via analysis of variance and Tukey post hoc comparisons. Multiple regression analysis was performed to estimate the relationship between rSO_2 and MAP, HR, SpO_2, SaO_2, PaO_2, or $PaCO_2$. For multiple regression analysis, rSO_2 data were averaged. When statistical significances were obtained after the multiple regression analysis, we performed linear regression analysis. Values are represented as means ± SDs; a p value < 0.05 was considered statistically significant.

Results

Of 56 eligible patients, two patients failed to meet the inclusion criteria, and 13 patients developed the protocol fault such as data acquisition failure ($n = 8$), position of blood pressure transducer error ($n = 2$), and blood pressure measurement failure (bending of the arterial catheter) ($n = 3$). Therefore, we enrolled 41 patients (Fig. 1). Patients' age, height, weight, body mass index (BMI) were 67 ± 6 yr., 164.8 ± 6.0 cm, 64.4 ± 9.2 kg, and 23.7 ± 2.9 kg/m^2, respectively. One patient has BMI over 30 kg/m^2 (30.6 kg/m^2). No patients have comorbidities such as chronic obstructive pulmonary disease, heart failure, or uncontrolled hypertension. BIS before anesthesia was 93 ± 6. Propofol was infused at 2.8 ± 0.5 μg/ml and remifentanil was infused at 0.37 ± 0.10 μg/kg/min. BIS was maintained at 44 ± 6 during the study period. Body temperature before anesthesia was 36.3 ± 0.4 °C, and was maintained at 36.5 ± 0.5 °C during the study period.

Mean arterial blood pressure before anesthesia was 95 ± 9 mmHg. There were 8 patients who developed hypotension (MAP below 60 mmHg) after the induction of anesthesia. They were treated with ephedrine 5 mg and phenylephrine 0.05 mg. As shown in Fig. 2a, MAP decreased to 67 ± 10 mmHg before the pneumoperitoneum, and increased significantly after the pneumoperitoneum (81 ± 13 mmHg). After the Trendelenburg position, MAP slightly increased by 3 mmHg but the change was not statistically significant. Then it decreased significantly at 30, 45, and 60 min after the Trendelenburg position

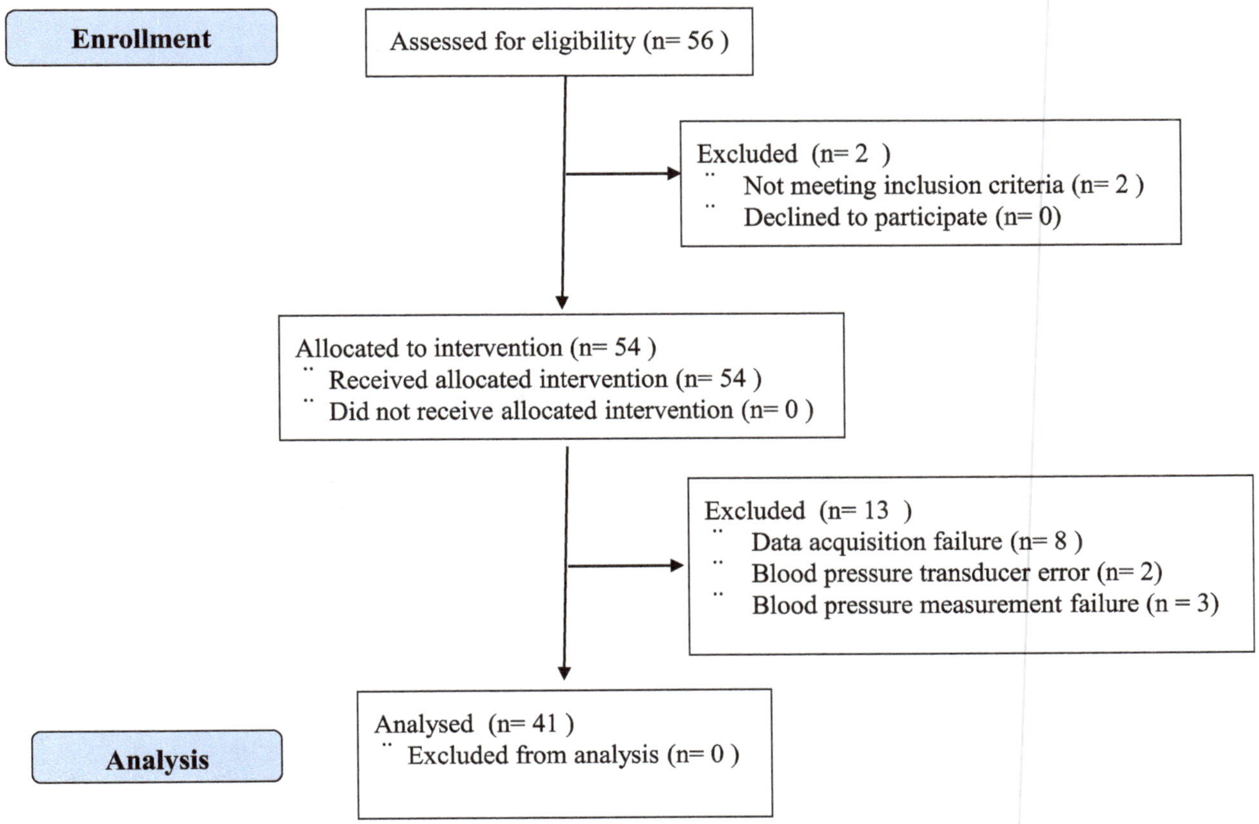

Fig. 1 CONSORT diagram

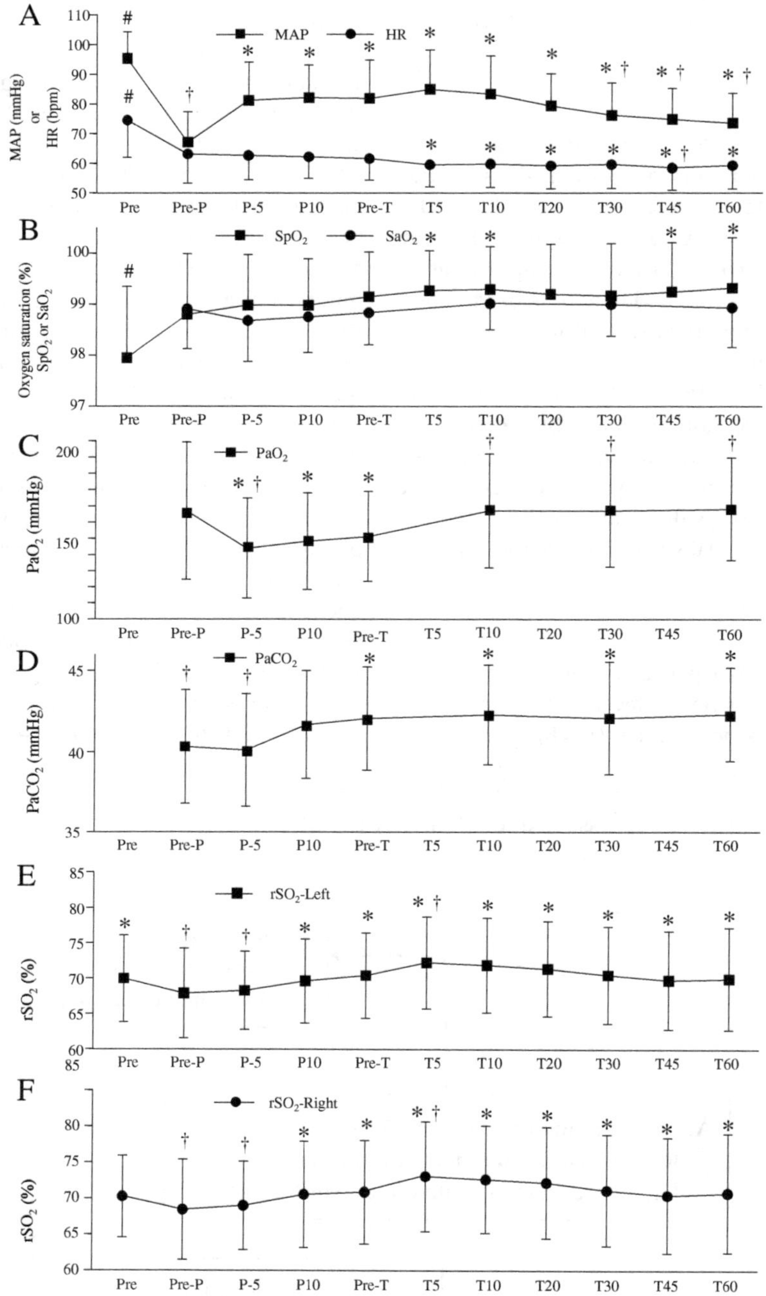

Fig. 2 **a** Changes in mean arterial blood pressure (MAP) and heart rate (HR). **b** Changes in percutaneous (SpO_2) and arterial (SaO_2) oxygen saturation. **c** Changes in arterial oxygen tension (PaO_2). **d** Changes in carbon dioxide tension ($PaCO_2$). **e** Changes in left cerebral regional oxygen saturation (rSO_2). **f** Changes in right cerebral regional oxygen saturation (rSO_2). Pre: before the induction of anesthesia, Pre-P: just before the pneumoperitoneum, P-5, 10: 5, 10 min after the pneumoperitoneum, Pre-T: just before the Trendelenburg position (approximately 15 min after the pneumoperitoneum), T-5, 10, 20, 30, 45, 60: 5, 10, 20, 30, 45, 60 min after the Trendelenburg position. * $P < 0.05$, compared with Pre-P, † $p < 0.05$, compared with Pre-T, # $P < 0.05$, compared with other time points

compared with that before the Trendelenburg position. Heart rate before anesthesia was 75 ± 12 beats/min. It decreased to 63 ± 10 beats/min before the pneumoperitoneum. Heart rate from 10 min to 60 min after the Trendelenburg position significantly decreased compared with that at before pneumoperitoneum (Fig. 2a). SpO_2 before anesthesia (Pre) was 98.0 ± 1.4%, and increased to 99.0 ± 1.0% throughout the study period (Fig. 2b). SaO_2 did not change in this study (Fig. 2b).

PaO_2 before the pneumoperitoneum was 167.4 ± 43.9 mmHg. PaO_2 decreased after the pneumoperitoneum, and increased after the Trendelenburg position. $PaCO_2$ before the pneumoperitoneum was 40.3 ± 3.5 mmHg (Fig.2c). $PaCO_2$ slightly but significantly increased after the pneumoperitoneum. $PaCO_2$ remained high level during the pneumoperitoneum combined with the Trendelenburg position (Fig.2d).

Before general anesthesia, left (Fig.2e) and right (Fig.2f) rSO_2 were 70.0 ± 6.2% and 70.3 ± 5.6%, respectively. Before the pneumoperitoneum, left and right rSO_2 decreased to 67.9 ± 6.3% and 68.5 ± 7.0%. Ten min after the pneumoperitoneum, left and right rSO_2 significantly increased to 69.6 ± 5.9% and 70.6 ± 7.4%. While patients were in the Trendelenburg position, left and right rSO_2 significantly increased temporarily (5 min after the Trendelenburg position), and decreased to the baseline value afterwards but the change was not statistically significant.

Multiple regression analysis showed that change of rSO_2 was correlated with MAP ($p < 0.05$) and $PaCO_2$ ($p < 0.0001$) (Table 1). Linear regression analysis revealed that $rSO_2 = 65.717 + 0.0558 \times MAP$, r = 0.1141 (95% confidence interval; 0.0059–0.2197), and $rSO_2 = 45.3682 + 0.60127 \times PaCO_2$, r = 0.3059 (95% confidence interval; 0.2037–0.4015).

Table 1 Multiple regression analysis between rSO_2 and MAP, HR, SpO_2, SaO_2, PaO_2, or $PaCO_2$

	Unstandardized coefficients		Standardized coefficients	t	p-value
	B	SE	β		
	83.0782	70.0290			
MAP	0.07342	0.03057	0.1364	2.40144	0.0170
HR	0.01319	0.04505	0.0168	0.29271	0.7700
SpO_2	−0.6075	0.55434	−0.0803	1.09593	0.2741
SaO_2	0.13072	0.75372	0.0144	0.17343	0.8624
PaO_2	0.01468	0.01322	0.0813	1.1022	0.2679
$PaCO_2$	0.61094	0.11081	0.3222	5.51332	0.0000

Change of rSO_2 was correlated with MAP ($p < 0.05$) and $PaCO_2$ ($p < 0.0001$)

rSO_2 cerebral regional tissue oxygen saturation, *MAP* mean arterial blood pressure, *HR* heart rate, *SpO_2* percutaneous arterial oxygen saturation, *SaO_2* arterial oxygen saturation, *B* regression coefficient, *SE* standard error, *β* standardized partial regression coefficient

Discussion

We found in the present study that rSO_2 increased after the pneumoperitoneum and further increased temporarily after the steep Trendelenburg position, and decreased afterwards. These changes were along with the alteration of MAP and $PaCO_2$. However, the changes did not correlate with the changes of HR, PaO_2, or SaO_2.

The cerebral perfusion pressure is regarded as MAP minus central venous pressure (or intracranial pressure) [3]. A previous study reported that central venous pressure increased by 2–5 mmHg during the pneumoperitoneum [8, 9]. On the other hand, another previous study reported that MAP did not change after the pneumoperitoneum [9]. Thus, cerebral perfusion pressure should slightly decrease after the pneumoperitoneum. Contrary to the previous study [9], another study reported that pneumoperitoneum with a consequent increase in intracranial pressure produced systemic hypertension. [10]. Our study concurs with the latter study that MAP increased after the pneumoperitoneum. In patients in this study, cerebral autoregulation should be intact. Owing to the cerebral autoregulation, the cerebral blood flow is maintained constantly within a wide range of cerebral perfusion pressure. It is reasonable to assume that cerebral perfusion pressure remained normal level after the pneumoperitoneum. rSO_2 reflects cerebral perfusion [11]. Therefore, we assumed that rSO_2 would be unchanged after the pneumoperitoneum. However, rSO_2 increased after the pneumoperitoneum in this study. In steady state, cerebral blood flow is maintained constant with static cerebral autoregulation [4]. In acute change in blood pressure, cerebral blood flow is compensatory adjusted by dynamic cerebral autoregulation [12, 13]. However, there is a time lag between the rise in blood pressure and the activation of dynamic cerebral autoregulation [14]. If blood pressure increased suddenly, cerebral blood flow may increase transiently. As a result, rSO_2 increased.

After the Trendelenburg position combined with CO_2 pneumoperitoneum, rSO_2 increased initially. Some studies reported that central venous pressure increased by 10–16 mmHg during the Trendelenburg position combined with CO_2 pneumoperitoneum [15–17]. On the other hand, blood pressure also increased by 10–15 mmHg during the Trendelenburg position combined with CO_2 pneumoperitoneum in the previous studies [2, 15, 17]. In agreement with those studies, we observed that MAP increased by 16–18 mmHg at 5–10 min after the Trendelenburg position combined with CO_2 pneumoperitoneum compared with that before the pneumoperitoneum. Change in cerebral perfusion pressure immediately after the Trendelenburg position was 16–18 mmHg (MAP change) minus 10–16 mmHg (assumed CVP change) [15–17]. The value was 0–8 mmHg. Whereas change in cerebral perfusion pressure after pneumoperitoneum was 14 mmHg (MAP change) minus 2–5 mmHg (assumed CVP change) [8, 9]. The value was 9–12 mmHg. Therefore, it is assumed that the cerebral perfusion pressure did not increase after the Trendelenburg position compared with that at the CO_2 pneumoperitoneum. Cerebral perfusion pressure was not involved in the transient increase in rSO_2 just after the Trendelenburg position combined with CO_2 pneumoperitoneum. Schramm et al. reported that cerebral autoregulation deteriorated with Trendelenburg position combined with pneumoperitoneum [18]. Garrett et al. [19] reported that the cerebral blood flow velocity decreased when the posture was changed from the supine to the seated position. Postural change influences cerebral blood flow. Based on those previous studies, cerebral blood flow increased temporarily when the posture was changed from the supine to the Trendelenburg position. Due to transient increase in cerebral blood flow, rSO_2 initially increased after the Trendelenburg position combined with CO_2 pneumoperitoneum.

Cerebral blood flow varies with $PaCO_2$. We recently reported that changes in rSO_2 significantly correlated with changes in $PaCO_2$. [20]. Abdominally insufflated carbon dioxide is absorbed into systemic circulation and is exhaled with ventilation. We attempted to adjust tidal volume and respiratory rate to maintain $PaCO_2$ at 40 ± 5 mmHg. However, $PaCO_2$ increased significantly after the pneumoperitoneum. Thus, rSO_2 increased along with the rise in $PaCO_2$. rSO_2 gradually decreased after the pneumoperitoneum combined with the Trendelenburg position. Nevertheless, $PaCO_2$ remained high level during the pneumoperitoneum combined with the Trendelenburg position. Although there was a correlation between rSO_2 and $PaCO_2$, $PaCO_2$ may be less involved in the change of rSO_2. On the other hand, MAP was observed highest at 5 min after the Trendelenburg position (T5 in the Fig. 2a) and it decreased thereafter. Head-down position in combination with a pneumoperitoneum impairs cerebral autoregulation over time [18]. It is likely that rSO_2 changes with alterations in mean blood pressure rather than change of $PaCO_2$.

Cerebral oxygenation can be monitored by rSO_2 [21]. Cerebral oxygenation may influence the change of rSO_2 in this study. According to the manufacturer, rSO_2 reflects 25% arterial and 75% venous portion of blood. If cerebral oxygen consumption decreased, venous blood oxygen could be increased. As a result, rSO_2 may have increased. However, BIS was unchanged after the induction of anesthesia. There were no factors that involved the decline in cerebral oxygen consumption after the pneumoperitoneum. Furthermore, PaO_2 was significantly decreased after pneumoperitoneum. Therefore, oxygenation status was unlikely to participate in the rise of rSO_2.

In this study, data before anesthesia were obtained under room air breathing and other data were measured under oxygen inspiration. Therefore, arterial oxygen saturation before anesthesia was significantly lower than that after the induction of anesthesia. However, rSO_2 before anesthesia was significantly higher than that after the induction of anesthesia. Mean arterial blood pressure also declined after the induction of anesthesia. In addition, cerebral metabolic rate decreases after the induction of anesthesia that results in decrease in cerebral blood flow [22]. This phenomenon may indicate that rSO_2 is firmly affected by MAP and cerebral blood flow rather than arterial oxygenation status in this study situation.

Cerebral autoregulation, which is expected to keep cerebral blood flow constant, mainly depends on cerebral perfusion pressure [4]. If cerebral perfusion pressure were too low (below the lower limit of autoregulation), cerebral blood flow might depend on MAP [23]. When the cerebral perfusion pressure was below the lower limit of autoregulation, cerebral blood flow should have been changed directly with the fluctuation of MAP. In this situation, rSO_2 altered along with the change of MAP though decrease in blood pressure below the lower limit of autoregulation was not observed in this study. Nevertheless, individual variation in MAP while anesthetized and the lower limit of autoregulation might make the rSO_2-MAP relationship different for different individuals.

In this study, PaO_2 decreased after pneumoperitoneum. A previous study suggested that pneumoperitoneum elevated diaphragm that can lead to basilar atelectasis, with resulting right to left shunt formation [24]. Atelectasis caused by pneumoperitoneum may contribute to the decrease of PaO_2. After the Trendelenburg position, PaO_2 increased. Some studies reported that peak and mean airway pressure increased after the Trendelenburg position [25, 26]. Elevated airway pressure may have contributed to reduce atelectasis. As a result, PaO_2 increased.

This study has some limitations. First, we did not measure central venous pressure because central venous catheterization is an invasive method and not always necessary for robotic-assisted endoscopic prostatic surgery. In many studies, central venous pressure was increased after pneumoperitoneum [8, 9] and the Trendelenburg position combined with pneumoperitoneum. [15–17] Therefore, the present study was based on an assumption that central venous pressure increased in this study. Second, cerebral blood flow was not measured. Transcranial Doppler can be utilized to assess the cerebral blood flow. However, due to the protection pads that supported the patient during the surgery, there was no space on the patient's head for the Doppler probe attachment. Third, extracranial contamination affects rSO_2. Davie et al. reported that the extracranial contamination potentially affected rSO_2 [27]. They also indicated that forehead skin blood made an impact on rSO_2 [27]. Trendelenburg position may cause venous stasis, which could result in the increase of venous portion of blood. Therefore, Trendelenburg position may have affected the relative arterial and venous content of the forehead skin blood. Extracranial contamination might have influenced rSO_2 in this study.

Conclusions

In conclusion, pneumoperitoneum and the Trendelenburg position in robotic-assisted endoscopic prostatic surgery did not aggravate cerebral oxygenation. Changes in rSO2 were associated with the alteration of MAP and PaCO2, but did not correlate with the changes of HR, PaO2, or SaO2, indicating that arterial blood pressure is the critical factor in the cerebral oxygenation.

Abbreviations

BIS: Bispectral index; HR: Heart rate; MAP: Mean arterial blood pressure; $PaCO_2$: Arterial carbon dioxide tension; PaO_2: Arterial oxygen tension; rSO_2: Cerebral regional tissue oxygen saturation; SaO_2: Arterial oxygen saturation; SpO_2: Percutaneous arterial oxygen saturation

Acknowledgements

Not applicable

Authors' contributions

TM conducted the study, acquired the data, and wrote the draft of manuscript. TI designed the study, analyzed and interpreted the data, wrote the manuscript, and is the corresponding author. NS acquired the data, reviewed the analysis, interpreted the data, and revised the manuscript. MK interpreted the data, and revised the manuscript. KM interpreted the data, and revised the manuscript. TM interpreted the data, and revised the manuscript. All authors read and approved the final manuscript.

Author details

[1]Department of Anesthesiology, Faculty of Medicine, University of Yamanashi, Chuo, Yamanashi, Japan. [2]Surgical Center, University of Yamanashi Hospital, University of Yamanashi, 1110 Shimokato, Chuo, Yamanashi 409-3898, Japan.

References

1. Halverson A, Buchanan R, Jacobs L, Shayani V, Hunt T, Riedel C, et al. Evaluation of mechanism of increased intracranial pressure with insufflation. Surg Endosc. 1998;12:266–9.
2. Kalmar AF, Foubert L, Hendrickx JF, Mottrie A, Absalom A, Mortier EP, et al. Influence of steep Trendelenburg position and CO_2 pneumoperitoneum on cardiovascular, cerebrovascular, and respiratory homeostasis during robotic prostatectomy. Br J Anaesth. 2010;104:433–9.
3. Munis JR, Lozada LJ. Giraffes, siphons, and starling resistors. Cerebral perfusion pressure revisited. J Neurosurg Anesthesiol. 2000;12:290–6.
4. Paulson OB, Strandgaard S, Edvinsson L. Cerebral autoregulation. Cerebrovasc Brain Metab Rev. 1990;2:161–92.
5. Tzeng YC, Ainslie PN. Blood pressure regulation IX: cerebral autoregulation under blood pressure challenges. Eur J Appl Physiol. 2014;114:545–59.
6. Ali AM, Green D, Zayed H, Halawa M, El-Sakka K, Rashid HI. Cerebral monitoring in patients undergoing carotid endarterectomy using a triple assessment technique. Interact Cardiovasc Thorac Surg. 2011;12:454–7.
7. Park EY, Koo BN, Min KT, Nam SH. The effect of pneumoperitoneum in the steep Trendelenburg position on cerebral oxygenation. Acta Anaesthesiol Scand. 2009;53:895–9.
8. Andersson L, Wallin CJ, Sollevi A, Odeberg-Wernerman S. Pneumoperitoneum in healthy humans does not affect central blood volume or cardiac output. Acta Anaesthesiol Scand. 1999;43:809–14.
9. Hänel F, Blobner M, Bogdanski R, Werner C. Effects of carbon dioxide pneumoperitoneum on cerebral hemodynamics in pigs. J Neurosurg Anesthesiol. 2001;13:222–6.
10. Ben-Haim M, Mandeli J, Friedman RL, Rosenthal RJ. Mechanisms of systemic hypertension during acute elevation of intraabdominal pressure. J Surg Res. 2000;91:101–5.
11. Rigamonti A, Scandroglio M, Minicucci F, Magrin S, Carozzo A, Casati A. A clinical evaluation of near-infrared cerebral oximetry in the awake patient to monitor cerebral perfusion during carotid endarterectomy. J Clin Anesth. 2005;17:426–30.
12. Kurazumi T, Ogawa Y, Yanagida R, Morisaki H, Iwasaki KI. Dynamic cerebral autoregulation during the combination of mild hypercapnia and cephalad fluid shift. Aerosp Med Hum Perform. 2017;88:819–26.
13. Zhang R, Zuckerman JH, Giller CA, Levine BD. Transfer function analysis of dynamic cerebral autoregulation in humans. Am J Phys. 1998;274:H233–41.
14. Chiu CC, Yeh SJ. Assessment of cerebral autoregulation using time-domain cross-correlation analysis. Comput Biol Med. 2001;31:471–80.
15. Choi SH, Lee SJ, Rha KH, Shin SK, Oh YJ. The effect of pneumoperitoneum and Trendelenburg position on acute cerebral blood flow-carbon dioxide reactivity under sevoflurane anaesthesia. Anaesthesia. 2008;63:1314–8.
16. Doe A, Kumagai M, Tamura Y, Sakai A, Suzuki K. A comparative analysis of the effects of sevoflurane and propofol on cerebral oxygenation during steep Trendelenburg position and pneumoperitoneum for robotic-assisted laparoscopic prostatectomy. J Anesth. 2016;30:949–55.
17. Kalmar AF, Dewaele F, Foubert L, Hendrickx JF, Heeremans EH, Struys MM, et al. Cerebral haemodynamic physiology during steep Trendelenburg position and CO_2 pneumoperitoneum. Br J Anaesth. 2012;108:478–84.
18. Schramm P, Treiber AH, Berres M, Pestel G, Engelhard K, Werner C, et al. Time course of cerebrovascular autoregulation during extreme Trendelenburg position for robotic-assisted prostatic surgery. Anaesthesia. 2014;69:58–63.
19. Garrett ZK, Pearson J, Subudhi AW. Postural effects on cerebral blood flow and autoregulation. Phys Rep. 2017;5:e13150.
20. Ishiyama T, Kotoda M, Asano N, Ikemoto K, Shintani N, Matsuoka T, et al. Effects of hyperventilation on cerebral oxygen saturation estimated using near-infrared spectroscopy: a randomised comparison between propofol and sevoflurane anaesthesia. Eur J Anaesthesiol. 2016;33:929–35.
21. Aliane J, Duale C, Guesmi N, Baud C, Rosset E, Pereira B, et al. Compared effects on cerebral oxygenation of ephedrine vs phenylephrine to treat hypotension during carotid endarterectomy. Clin Exp Pharmacol Physiol. 2017;44:739–48.
22. Conti A, Iacopino DG, Fodale V, Micalizzi S, Penna O, Santamaria LB. Cerebral haemodynamic changes during propofol-remifentanil or sevoflurane anaesthesia: transcranial Doppler study under bispectral index monitoring. Br J Anaesth. 2006;97:333–9.
23. Pater PM, Drummond JC. Cerebral physiology and the effects of anesthetic drugs. In: Miller RD, editor. Miller's Anesthesia, vol. 1. 7th ed. Philadelphia: Churchill Livingstone; 2010. p. 305–39.
24. Haydon GH, Dillon J, Simpson KJ, Thomas H, Hayes PC. Hypoxemia during diagnostic laparoscopy: a prospective study. Gastrointest Endosc. 1996;44:124–8.
25. Assad OM, El Sayed AA, Khalil MA. Comparison of volume-controlled ventilation and pressure-controlled ventilation volume guaranteed during laparoscopic surgery in Trendelenburg position. J Clin Anesth. 2016;34:55–61.
26. Kim MS, Soh S, Kim SY, Song MS, Park JH. Comparisons of pressure-controlled ventilation with volume guarantee and volume-controlled 1:1 equal ratio ventilation on oxygenation and respiratory mechanics during robot-assisted laparoscopic radical prostatectomy: a randomized-controlled trial. Int J Med Sci. 2018;15:1522–9.
27. Davie SN, Grocott HP. Impact of extracranial contamination on regional cerebral oxygen saturation: a comparison of three cerebral oximetry technologies. Anesthesiology. 2012;116:834–40.

4

A small dose of remifentanil pretreatment suppresses sufentanil-induced cough during general anesthesia induction

Wendong Lin[1], Jiehao Sun[1] and Shuying Fu[2*]

Abstract

Background: Intravenous use of sufentanil can elicit cough. This study aimed to evaluate the inhibitory effect of pre-injection of a mall dose of remifentanil on sufentanil-induced cough during the induction of general anesthesia.

Methods: This prospective, randomized, controlled trial was conducted from January 10, 2019 to March 01, 2019. A total of 100 patients undergoing elective surgery under general anesthesia were enrolled, and at last 84 patients were included and randomly allocated into two equal size groups ($n = 42$): Patients in the Remifentanil group (R group) received an intravenous infusion of remifentanil 0.3 μg/kg (diluted to 2 ml) 1 min before sufentanil injection; patients in the Control group (C group) received 2 ml of normal saline (NS) at the same time point. Injections of patients in both groups were completed within 5 s. Then, sufentanil 0.5 μg/kg was injected within 5 s and the number of coughs that occurred within 1 min after sufentanil injection were recorded. One minute after sufentanil injection, etomidate 0.3 mg/kg and cisatracurium 0.15 mg/kg were given for general anesthesia induction irrespective of the presence or absence of cough. The mean arterial pressure (MAP) and heart rate (HR) at time points just before remifentanil pretreatment administration (T0), 3 min after administration (T1), 1 min after intubation (T2), and 3 min after intubation (T3) were recorded.

Results: The incidence of cough in patients in the R group and C group was 4.8 and 31%, respectively. Compared with group C, the incidence and severity of cough in group R was significantly lower ($P < 0.01$). No significant differences were observed in MAP and HR at the time of general anesthesia induction between the two groups ($P > 0.05$).

Conclusion: Pretreatment with a small dose of remifentanil effectively and safely reduced the incidence and severity of cough induced by sufentanil during anesthesia induction and can be used as an alternative treatment to inhibit coughing caused by sufentanil.

Keywords: Remifentanil, Sufentanil, General anesthesia, Cough

* Correspondence: fushuying2007@sina.com
[2]Department of Anesthesiology, The Second Affiliated Hospital and Yuying Children's Hospital of Wenzhou Medical University, Wenzhou 325000, China

Background

Sufentanil has been commonly used for the induction of general anesthesia because of its strong analgesic properties [1]. However, the intravenous use of sufentanil can elicit cough [1, 2].

This side effect may increase intracranial, intraocular, and intraabdominal pressure, which may endanger patients with a cerebral aneurysm, open eye injury or abdominal aortic aneurysm.

Various agents have been used for cough suppression prior to induction of general anesthesia including: 1- intravenous opioid such as fentanyl, 2- intramuscular morphine, 3-dexmedetomidine, 4- magnesium sulfate, 5- terbutaline, 6- lidocaine, and 7- dezocine [1, 3–8].

However, because of their more or less potential additional side effects, long onset time, long duration, inconvenience to get, they were somewhat limited in clinical use.

Remifentanil is an opioid that has both short onset time and short duration and is also readily available.

The use of remifentanil for cough suppression has previously been documented [9–13]. Remifentanil has shown effective cough suppression, however, in few studies, remifentanil has been used prior to the induction of general anesthesia to prevent opioid-induced cough.

Therefore, in this study, we evaluated the effects of remifentanil on the incidence and severity of sufentanil-induced cough during the induction of general anesthesia, thereby aiming to assess whether a small dose of remifentanil could be used as an treatment to inhibit sufentanil-induced cough.

Methods

CONSORT guidelines

This study adheres to CONSORT guidelines.

Participants

This study passed the ethical review by the Ethics Committee of the First Affiliated Hospital of Wenzhou Medical University (2018–150) (Wenzhou, China), and was registered at the Chinese Clinical Trial Registry (ChiCTR1900020587, January 9, 2019). Written informed consent was obtained from all patients.

One hundred patients were screened, and a total of 84 patients scheduled for elective surgery under general anesthesia (aged 20–70 years), classified as ASA I or II, were selected (shown as Fig. 1).

Exclusion criteria were: smoking; Body Mass Index (BMI) over 28; increased intracranial, intraabdominal or intraocular pressure before operation; a history of

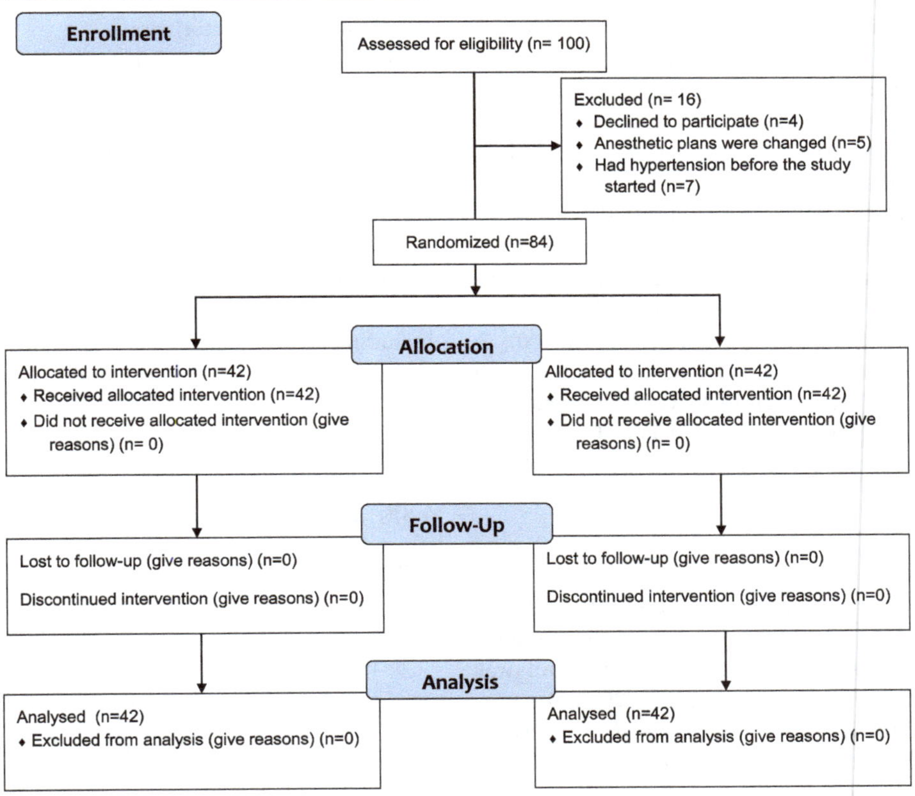

Fig. 1 Flow of participants through the study

respiratory diseases, such as asthma, chronic cough, and upper respiratory tract infection within two weeks; a history of other systemic diseases, including gastroesophageal reflux, hypertension, diabetes, heart disease, impaired kidney or liver function; a history of chronic administration of opioids, cough-causing medications, such as angiotensin-converting-enzyme inhibitors (ACE-inhibitors), and anti-cough medications, such as bronchodilators and steroid therapy.

Anesthesia and research procedure

The trial was conducted from January 10, 2019 to March 01, 2019 at The First Affiliated Hospital of Wenzhou Medical University (Wenzhou, China). None of the patients received any premedication. In brief, a 20-gauge cannula was inserted into the dorsum of the hand of each patient and connected to a T-connector for drug administration. Standard ASA monitors were attached, including non-invasive arterial pressure, electrocardiography, and pulse oxygen saturation (SPO_2). The 84 patients were randomly and equally divided into two groups: R group for remifentanil 0.3 µg/kg (diluted to 2 ml) intravenous infusion; C group for 2 ml of NS. All patients were given oxygen via a face mask (6 L/min) before the induction of anesthesia. Injections of both two groups (remifentanil or saline) were completed within 5 s. One minute after injection, each patient was given a sufentanil bolus of 0.5 µg/kg within 5 s.

The number of coughs that occurred within 1 min after sufentanil injection were recorded and the severity was graded depending on the cough times (mild, 1–2; moderate, 3–4; and severe, ≥5).

One minute after the injection of sufentanil, etomidate 0.3 mg/kg and cisatracurium 0.15 mg/kg were given for the induction of general anesthesia irrespective of the presence or absence of cough. MAP and HR immediately before remifentanil or NS administration (T0), 3 min after administration (T1), 1 min after intubation (T2), and 3 min after intubation (T3) were recorded.

Throughout the experiment, side effects of remifentanil, such as muscle rigidity or other unintended effects were also recorded.

Statistical analysis

Sample size estimates were done using PASS 11 software (PASS, Kaysville, UT, USA). In our pilot study, the incidence of cough elicited by 0.5 µg/kg of sufentanil was 30% (6/20), which was reduced to 5% (1/20) after pretreatment with remifantanil. To achieve 80% statistical power with $\alpha = 0.05$, each group would require no less than 32 patients. To account for drop-outs, we recruited 50 patients per group.

Using a computer generated random-number sequence, patients were randomly and equally divided into two groups by. Random allocation sequences were collected, participants were enrolled and assigned to interventions and outcomes were assessed. Both remifentanil (0.3 µg/kg, diluted to 2 ml) and NS were injected in a volume of 2 ml. After assignment, both participants and investigators were blinded to interventions.

Data were analyzed by SPSS software 22.0 (IBM Corp, Armonk, NY, USA). The normality of measurement data distribution was tested by the Shapiro-Wilk test. Measurement data of normal distribution (age, BMI, etc.) were presented as the mean ± standard deviation and were analyzed by Student's t test. Measurement data of non-normal distribution were presented as the median (Q1, Q3) and analyzed by the Mann–Whitney U test. Categorical data were presented as absolute and relative effect sizes, and assessed by the Chi-square test or Fisher's exact test as appropriate. Grade data (the severity of coughs) were analyzed by Mann–Whitney U test. Continuous variables at different time points were compared by using repeated measures design analysis of variance. $P < 0.05$ was considered statistically significant.

Results

Demographic characteristics

This trial was conducted from January 10, 2019 to March 01, 2019. A total of 100 eligible patients were screened among which 84 patients participated in our study and were included in the final analyses (four patients declined participation; seven patients had unacceptable hypertension before the start of the study; the anesthetic plans of five patients changed before the study started) (Fig. 1).

ASA physical status and demographic characteristics, including gender, age, and the BMI of patients in the two groups were similar ($P > 0.05$, Table 1).

Incidence and severity of cough

The incidence in group C was 31% and in group R was 4.8%. Both the incidence and severity of cough in

Table 1 Demographic data

Group	Gender (M/F)	Age (yr)	ASA class (I/II)	BMI (kg/m^2)
Group C(n = 42)	16/26	43.6 ± 11.4	16/26	22.5 ± 1.9
Group R(n = 42)	18/24	45.6 ± 11.0	11/31	22.9 ± 2.9
P value	0.657	0.414	0.243	0.449

Values are expressed as the mean ± standard deviation or as number of cases. No statistical differences were observed between groups in gender, age, ASA class or BMI.
R = remifentanil, C = control; M = male, F = female; ASA = American Society of Anesthesiologists physical status; BMI = body mass index.

Group R were significantly lower than those in Group C ($p < 0.01$, Table 2).

Hemodynamic data changes

There was no statistical difference in the data of HR and MAP between two groups at four corresponding time points ($p > 0.05$, Table 3 and Table 4).

Side effects or unintended effects

In both groups, none of the patients showed signs of apnea, muscle rigidity or other unintended effects.

Discussion

In this study, we demonstrated that pretreatment with remifentanil at a small dose of 0.3 μg/kg reduced the incidence and severity of sufentanil-induced cough without influencing the hemodynamics during anesthetic induction. The incidence of cough was 31% in patients in group C and decreased to 4.8% in patients in Group R.

Coughing following the administration of opioid drugs during general anesthesia induction is often reported. In this study, the incidence of cough induced by sufentanil was 31%. In an study by Agarwal et al. [2] sufentanil 0.3 μg/kg injected over 5 s elicited cough in 15.8% of patients, while in another study by Li et al. [14] the incidence of cough was 37% after the injection of sufentanil 0.5 μg/kg within 3 s. With a high dose of sufentanil (1 μg/kg), the incidence of sufentanil-induced cough could be up to 45.8% [1]. The various incidence among different studies might be due to the different doses of sufentanil used and the differences in concentrations, administration rate, race and age [1, 15].

Various mechanisms have been proposed to explain opioid-induced cough. A plumonary chemoreflex mediated by either vagal C-fiber receptors close to pulmonary vessels or irritant receptors may play a role in opioid-induced cough [16]. Opioid-induced histamine release [17] and muscle rigidity leading to sudden closure of the vocal cords or supraglottic obstruction by soft tissue [18] may be another possible casual factor for cough. In addition, in several studies, it was demonstrated that opioid receptor dualism might be an important mechanism of opioid-induced cough [3, 8, 19].

Various pretreatments with drugs, such as lidocaine, terbutaline, dezocine, dexmedetomidine, and magnesium sulfate have been reported to reduce the incidence of opioid-induced cough [1, 5, 6, 8, 20], however these drugs might add side effects and potential risks. In a study by He et al. [5], an injection with dexmedetomidine 0.5 μg/kg or 1.0 μg/kg over 10 min inhibited cough induced by the subsequent fentanyl (4 μg/kg) intravenous injection. However, this dose of dexmedetomidine has the potential to cause bradycardia and hypotension. Furthermore, an injection that is too slow may cause an issue. In another study [1], 30 or 50 mg/kg of $MgSO_4$ inhibited cough induced by a subsequent injection with 1.0 μg/kg sufentanil, however several patients dropped out of the study due to an obvious burning sensation during the injection of $MgSO_4$. In addition, the injection of $MgSO_4$ could increase plasma levels of magnesium. Furthermore, inhalation of terbutaline (5 mg in 2 ml NS, via a jet nebulizer) fifteen minutes before bolus fentanyl (5 μg/kg, iv) has been reported to inhibit cough [6], however the inaccessibility of terbutaline, long operating time, and complicated operations are some limitations of this approach. The injection of lidocaine 0.5 mg/kg has been proven effective to suppress fentanyl-induced cough [20], however the inhibition of cardiac function may be a potential risk. Dezocine 0.1 mg/kg 2 min prior to the administration

Table 3 Changes of MAP

Groups	MAP (mm Hg)			
	T0	T1	T2	T3
Group C	94.9 ± 13.8	76.2 ± 12.9	93.9 ± 20.4	82.0 ± 17.0
Group R	99.0 ± 12.7	78.7 ± 13.3	95.0 ± 16.5	84.7 ± 15.5
P value	$P = 0.322$			

Table 2 Incidence and severity of sufentanil induced cough

Groups	Incidence of cough (n(%))	Severity of cough (n(%))			
		None	Mild	Moderate	Severe
Group C(n = 42)	31	69	7.1	4.8	19
Group R(n = 42)	4.8	95.2	2.4	0	2.4
P value	0.002*	0.002*			

Values are expressed as frequency.
Both the incidence and severity of cough in patients in Group R were significantly lower compared to those in patients in Group C ($P < 0.01$).
R = remifentanil; C = control. The severity of cough was graded as mild (1, 2), moderate (2, 3), or severe (> 5) based on the number of cough observed in 60s after sufentanil injection. *Indicates $P < 0.01$ compared with patients in Group C.

Table 4 Changes of HR

Groups	HR (bpm)			
	T0	T1	T2	T3
Group C	80.0 ± 18.2	68.6 ± 16.9	77.0 ± 19.0	67.7 ± 15.2
Group R	78.9 ± 11.3	67.9 ± 11.0	77.8 ± 13.1	70.5 ± 10.9
P value	$P = 0.886$			

Values are expressed as mean ± standard deviation.
There were no significant differences in ether MAP or HR between the two groups.
R = remifentanil, C = control; T0, time before administration of remifentanil or normal saline; T1: 3 min after administration; T2: 1 min after intubation; T3: 3 min after intubation; MAP: mean arterial pressure; HR: heart rate.

of intravenous sufentanil (0.5 μg/kg) can also effectively suppress fentanyl-induced cough [8], however in short surgeries, the excessive sedation time of this dose of dezocine may be a problem.

In several other studies, a pre-emptive small dose of the opioids was used to inhibit opioid-induced cough, which could avoid the additional side effects or potential risks of other types of drugs. Hung et al. [4] reported that a pre-emptive small dose of fentanyl (25 μg) significantly reduced cough induced by a subsequent injection of 125 μg fentanyl, and Phua et al. [3] showed that intramuscular morphine pretreatment 1 h before general anesthesia induction could also decrease the incidence of fentanyl-induced cough. However, either fentanyl or morphine has limitations because of long onset or long duration time.

In the current study, we found that remifentanil, an opioid that is readily available, with both short onset and duration time, could decrease the incidence and severity of sufentanil-induced cough during anesthetic induction.

It is not yet clear how small doses of opioids inhibit the cough caused by opioids themselves. In a study by Hung et al. [4], a pre-emptive small dose of fentanyl (25 μg) significantly reduced cough induced by a subsequent injection with 125 μg fentanyl, and this phenomenon was thought to be associated with the lower plasma concentration fluctuation of fentanyl.

However, in the current study, we found that a pre-emptive small dose of 0.3 μg/kg remifentanil reduced cough induced by a subsequent injection with 0.5 μg/kg sufentanil. However, what was used as a pretreatment was another opioid, remifentanil, not sufentanil itself. Hence, the theory of fluctuations in the sufentanil plasma concentration mentioned above seems unlikely.

We hypothesized that opioid receptor dualism may be a possible mechanism to partly explain this phenomenon. One of the common and useful side-effects of opioid analgesics is suppression of the cough reflex, which is the basis of their use in oral cough suppressants [3]. Sufentanil, fentanyl, and remifentanil infusion before recovery from general anesthesia have previously been reported to suppress coughing during extubation [9, 21, 22]. Opioids may inhibit the cough reflex by a direct effect on the cough center in the medulla, at doses lower than those required for analgesia [3]. Therefore, we suggested that the anti-tussive effect of pre-emptive remifentanil in the present study might be related to a centrally-acting effect. The low priming dose of remifentanil might initially exert a central anti-tussive effect and then inhibit the cough-inducing effect of a subsequent large dose of sufentanil. This hypothesis was partly supported by the study of Phua et al. [3] in which the incidence of fentanyl-induced cough was reduced by intramuscular morphine pretreatment 1 h before general anesthesia induction. However, this speculation lacks definitive evidence, and therefore additional studies are warranted to verify this hypothesis, and to reveal the underlying mechanism of action.

Given that remifentanil has a respiratory depressive effect, possible apnea-related absence of cough after remifentanil administration must be considered. It is also possible that the dose of remifentanil caused a transient apnea that resulted in an absence of coughing. For example, Remifentanil took 50–60 s to reach the effect point, and the apnea took 40–50 s, which partially or even completely covered the observation time after sufentanil administration.

Remifentanil may induce muscle rigidity and blood pressure and HR decline [15]. In a study performed by Shen et al. [15], three patients in the rernifenranil group showed muscle rigidity. and one patient had significant bradycardia that required treatment with atropine. However, in our study, none of the patients showed such adverse reactions, which might be due to the very low dose of remifentanil that was used.

Our study has several limitations. Few studies have shown the number doses of remifentanil that are used to suppress cough caused by opioids, therefore, we used a dose of remifentanil that was close to the dose of fentanyl used in the study of Hung et al. [4] in which a pre-emptive small dose of fentanyl (25 μg) was used to reduce cough induced by a subsequent injection with125 μg fentanyl. Thus, we used a single dose of remifentanil, and therefore do not know whether different doses, such as 0.1 μg/kg, 0.2 μg/kg, 0.4 μg/kg would be effective in suppressing the sufentanil-induced cough reflex. Additional studies will need to be performed to explore the relationship between dose and the cough suppressing effect of remifentanil.

Conclusion

In conclusion, pretreatment with a small dose of remifentanil effectively and safely suppresses the incidence and severity of sufentanil-induced cough during the induction of general anesthesia, and may be used as an alternative treatment to inhibit sufentanil-induced cough.

Abbreviations

ACE: Angiotensin-converting-enzyme; ASA: American Society of Anesthesiologists; BMI: Body mass index; HR: Heart rate; IV: Intravenous; MAP: Mean arterial pressure; NS: Normal saline; SPO_2: Pulse oxygen saturation; SPSS: Statistical Product for Social Sciences

Acknowledgements

We would like to thank Dongqi Zhang from The First Affiliated Hospital of Wenzhou Medical University for assistance of data collection.

Authors' contributions

WL performed the trial and wrote the manuscript. JS assisted with trial conduct and data analysis. SF designed the study and revised the manuscript. All authors read and approved the final manuscript.

Author details
[1]Department of Anesthesiology, The First Affiliated Hospital of Wenzhou Medical University, Wenzhou 325000, China. [2]Department of Anesthesiology, The Second Affiliated Hospital and Yuying Children's Hospital of Wenzhou Medical University, Wenzhou 325000, China.

References

1. An L, Gui B, Su Z, Zhang Y, Liu H. Magnesium sulfate inhibits sufentanil-induced cough during anesthetic induction. Int J Clin Exp Med. 2015;8(8):13864–8.
2. Agarwal A, Gautam S, Nath SS, Gupta D, Singh U. Comparison of the incidence and severity of cough induced by sufentanil and fentanyl: a prospective, randomised, double-blind study. ANAESTHESIA. 2007;62(12):1230–2.
3. Phua WT, Teh BT, Jong W, Lee TL, Tweed WA. Tussive effect of a fentanyl bolus. Canadian Journal Of Anaesthesia = Journal Canadien D'anesthesie. 1991 1991-04-01;38(3):330–4.
4. Hung KC, Chen CW, Lin VCH, Weng HC, Hsieh SW. The effect of pre-emptive use of minimal dose fentanyl on fentanyl-induced coughing. ANAESTHESIA [Article]. 2010;65(1):4–7.
5. He L, Xu J, Dai R. Dexmedetomidine reduces the incidence of fentanyl-induced cough: a double-blind, randomized, and placebo-controlled study. UPSALA J MED SCI. 2012;117(1):18–21.
6. Lui PW, Hsing CH, Chu YC. Terbutaline inhalation suppresses fentanyl-induced coughing. CANADIAN JOURNAL OF ANAESTHESIA-JOURNAL CANADIEN D ANESTHESIE. [Article]. 1996;43(12):1216–9.
7. Guler G, Aksu R, Bicer C, Tosun Z, Boyaci A. Comparison of the effects of ketamine or lidocaine on fentanyl-induced cough in patients undergoing surgery: a prospective, double-blind, randomized, placebo-controlled study. CURRENT THERAPEUTIC RESEARCH-CLINICAL AND EXPERIMENTAL. [Article]. 2010;71(5):289–97.
8. Liu XS, Xu GH, Shen QY, Zhao Q, Cheng XQ, Zhang J, et al. Dezocine prevents sufentanil-induced cough during general anesthesia induction: a randomized controlled trial. PHARMACOL REP [Journal Article; Randomized Controlled Trial; Research Support, Non-US Gov't] 2015 2015-02-01;67(1):52–55.
9. Cho HB, Kim JY, Kim DH, Kim DW, Chae YJ. Comparison of the optimal effect-site concentrations of remifentanil for preventing cough during emergence from desflurane or sevoflurane anaesthesia. J INT MED RES. [Comparative Study; Journal Article; Randomized Controlled Trial]. 2012 2012-01-20;40(1):174–183.
10. Jun NH, Lee JW, Song JW, Koh JC, Park WS, Shim YH. Optimal effect-site concentration of remifentanil for preventing cough during emergence from sevoflurane-remifentanil anaesthesia. ANAESTHESIA. [Journal Article; Randomized Controlled Trial]. 2010 2010-09-01;65(9):930–935.
11. Kim H, Choi SH, Choi YS, Lee JH, Kim NO, Lee JR. Comparison of the antitussive effect of remifentanil during recovery from propofol and sevoflurane anaesthesia. ANAESTHESIA. [Comparative Study; Journal Article; Randomized Controlled Trial]. 2012 2012-07-01;67(7):765–770.
12. Lee B, Lee JR, Na S. Targeting smooth emergence: the effect site concentration of remifentanil for preventing cough during emergence during propofol-remifentanil anaesthesia for thyroid surgery. Br J Anaesth. [Clinical Trial; Journal Article; Research Support, Non-U.S. Gov't]. 2009 2009-06-01;102(6):775–778.
13. Yoo JY, Kim JY, Kwak HJ, Lee DC, Kim GW, Lee SY, et al. - Effect-site concentration of remifentanil for preventing cough during emergence in elderly patients undergoing nasal surgery: a comparison with adult patients. - Clin Interv Aging 2016 Sep 12;11:1247–1252. doi: https://doi.org/10.2147/CIA.S108705 . eCollection 2016.(- 1178-1998 (Electronic); - 1176-9092 (Linking)).
14. Li J, Li K. Effects of pre-inhalation of salbutamol on cough reflex induced by Sufentanil. In: Sadeghian SH, Mehta U, Rajbongshi P, ^editors. AER-Advances in Engineering Research; 2016. p. 237–9.
15. Shen J, Xu J, Zhou Z, Liu H, Yang J. Effect of equivalent doses of fentanyl, Sufentanil, and remifentanil on the incidence and severity of cough in patients undergoing abdominal surgery: a prospective, randomized, double-blind study. Current therapeutic research-clinical and experimental [article]. 2008;69(6):480–7.
16. Böhrer H, Fleischer F, Werning P. Tussive effect of a fentanyl bolus administered through a central venous catheter. ANAESTHESIA. 1990 1990-01-01;45(1):18–21.
17. Karlsson JA, Sant'Ambrogio G, Widdicombe J. Afferent neural pathways in cough and reflex bronchoconstriction. Journal Of Applied Physiology (Bethesda, Md.: 1985). 1988 1988-09-01;65(\):1007–1023.
18. Benthuysen JL, Smith NT, Sanford TJ, Head N, Dec-Silver H. Physiology of alfentanil-induced rigidity. ANESTHESIOLOGY. 1986 1986-04-01;64(4):440–446.
19. Ai Q, Hu Y, Wang Y, Wu S, Qin Z, Wang J, et al. Pentazocine pretreatment suppresses fentanyl-induced cough. PHARMACOL REP. [Journal Article; Randomized Controlled Trial]. 2010 2010-07-01;62(4):747–750.
20. Pandey CK, Raza M, Ranjan R, Singhal V, Kumar M, Lakra A, et al. Intravenous lidocaine 0.5 mg.Kg(−1) effectively suppresses fentanyl-induced cough. CANADIAN JOURNAL OF ANAESTHESIA-JOURNAL CANADIEN D ANESTHESIE [Article]. 2005;52(2):172–5.
21. Yoo YC, Na S, Jeong JJ, Choi EM, Moon BE, Lee JR. Dose-dependent attenuation by fentanyl on cough during emergence from general anesthesia. ACTA ANAESTH SCAND [Article]. 2011;55(10):1215–20.
22. Lee JY, Lim BG, Park HY, Kim NS. Sufentanil infusion before extubation suppresses coughing on emergence without delaying extubation time and reduces postoperative analgesic requirement without increasing nausea and vomiting after desflurane anesthesia. Korean J Anesthesiol [Journal Article] 2012 2012-06-01;62(6):512–517.

5

Comparison of emergence agitation between succinylcholine and rocuronium-sugammadex in adults following closed reduction of a nasal bone fracture

Seok-Jin Lee, Tae-Yun Sung* and Choon-Kyu Cho

Abstract

Background: Sugammadex allows rapid recovery from rocuronium-induced neuromuscular blockade. Succinylcholine is often used for brief surgeries but is associated with myalgia, headache, histamine release, and increased lactate levels. Thus, we hypothesized that succinylcholine may affect emergence agitation (EA) and compared the effects of succinylcholine and rocuronium-sugammadex on EA in patients undergoing closed reduction of a nasal bone fracture under general anesthesia.

Methods: Forty-two patients were prospectively enrolled and allocated randomly to the succinylcholine group (group SC) or the rocuronium-sugammadex group (group RS; each $n = 21$). Neuromuscular block and its reversal were achieved with succinylcholine and normal saline in group SC, whereas rocuronium and sugammadex were administered in group RS. After surgery, the incidence of EA as a primary outcome, the incidence of dangerous EA, and duration of EA as secondary outcomes were compared.

Results: The incidence of EA was higher in group SC than in group RS (90.5% vs. 47.6%, respectively; relative risk [RR] 4.3; 95% confidence interval [CI] 1.2 to 15.7; $P = .006$). The incidence of dangerous EA increased in group SC compared to group RS (33.3% vs. 4.8%, respectively; RR 2.1; 95% CI 1.3 to 3.4; $P = .045$). The duration of agitation was longer in group SC than in group RS [106.5 (65.1) vs. 40.4 (26.0) sec; mean difference 66.1 s; 95% CI 31.0 to 101.1; effect size 1.3; $P = .001$).

Conclusion: Succinylcholine increases the incidence, severity, and duration of EA compared to rocuronium-sugammadex in patients undergoing closed reduction of a nasal bone fracture.

Keywords: Emergence agitation, Rocuronium, Succinylcholine, Sugammadex

* Correspondence: unt1231@naver.com
Department of Anaesthesiology and Pain Medicine, Konyang University Hospital, Myunggok Medical Research Center, Konyang University College of Medicine, 158, Gwangeodong-ro, Seo-gu, Daejeon 35365, South Korea

Background

Despite a short surgical duration, general anesthesia is preferred for closed reduction of a nasal bone fracture due to extreme pain during the reduction manipulation, aspiration concerns, and better patient satisfaction with general anesthesia compared to local anesthesia [1]. However, closed reduction of a nasal bone fracture under general anesthesia is commonly associated with emergence agitation (EA) [2, 3].

Succinylcholine is a depolarizing neuromuscular blocking agent with a rapid onset time and a short duration of action; thus, it has been used for rapid sequence induction or short-duration procedures, such as closed reduction of a nasal bone fracture, despite its numerous side effects [2–5]. However, because sugammadex rapidly and effectively reverses any depth of steroidal neuromuscular blocking agent-induced neuromuscular blockade [6], the necessity for succinylcholine is controversial [7].

A case report suggested that rocuronium-sugammadex reduces the severity of agitation following electroconvulsive therapy by decreasing the increase in plasma lactate level compared to succinylcholine [8]. Additionally, succinylcholine can result in myalgia, headache, histamine release, increased intraocular pressure, and activation of the electroencephalogram [5, 9].

We hypothesized that succinylcholine would negatively affect EA and that rocuronium-sugammadex would reduce the incidence of EA compared to succinylcholine. Therefore, we designed this study to compare the effects of succinylcholine and rocuronium-sugammadex on EA in adult patients undergoing closed reduction of a nasal bone fracture.

Methods

We conducted this randomized prospective double-blind study after receiving approval from the Institutional Review Board of Konyang University Hospital, Daejeon, Korea (October 2017; KYUH 2017–07–020-001) and obtained written informed consent from all participants. The study was registered with the Korean Clinical Research Information Service (https://cris.nih.go.kr, permit number: KCT0002673) and adhered to CONSORT checklist. Subjects included patients aged 20–65 years with American Society of Anesthesiologists physical status classification I–II who underwent general anesthesia for closed reduction of a nasal bone fracture. We excluded patients who were contraindicated to any of the study drugs (e.g., hyperkalemia, renal failure [glomerular filtration rate < 30 mL/min], hepatic dysfunction, severe burn or trauma, neuromuscular disease, personal history or family history of malignant hyperthermia), history of an allergic reaction to any of the study drugs, body mass index ≥30 kg/m^2, presence of unstable vital signs, and any other fracture or injury requiring a combined operation in addition to reduction of a nasal bone fracture. Patients were allocated randomly (allocation ratio 1:1) to one of two groups (succinylcholine group: group SC or the rocuronium + sugammadex group; group RS) using a random number table generated using online randomization software (www.randomizer.org).

All patients fasted at least 8 h and received no premedication before the induction of anesthesia. Patients were blinded to their group allocation. All patients were monitored in the operating room using routine monitoring, including non-invasive automated blood pressure, pulse oximetry, electrocardiography, bispectral index (BIS; BIS VISTA™ monitor; Aspect Medical Systems, Norwood, MA, USA), and neuromuscular train-of-four (TOF) by acceleromyography (TOF-Watch SX®; Organon Ltd., Dublin, Ireland) on the adductor pollicis muscle. Preoxygenation was conducted with tidal volume breathing for 2 min using 8 L/min of 100% oxygen, and then anesthesia was induced with 2 mg/kg propofol and 1 μg /kg fentanyl. Succinylcholine (1 mg/kg) in group SC or rocuronium (0.6 mg/kg) in group RS was administered as a neuromuscular blocking agent to facilitate endotracheal intubation. After loss of consciousness and before administering the succinylcholine or rocuronium, the acceleromyograph was calibrated automatically in CAL-2 mode, and TOF stimulation was then initiated. Intubation was performed after confirming the disappearance of fasciculation or complete depression of the first twitch (T1) of the TOF in group SC, and after confirming a TOF count of zero in group RS. After intubation, volume-controlled mechanical ventilation was initiated at a tidal volume of 8 ml/kg and a respiratory rate of 12 breaths/min; then, the respiratory rate was adjusted to maintain an end-tidal carbon dioxide concentration of 30–40 mmHg. Anesthesia was maintained with 1.5–5 vol% of end-tidal concentration of sevoflurane and 50% nitrous oxide (N_2O) to maintain the BIS at 40–60. Before the end of surgery, 0.3 mg ramosetron was injected intravenously to prevent postoperative nausea and vomiting in all patients. All events during the maintenance of anesthesia, such as patient-ventilator dyssynchrony (PVD), were recorded. PVD was denoted by significant changes in the volume, pressure and flow graphic waveforms of the ventilator [10].

At the end of the surgery, intranasal packing and a nasal splint were applied and 2 or 4 mg/kg sugammadex (Bridion®; MSD, Seoul, Korea) plus normal saline (total volume = 5 mL) was intravenously injected to reverse the neuromuscular blockade based on neuromuscular monitoring in group RS, whereas 5 mL normal saline was injected in group SC.

The study drugs were prepared and anesthesia was induced by an anesthesiologist who knew the patient allocation but was not involved in data collection. Data collection in the operating room was performed by another anesthesiologist who entered the operating room immediately after induction of anesthesia and was blinded to the patient allocations. The TOF monitor was covered with a surgical towel and exposure was only permitted to the anesthesiologist who prepared the study drugs. Preparation of the study drugs was masked to the data-collecting anesthesiologist using an opaque partition between the two anesthesiologists.

The same extubation criteria were applied to the groups; BIS ≥80, tidal volume ≥ 5 ml/kg, and respiratory rate 10–25 rate/min during spontaneous breathing, except TOF ratio ≥ 0.9 in group RS. Duration of anesthesia and surgery were defined as the time from induction of anesthesia to extubation and the time from packing intranasal Bosmin®-soaked gauze (1 mg/mL epinephrine solution; Je Il Pharm, Seoul, Korea) to complete the nasal splint after applying intranasal packing with saline-soaked Merocel® (polyvinyl acetate sponge, Medtronic Xomed, Jacksonville, FL, USA).

Emergence was defined as the time interval from discontinuation of the inhalational anesthetic to 5 min after extubation. The Ricker Sedation-Agitation Scale (RSAS) was used to assess EA [11], and the maximum score was recorded: 1 = unarousable, 2 = very sedated, 3 = sedated, 4 = calm and cooperative, 5 = agitated and calm to verbal instruction, 6 = very agitated, requiring restraint; 7 = pulling at the tracheal tube, trying to remove catheters, or striking the staff. RSAS ≥5 and = 7 were defined as EA and dangerous EA, respectively. The duration of any EA was measured. During emergence, time to first spontaneous respiration, time to first awakening response, such as eye opening to a verbal command or grimacing, and time to extubation were measured and recorded.

Postoperative pain and the sense of suffocation were recorded in the post-anesthetic care unit (PACU) on a 0–10 numeric rating scale (NRS, 0 = no sense of pain/suffocation, 10 = worst sense of pain/suffocation imaginable). In case of a NRS for pain > 4, 0.5 mg/kg fentanyl was injected intravenously and the patient was re-evaluated 10 min later. If a patient complained of nausea or vomiting, 10 mg metoclopramide was injected intravenously. Any complications, such as bitter taste, dizziness, headache, shivering, or respiratory depression, were also evaluated and recorded by the data-collecting anesthesiologist.

The primary outcome was incidence of EA (RSAS ≥5). The secondary outcomes were incidence of dangerous EA (RSAS = 7) and duration of EA. Other outcomes were frequency of PVD, time to first spontaneous respiration, time to first awakening response, time to extubation, NRS for postoperative pain and sense of suffocation, requirement for analgesics and/or antiemetics, and adverse events.

Statistical analysis

In a pilot study, the incidence of EA was 92.0% in group SC (n = 12). A sample size of 19 patients per group was required to detect a 50% reduction in the incidence of EA with a power of 0.8 and a two-sided α-value of 0.05. Thus, we enrolled 21 patients per group considering potential dropout. The statistical analysis was conducted using SPSS software (ver. 18.0 for Windows; SPSS Inc., Chicago, IL, USA). The distribution of the numerical data was assessed with the Kolmogorov–Smirnov test. Continuous variables are presented as mean (standard deviation) or median and interquartile range, and were analyzed using Student's t-test or the Mann–Whitney U-test where appropriate. Categorical variables were expressed as numbers (%) or numbers and analyzed by the χ^2 test or Fisher's exact test as appropriate. A P-value < .05 was considered significant.

Results

In total, 46 patients were assessed for eligibility (28 November 2017 to 17 April 2018), and 4 were excluded; 3 patients had another fracture in addition to the nasal bone fracture and 1 patient refused to participate in the study. Consequently, 42 patients were randomly allocated to group SC or RS and analyzed (Fig. 1).

The demographic data were comparable between the two groups (Table 1).

The incidence of EA was significantly higher in group SC than group RS (90.5% [19/21] vs. 47.6% [10/21], respectively; relative risk [RR] 4.3; 95% CI 1.2 to 15.7; P = .006; Table 2). The incidence of dangerous EA was also significantly higher in group SC than group RS (33.3% [7/21] vs. 4.8% [1/21], respectively; RR 2.1; 95% CI 1.3 to 3.4; P = .045; Table 2). The duration of agitation was significantly more prolonged in group SC than group RS [106.5 (65.1) sec vs. 40.4 (26.0) sec, respectively; mean difference 66.1 s; 95% CI 31.0 to 101.1; effect size 1.3; P = .001; Table 2). During surgery, PVD was more frequent in group SC than group RS (23.8% [5/21] vs. 0% [0/21], respectively; RR 2.3; 95% confidence interval [CI] 1.6 to 3.3; P = .048; Table 2). Time to spontaneous respiration, time to first awakening response, and time to extubation did not differ between the groups (Table 2). In the PACU, the NRS for pain, the NRS for sense of suffocation, and the requirement for analgesics and/or an antiemetic drug did not differ between the groups (Table 2).

The rate of adverse events was also similar between the groups (Table 3).

Discussion

This study demonstrated that neuromuscular blockade using succinylcholine and spontaneous recovery of neuromuscular function is associated with more

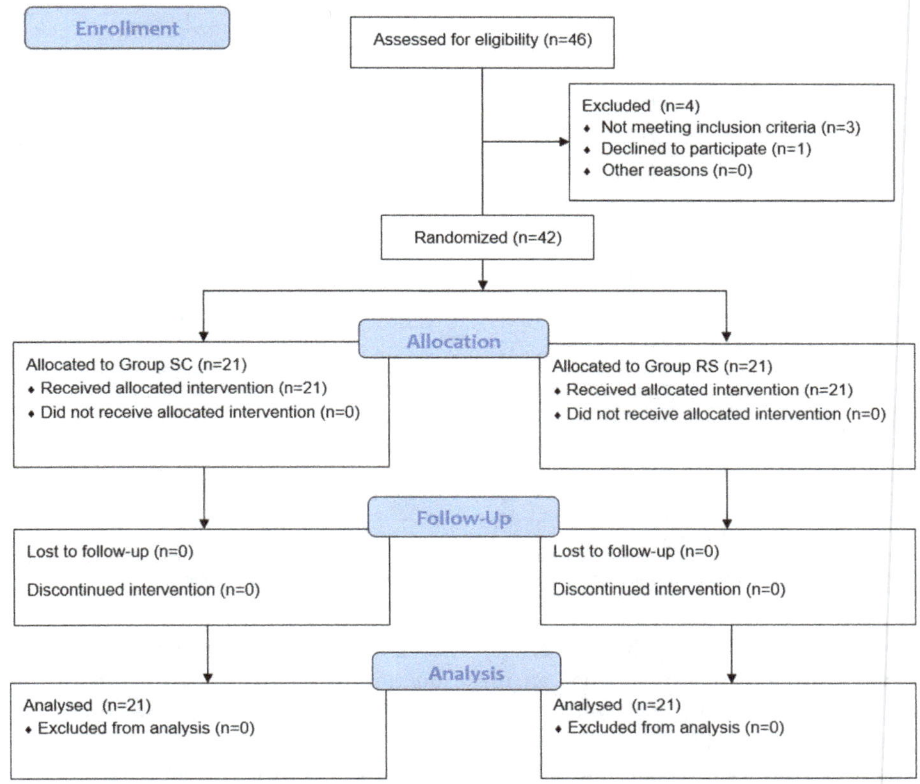

Fig. 1 Flow chart. Group SC: succinylcholine group; Group RS: rocuronium + sugammadex group

frequent, dangerous, and longer EA compared to that encountered after administering rocuronium-induced neuromuscular blockade with reversal by sugammadex in adult patients undergoing closed reduction of a nasal bone fracture.

Table 1 Demographic data and surgical details

	Group SC ($n = 21$)	Group RS ($n = 21$)
Age, yr	35.3 (14.5)	36.2 (14.2)
Gender (male), *n* (%)	14 (66.7)	14 (66.7)
Height, cm	169.8 (4.8)	167.7 (7.3)
Weight, kg	71.8 (11.0)	66.7 (5.6)
ASA (I/II), *n*	11/10	12/9
Intraoperative fluids, ml	100 [100–150]	150 [100–150]
Duration of surgery, min	17.6 (4.8)	16.5 (3.5)
Duration of anesthesia, min	32.4 (5.1)	32.3 (4.5)
Sugammadex (dose), *n* (%)		
2 mg/kg	NA	9 (42.9)
4 mg/kg	NA	12 (57.1)

Values are mean (standard deviation), median [IQR; interquartile range], numbers (%), or numbers
Group SC succinylcholine group, *Group RS* rocuronium + sugammadex group, *AS* American Society of Anesthesiologists physical status classification, *NA* not applicable

Several studies have investigated the prevention of EA by comparing inhalation anesthetics and intravenous anesthetics or by using analgesics or sedatives [3, 12–16]; potent analgesics (remifentanil, fentanyl, nefopam), *N*-methyl-D-aspartate receptor antagonists (ketamine, magnesium sulfate, and tramadol), α2-aderenoreceptor agonists (clonidine and dexmedetomidine), and propofol have a protective effect on EA, while inhalation anesthetics with low blood/gas partition coefficients (sevoflurane and desflurane), doxapram, and benzodiazepine premedication increase the risk of EA.

To our knowledge, this is the first randomized controlled study to compare the effects of different kinds of neuromuscular blocking agents with reversal on EA after general anesthesia. Our results suggest that different types of neuromuscular blocking agents (depolarizing vs. nondepolarizing) and/or reversal (spontaneously vs. by sugammadex) may affect the characteristics of EA.

EA is more common following closed reduction of a nasal bone fracture than following other surgeries [2, 3, 15]. We speculate that the use of sevoflurane as an inhalation anesthetic agent with low blood-gas solubility is a causative factor in the relatively high incidence of EA after this surgery. Closed reduction of a nasal bone fracture is a short-duration surgery, so inhalation anesthetics

Table 2 Intraoperative and recovery data

	Group SC ($n = 21$)	Group RS ($n = 21$)	Mean difference or RR (95% CI)	*P*
In operating room				
Patient-ventilator dyssynchrony, *n* (%)	5 (23.8)	0 (0)	2.3 (1.6 to 3.3)	0.04
Emergence agitation, *n* (%)	19 (90.5)	10 (47.6)	4.3 (1.2 to 15.7)	0.01
Dangerous emergence agitation, *n* (%)	7 (33.3)	1 (4.8)	2.1 (1.3 to 3.4)	0.04
Duration of agitation, sec	106.5 (65.1)	40.4 (26.0)	66.1 (31.0 to 101.1)	0.001
Time to spontaneous respiration, min	5.9 (2.1)	5.6 (2.0)	0.3 (−0.9 to 1.6)	0.60
Time to first awakening response, min	6.9 (1.7)	7.1 (1.7)	−0.3 (−1.4 to 0.7)	0.54
Time to extubation, min	8.3 (1.7)	7.4 (1.7)	0.9 (−0.1 to1.9)	0.09
In PACU				
NRS for pain	2.8 (2.4)	3.5 (2.4)	−0.7 (−2.2 to 0.7)	0.34
NRS for sense of suffocation	7.1 (2.0)	6.5 (2.6)	0.6 (−0.8 to 2.1)	0.39
Fentanyl, *n* (%)	3 (14.3)	5 (23.8)	NA	0.70
Metoclopramide, *n* (%)	0	1 (4.8)	NA	> 0.99

Values are mean (standard deviation), numbers (%) or numbers
Group SC succinylcholine group, *Group RS* rocuronium + sugammadex group, *RR* relative risk, *CI* confidence interval, *NRS* numerical rating scale (0 = no sense of pain/suffocation, 10 = worst sense of pain/suffocation imaginable), *NA* not applicable, *PACU* post-anesthesia care unit

permitting rapid recovery after surgery have been favored [2, 3]. However, inhalation anesthesia has an increased incidence of EA compared with total intravenous anesthesia [15, 17]. Additionally, sevoflurane anesthesia causes increases in brain lactate and glucose concentrations, and elevated brain lactate and glucose concentrations are positively correlated with the EA score [18]. Another factor that may increase EA is intranasal packing because packing can lead to an abrupt sense of suffocation when a patient's consciousness is restored. A previous study [17] on adults undergoing nasal surgery found that intranasal packing following nasal surgery was not a risk factor for EA; the authors explained that nasal obstruction by nasal packing had little influence on their patients' breathing because patients who undergo nasal surgery are chronic mouth breathers due to their nasal disease. However, that study did not include patients undergoing closed reduction of a nasal bone fracture [17]. Most patients who require closed reduction of a nasal bone fracture are not chronic mouth breathers because their fracture resulted from acute trauma [1]. This is supported by the NRS scores in the PACU of our patients: although previous studies [15, 17, 19] have demonstrated that pain is one of the most important risk factors for EA in adults, scores for suffocation were substantially higher than pain scores in both study groups (Table 2).

Table 3 Adverse events

	Group SC ($n = 21$)	Group RS ($n = 21$)	*P*
Headache	2 (9.5)	5 (23.8)	0.41
Dizziness	2 (9.5)	0 (0)	0.48
Bitter taste	2 (9.5)	0 (0)	0.48
Myalgia	1 (4.8)	0 (0)	> 0.99
Dry mouth	1 (4.8)	0 (0)	> 0.99
Shivering	0 (0)	1 (4.8)	> 0.99
Nausea	0 (0)	1 (4.8)	> 0.99
Vomiting	0 (0)	0 (0)	NA

Values are numbers (%)
Group SC succinylcholine group, *Group RS* rocuronium + sugammadex group, *NA* not applicable

In the present study, succinylcholine had a more negative association with EA in terms of incidence, severity, and duration, compared to rocuronium-sugammadex. Although the precise mechanism of EA is unclear, possible explanations are as follows. First, EA may be related to metabolic changes because the use of succinylcholine increases lactate and potassium concentrations compared to rocuronium-sugammadex [8, 20]. An increase in brain lactate level could indicate greater neuronal activity and is linked with a tendency to manifest EA [18]. Increased potassium level may affect potassium channels in the lateral nucleus of the amygdala, which is associated with regulating stress-induced behavior [21]. Second, although the succinylcholine and rocuronium doses used in this study correspond to the typical doses recommended to facilitate intubation, the different depth of neuromuscular block between the groups may have affected EA. The duration of a complete succinylcholine block (dose of 1 mg/kg) in a patient with normal plasma cholinesterase is 3–7 min and the duration of action for rocuronium (dose of 0.6 mg/kg) is 35–45 min [5, 9]. In our study, the difference in duration of action between the two neuromuscular blocking agents resulted in more frequent PVD in group SC than in group RS (23.8% vs.

0%, respectively). Rocuronium provided deep or moderate depth of neuromuscular block in all patients in group RS until the end of surgery on TOF monitoring. Insufficient neuromuscular block in group SC may increase the administration of sevoflurane to suppress PVD. Moreover, although we adjusted the concentration of sevoflurane according to an equal BIS of 40–60 in both groups, the shallow depth of the neuromuscular block in group SC increased electromyographic (EMG) activity, which can result in an increased concentration of sevoflurane to decrease the BIS, regardless of the actual level of sedation [22]. However, different concentrations of sevoflurane and resulting depths of anesthesia did not affect the EA [23]. Third, succinylcholine can increase intraocular and intragastric pressure, cause flushing due to histamine release, and have undesirable autonomic effects [9]. It is not known exactly how these factors affect the occurrence of EA, but it is likely that they had a negative effect on EA.

In the present study, the incidence of EA in group SC was higher than in a previous study of closed reduction of nasal bone fracture, despite the use of the same neuromuscular blocking agent (succinylcholine) and the same inhalation anesthetics (sevoflurane-N_2O) [3]. This difference might be related to the use of different EA assessment parameters. In the previous study [3], the authors reported an EA incidence of 45.0% using Aono's scale [24] and EA was defined when the Aono score was ≥3. In other words, they did not include cases as EA when the Aono score was 2. Aono's scale defines 2 as "not calm, but could be easily calmed", which is very similar to a RSAS of 5 (= agitated and calm to verbal instruction), which we used to consider EA in our study. If an Aono's score of 2 were to be considered EA, the incidence of EA would be 95.0%, which is comparable to the 90.5% in our study.

The use of rocuronium-sugammadex reduces the frequency of headache and myalgia following electroconvulsive therapy compared to succinylcholine [4]. However, adverse events were comparable between the two groups in our study. The reason for the discordance in the results of adverse events may be mainly attributed to the different interventions (electroconvulsive therapy vs. closed reduction of a nasal bone fracture); it might also be related to the fact that our study was not fully powered to detect differences in adverse events.

Although rocuronium-sugammadex has several advantages over succinylcholine (e.g., predictable reversal of any depth of rocuronium-induced neuromuscular block, reduced incidence of PVD during mechanical ventilation, reduced incidence and severity of EA, etc.), sugammadex is significantly more expensive. A systemic review of rocuronium-sugammadex and succinylcholine failed to produce an estimate cost-effectiveness due to a lack of underlying relevant clinical data [25]. Conclusive pharmacoeconomic assessment of these drugs may require further clinical studies.

This study had several limitations. First, objective neuromuscular monitoring was not included in the extubation criteria of group SC because tetanic fade does not occur at a clinically appropriate concentration of succinylcholine [26]. Although clinically significant residual neuromuscular block was not observed in this study, there was the possibility of residual neuromuscular block in some patients who received succinylcholine because succinylcholine has high interpatient variability in duration of action (range 1.3–44 min) [27]. Incomplete recovery of neuromuscular function may be partly attributed to the high incidence of EA in group SC by causing distress and agitation during emergence. Second, the blood concentration of carbon dioxide was not measured in this study. A decrease in cerebral blood flow due to hypocarbia, and acidosis due to hypercarbia, may alter consciousness and contribute to the occurrence of EA [28]. However, in this study, the end-tidal carbon dioxide was adjusted from 30 to 40 mmHg in both groups; therefore, the effect of blood carbon dioxide on EA would be similar in both groups. Finally, it is unclear whether the results of this study are due to an EA-preventive effect of rocuronium-sugammadex or an EA-inducing effect of succinylcholine, or both. However, considering that rocuronium or sugammadex intrinsically has no analgesic or sedative effects that could contribute to reduce the incidence of EA, the results of this study may be mainly due to the EA-inducing effect of succinylcholine. On the other hand, even if rocuronium-sugammadex has intrinsic efficacy in preventing EA, it is also uncertain which of the two mainly contributed to reducing the incidence of EA. Further studies using rocuronium with different kinds of reversal agents (e.g., antiacetylcholinesterase vs. sugammadex vs. spontaneous recovery) or different kinds of neuromuscular blocking agents (e.g., rocuronium vs. vecuronium) with reversal by sugammadex are needed.

Conclusion

Rocuronium-induced neuromuscular block and recovery using sugammadex are effective for decreasing the incidence, severity, and duration of EA compared to succinylcholine following closed reduction of a nasal bone fracture.

Abbreviations

EA: Emergence agitation; NA: Not applicable; NRS: Numerical rating scale; PACU: Post-anesthesia care unit; RS: Rocuronium-sugammadex; SC: Succinylcholine

Acknowledgements

Not applicable.

Authors' contributions

TYS designed the study, analyzed and interpreted the patient's data. TYS, SJL and CKC performed the investigation and data curation. TYS and SJL were major contributor in writing and revising the manuscript. All authors have read and approved the manuscript.

References

1. Al-Moraissi EA, Ellis E. Local versus general anesthesia for the management of nasal bone fractures: a systematic review and meta-analysis. J Oral Maxillofac Surg. 2015;73:606–15.
2. Lee YS, Baek CW, Kim DR, Kang H, Choi GJ, Park YH, et al. Comparison of hemodynamic response to tracheal intubation and postoperative pain in patients undergoing closed reduction of nasal bone fracture under general anesthesia: a randomized controlled trial comparing fentanyl and oxycodone. BMC Anesthesiol. 2016;16(1):115.
3. Kim YS, Chae YK, Choi YS, Min JH, Ahn SW, Yoon JW, et al. Comparative study of emergence agitation between sevoflurane and propofol anesthesia in adults after closed reduction of nasal bone fracture. Korean J Anesthesiol. 2012;63(1):48–53.
4. Saricicek V, Sahin L, Bulbul F, Ucar S, Sahin M. Does rocuronium-sugammadex reduce myalgia and headache after electroconvulsive therapy in patients with major depression? J ECT. 2014;30:30–4.
5. Lee C. Goodbye suxamethonium! Anaesthesia. 2009;64:73–81.
6. Keating GM. Sugammadex: a review of neuromuscular blockade reversal. Drugs. 2016;76:1041–52.
7. Caldwell JE, Miller RD. Clinical implications of sugammadex. Anaesthesia. 2009;64(Suppl 1):66–72.
8. Postaci A, Tiryaki C, Sacan O, Ornek D, Kalyoncu M, Dikmen B. Rocuronium-sugammadex decreases the severity of post-electroconvulsive therapy agitation. J ECT. 2013;29:e2–3.
9. Orebaugh SL. Succinylcholine: adverse effects and alternatives in emergency medicine. Am J Emerg Med. 1999;17:715–21.
10. Mellott KG, Grap MJ, Munro CL, Sessler CN, Wetzel PA. Patient-ventilator dyssynchrony: clinical significance and implications for practice. Crit Care Nurse. 2009;29:41–55.
11. Riker RR, Picard JT, Fraser GL. Prospective evaluation of the sedation-agitation scale for adult critically ill patients. Crit Care Med. 1999;27:1325–9.
12. Polat R, Peker K, Baran I, Bumin AG, Gülöksüz TC, Dönmez A. Comparison between dexmedetomidine and remifentanil infusion in emergence agitation during recovery after nasal surgery: a randomized double-blind trial. Anaesthesist. 2015;64(10):740–6.
13. Jee YS, You HJ, Sung TY, Cho CK. Effects of nefopam on emergence agitation after general anesthesia for nasal surgery: a prospective, randomized, and controlled trial. Medicine. 2017;96:e8843.
14. Lee SJ, Choi SJ, In CB, Sung TY. Effects of tramadol on emergence agitation after general anesthesia for nasal surgery: a retrospective cohort study. Medicine. 2019;98(10):e14763.
15. Yu D, Chai W, Sun X, Yao L. Emergence agitation in adults: risk factors in 2,000 patients. Can J Anesth. 2010;57:843–8.
16. Dahmani S, Stany I, Brasher C, Lejeune C, Bruneau B, Wood C, et al. Pharmacological prevention of sevoflurane and desflurane-related emergence agitation in children: a meta-analysis of published studies. Br J Anaesth. 2010;104:216–23.
17. Kim HJ, Kim DK, Kim HY, Kim JK, Choi SW. Risk factors of emergence agitation in adults undergoing general anesthesia for nasal surgery. Clin Exp Otorhinolaryngol. 2015;8:46–51.
18. Jacob Z, Li H, Makaryus R, Zhang S, Reinsel R. Metabolomic profiling of children's brains undergoing general anesthesia with sevoflurane and propofol. Anesthesiology. 2012;117:1062–71.
19. Rim JC, Kim JA, Hong JI, Park SY, Lee JH, Chung CJ. Risk factors of emergence agitation after general anesthesia in adult patients. Anesth Pain Med. 2016;11(4):410–6.
20. Sabo D, Jahr J, Pavlin J, Philip B, Shimode N, Rowe E, et al. The increases in potassium concentrations are greater with succinylcholine than with rocuronium-sugammadex in outpatient surgery: a randomized, multicentre trial. Can J Anaesth. 2014;61(5):423–32.
21. McLott J, Jurecic J, Hemphill L, Dunn KS. Development of an amygdalocentric neurocircuitry-reactive aggression theoretical model of emergence delirium in posttraumatic stress disorder: an integrative literature review. AANA J. 2013;81:379–84.
22. Dahaba AA. Different conditions that could result in the bispectral index indicating an incorrect hypnotic state. Anesth Analg. 2005;101:765–73.
23. Frederick HJ, Wofford K, de Lisle DG, Schulman SRA. Randomized controlled trial to determine the effect of depth of anesthesia on emergence agitation in children. Anesth Analg. 2016;122:1141–6.
24. Aono J, Ueda W, Mamiya K, Takimoto E, Manabe M. Greater incidence of delirium during recovery from sevoflurane anesthesia in preschool boys. Anesthesiology. 1997;87(6):1298–300.
25. Chambers D, Paulden M, Paton F, Heirs M, Duffy S, Hunter JM, et al. Sugammadex for reversal of neuromuscular block after rapid sequence intubation: a systematic review and economic assessment. Br J Anaesth. 2010;105:568–75.
26. Jonsson M, Dabrowski M, Gurley DA, Larsson O, Johnson EC. Activation and inhibition of human muscular and neuronal nicotinic acetylcholine receptors by succinylcholine. Anesthesiology. 2006;104:724–33.
27. Dell-Kuster S, Levano S, Burkhart CS, Lelais F, Zemp A, Schobinger E, et al. Predictors of the variability in neuromuscular block duration following succinylcholine: a prospective, observational study. Eur J Anaesthesiol. 2015; 32:687–96.
28. Viswanath O, Kerner B, Jean YK, Soto R, Rosen G. Emergence delirium: a narrative review. J Anesthesiol Clin Sci. 2015;4:2.

6

Comparison of regional and local anesthesia for arteriovenous fistula creation in end-stage renal disease

Chen Gao[1], Chunyan Weng[2], Chenghai He[3*], Jingli Xu[2] and Liqiang Yu[1]

Abstract

Background: Arteriovenous fistulae (AVF) are the hemodialysis access modality of choice for patients with end-stage renal disease. However, they have a high early failure rate. Good vascular access is essential to manage long-term hemodialytic treatment, but some anesthesia techniques directly affect venous diameter as well as intra- and post-operative blood flow. The main purpose of this meta-analysis was to compare the results of regional and local anesthesia (RA and LA) for arteriovenous fistula creation in end-stage renal disease.

Methods: We conducted a systematic review and meta-analysis to synthesize evidence from 7 randomized controlled trials (565 patients) and 1 observational study (408 patients) with the aim of evaluating the safety and efficacy of RA versus LA in surgical construction of AVF.

Results: Pooled data showed that RA was associated with higher primary patency rates than LA (odds ratio [OR], 1.88; 95% confidence interval [CI]: 1.24–2.84; $P = 0.003$; $I^2 = 31\%$). Additionally, brachial artery diameter was significantly increased in the RA versus LA group (mean difference [MD], 0.83; 95% CI: 0.75–0.92; $P < 0.001$; $I^2 = 97\%$) and the need for intra- as well as post-operative pain killers was significantly less (RA, $P = 0.0363$; LA, $P = 0.0318$). Moreover, operation duration was significantly reduced using RA versus LA (MD, − 29.63; 95% CI: − 32.78 - -26.48; $P < 0.001$; $I^2 = 100\%$).

Conclusions: This meta-analysis suggests that RA is preferable to LA in patients with end-stage renal disease in guaranteeing AVF patency and increasing brachial artery diameter.

Keywords: Arteriovenous fistula, End-stage renal disease, Local anesthesia, Regional anesthesia, Meta-analysis, Systematic review

Background

The construction of arteriovenous fistulae (AVF) is an established form of therapy for patients with chronic renal failure. However, the primary failure rate for AVF creation under local anesthesia (LA) for hemodialysis is very high; approximately one third of AVF fail at an early stage [1]. General anesthesia (GA), regional anesthesia (RA), and local anesthetic infiltration are three acceptable anesthetic techniques used for the surgical construction of AVF; however, the choice of anesthetic technique may significantly affect early patency or long-term AVF outcomes.

General anesthesia is associated with increased cardiorespiratory complications in patients with end-stage

* Correspondence: hikiddhechenghai@163.com
[3]Department of Internal Medicine, The Affiliated Hospital of Hangzhou Normal University, 126 Wenzhou Road, Zhejiang, Hangzhou, China

renal disease. Thus, in such patients, RA, such as a brachial plexus block (BPB), or LA are favored for AVF creation. However, whilst both local anesthetic infiltration and RA avoid the risks associated with GA, only RA may be used to produce an associated sympathetic nerve block, which increases venous diameter and arterial flow intraoperatively, as well as in the early postoperative period.

Compared with LA, BPB is thought to improve local hemodynamic parameters. However, the effects of both techniques on fistula patency and failure rates are highly controversial. Therefore, we conducted a systematic review and meta-analysis to collect evidence from published randomized controlled trials (RCTs) and observational studies to assess the safety and efficacy of LA and RA in the surgical creation of AVF.

Methods

Electronic searches

This systematic review and meta-analysis followed the Preferred Reporting Items for Systematic Reviews and Meta-Analyses (PRISMA) statement recommendations. We searched the literature using PubMed, EMBASE, and Cochrane library databases, and included studies published from August 1951 to September 2017. The Medical Subject Headings (MESH) search query used were as follows: arteriovenous fistula OR (arteriovenous AND fistula) AND (anesthesia OR local anesthesia OR brachial plexus anesthesia OR regional anesthesia OR anesthesia OR regional anesthesia OR brachial plexus block OR brachial plexus anesthesia OR brachial plexus blockade OR local anesthesia OR conduction anesthesia OR infiltration anesthesia). We also reviewed the reference lists of eligible studies and reviews to identify any additional relevant studies. Disagreement over relevance was resolved by consensus.

Study selection

Study titles and abstracts were screened for eligibility by two independent reviewers. Eligible studies included open-label and double-blinded RCTs, as well as retrospective studies with adult open-label participants (≥ 18 years), that compared the efficacy of RA versus LA for AVF creation in end-stage renal disease. Studies meeting any of the following criteria were excluded: (a) animal-based studies; (b) studies not published in English; (c) abstracts, editorials, case reports, reviews, and case series.

The following data and outcomes were extracted and included in the study: (a) study characteristics (including: study design, sample size, follow-up duration, and publication year); (b) primary clinical outcomes (including: primary fistula patency rate, primary fistula failure rate, surgery duration, change in brachial artery diameter (mm), change in brachial artery blood flow rate (mL/min), and post-surgery comorbidities).

Data analyses and quality assessment

We used Review Manager software (RevMan version 5.3) to analyze the extracted data. Odds ratios (ORs) were calculated with 95% confidence intervals (CIs). Heterogeneity between ORs for the same outcomes across different studies were explored using the I^2 inconsistency test, which describes the percentage of total variation across studies due to heterogeneity as opposed to chance. A value of 0% indicates no observed statistical heterogeneity, whilst larger values signify more substantial heterogeneity.

The studies were assessed using the Cochrane risk of bias tool (Fig. 2) and the Newcastle-Ottawa Scale (Table 1). Disagreements between the two independent investigators were resolved via discussion.

Results

Details of the auto-selection process are outlined in Fig. 1. Overall, 8 studies, including 7 RCTs [2–8] and 1 retrospective study, [9] with a total of 955 patients, met the inclusion criteria. The characteristics of all included studies are provided in Table 2 Details of the quality assessments are provided in Fig. 2 and Table 1.

Clinical outcomes

In total, 7 studies, including 852 patients, [2, 3, 5–9] evaluated primary patency rates in RA versus LA; RA was associated with higher primary patency rates than LA (OR, 1.88; 95% CI: 1.24–2.84; $P = 0.003$; $I^2 = 31\%$; Fig. 3). The combined data from 3 trials, [6–8] including 284 patients, demonstrated that RA was associated with significantly increased brachial artery diameters compared to LA (mean difference (MD), 0.83; 95% CI: 0.75–0.92; $P < 0.001$; $I^2 = 97\%$). The combined data from 2 trials, [6, 8] including 144 patients, revealed that LA was associated with significantly reduced branchial artery blood flow compared to RA (MD, 47.5; 95% CI: 35.18–59.12; $P < 0.001$; $I^2 = 83\%$). Two trials, [4, 6] including 229 patients, reported data regarding operative times, demonstrating significantly longer operative times in RA versus LA (MD, – 29.63 min, 95% CI: – 32.78 - -26.48; $P < 0.001$; $I^2 = 100\%$). Details of the clinical outcomes are provided in Table 3.

Complications

The combined data from 3 trials, [3, 6, 9] including 594 patients, demonstrated no difference between RA and LA in terms of vascular access infection (MD, 0.68; 95% CI: 0.23–2.02; $P = 0.49$; $I^2 = 0\%$). Three trials, [2, 3, 6] including 163 patients, revealed no significant difference between RA and LA with respect to the incidence of

Table 1 Risk of bias assessment

Study	Selection	Comparability	Exposure	Total score
Solomonson, et al. 1994	**	**	***	7

fistula thrombosis (OR, 0.21; 95% CI: 0.03–1.27; $P = 0.09$; $I^2 = 0\%$). Observations after BPBs in 1 trial, [3] including 60 patients, found no significant differences in the blocks until six-weeks post fistula creation (OR, 0.19; 95% CI: 0.01–4.06; $P = 0.29$; $I^2 = 0\%$). One trial, [4] including 103 patients, found a significant difference in pain intensity experienced between RA and LA ($P = 0.0363$ versus $P = 0.0318$, respectively), and time to postoperative pain initiation was significantly longer following RA versus LA. Operative duration was significantly shorter ($P = 0.0007$) for RA (67.5 ± 8.9 min) than LA (134.7 ± 14.8 min).

Discussion

This meta-analysis included 955 patients from 8 studies (7 RCTs and 1 retrospective study). Combined data demonstrates that RA is associated with higher AVF primary patency rates and improved local blood flow compared with LA. Moreover, operation duration and the use of pain killers was significantly reduced with RA versus LA .

Axillary-approached BPB (RA) was preferable to LA. Arterial and venous dilation are crucial for AVF maturation [2] yet vascular surgery, such as local infiltration anesthesia, can easily lead to vessel spasm, impairing blood flow and potentially resulting in early fistula thrombosis. Comparatively, BPB can be performed using interscalene, supraclavicular, infraclavicular, and axillar approaches [4]. In a recent study, BPB was found to provide higher blood flow to the radial artery and AVF compared to infiltration anesthesia [3] given the sympatholytic effect, producing significant vasodilatation, decreased vascular resistance, [10] and increased local blood flow. This is consistent with other recent studies showing improvements in arterial blood flow and vasodilatation with RA. In a recent study by Nofal et al, [7] the overall mean AVF blood flow was 42.21 ml/min more in the BPB versus LA group. Similarly, a report by Malovrh [11] revealed a mean preoperative flow rate of 54.5 ml/min in BPB vessels with a successful outcome versus 24.1 ml/min in vessels that failed LA. In another

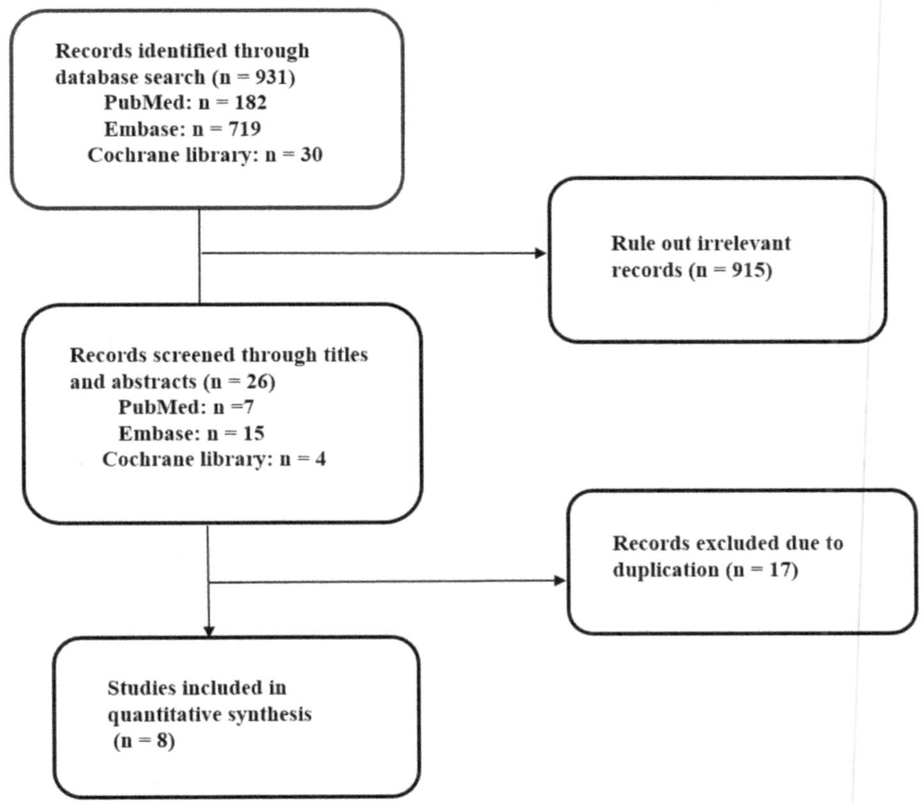

Fig. 1 Study selection flow diagram

Table 2 Summary of included studies and baseline characteristics of their populations

Study	Design and study arms	Sample size (*n*)	Age (M ± SD, years)	Sex (*n*)	Comorbidities (*n*)	Duration of follow up	Outcomes Examined
Mouquet, et al. 1989	RCT (BPB vs. LA or GA)	18	52 ± 16	Male (23); Female (13)	–	2 h; 3 days; 10 days	Brachial artery blood flow
Solomonson, et al. 1994	Retrospective study (BPB vs. LA or GA)	408	63 ± 14	Male (245); Female (163)	Infection (16); Neuropathy (9); Seizure (1); Cardiac event (17)	–	Fistula failure; Graft infection, neuropathy in the extremity receiving the fistula; Seizure; Cardiac arrest; MI; Death within 7 days
Lo Monte, et al. 2011	RCT (BPB vs. LA)	40	BPB, 66.15 ± 7.55; LA, 66 ± 7.49	Male (23); Female (17)	Diabetes (15); High blood pressure (13); Systemic lupus erythematosus (5); Glomerulonephritis (4); Autoimmune vasculitis (3);	100 days	PI ratio; Venous / arterial diameter; Vein diameter
Sahin, et al. 2011	RCT (BPB vs. LA)	60	BPB, 43.4 ± 10.7; LA, 46.8 ± 12.5	Male (34); Female (26)	Diabetes (24); Hypertension (27); Coronary artery Disease (21)	3 h; 7 days; 8 weeks	Radial artery flow; Fistula flow; Thrill presence
Shoshiashvili, et al. 2014	RCT (BPB vs. LA)	103	BPB, 60.1 ± 14; LA, 59.7 ± 13	Male (68); Female (35)	Arterial hypertension (87); Diabetes (18); Ischemic heart disease (9); Gastric ulcer (1); Hepatitis B (2); Hepatitis C (7); Osteoblastoma (1)	100 days	Intra-operative pain; Need for intraoperative pain killers; Need for postoperative pain killers; Duration of anesthesia (h); Attitude to the type of anesthesia; Pain intensity, night sleep; Limb immobility; Operation duration (min)
Meena, et al. 2015	RCT (BPB vs. LA)	60	BPB, 41.33 ± 12.906; LA, 47.7 ± 12.272	Male (46); Female (14)	Diabetes (8); Hypertension (21); Hypertension (14); IgA (15)	30 min 48 h; 2 weeks; 6 weeks	Vessel diameter; Peak systolic velocity; Mean diastolic velocity; Blood flow
Aitken, et al. 2016	RCT (BPB vs. LA)	126	60.8 ± 14.8	Male (79); Female (47)	Diabetes (34); Ischemic heart disease (48); Cerebrovascular accident (9); Hypertension (93) Obesity (41)	3 months	Brachial artery blood flow; Radiocephalic fistulae; Cephalic vein (wrist) diameter (mm); Brachiocephalic fistulae; Brachial artery diameter (mm); Cephalic vein (elbow) diameter (mm)
Nofal, et al. 2017	RCT (BPB vs. LA)	140	BPB, 39.52 ± 5.46; LA, 42.42 ± 5.41	Male (79); Female (61)	–	4 h; 1 week; 3 months	Radial artery internal diameter; Cephalic vein internal diameter

BPB brachial plexus block, *IgA* immunoglobulin A, *GA* general anesthesia, *LA* local anesthesia, *MI* myocardial infarction, *PI* pulsatility Index Ratio, *RCT* randomized controlled trial, *M ± SD* mean ± standard deviatio

study by Sahin et al, [3] improved blood flow in the radial artery was significantly greater post- versus pre-anesthesia. Moreover, post-anesthesia and immediately pre-surgery, radial artery blood flow was 56 ± 8.6 mL/min in the BPB group versus 40.7 ± 6.1 mL/min in the LA group ($P < 0.001$). Finally, Ebert et al [12] reported that both mean arterial and venous blood flow were increased (1.9 and 8.6 times, respectively) after BPB. Thus, we conclude that BPB anesthesia techniques in AVF construction can contribute to vessel dilation and reduced vasospasm via sympathectomy-like effects, increasing fistula blood flow, reducing fistula maturation time, and improving the success rates of vascular access procedures.

Arteriovenous fistulae operations can be performed under GA, LA, or RA. General anesthesia is associated with increased morbidity, [13] such as through cardiorespiratory complications in patients with end-stage renal disease, whilst LA is associated with complications such as vasospasm and pain and discomfort during surgery [10, 12, 14]. By comparison, RA (e.g. BPB), which is a targeted injection of LA to specifically block the motor and sensory nerves that supply the operative site, is less complicated than GA and safer than LA [15]. Moreover, BPB can be performed under ultrasound guidance, allowing for more accurate placement of the injection needle as well as more rapid onset and longer duration of the block, reduced vascular and neurological complications, and minimization of the volume of LA required [16, 17].

Pain control is also an important indicator of surgical success. Adequate pain control is extremely important in patients with end-stage renal disease with severe comorbidities [15]. The prospective, randomized, clinical

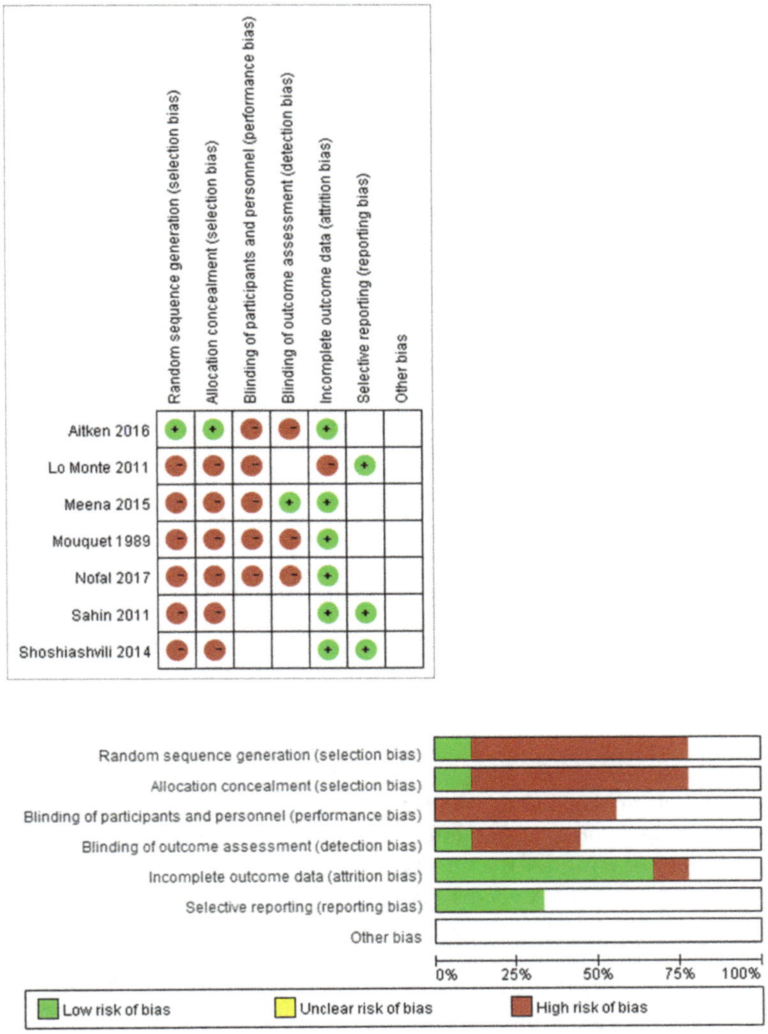

Fig. 2 Risk of bias assessment

study from Shoshiashvili et al [4] showed significantly different results between BPB and LA groups in terms of pain intensity. The need for intra- as well as post-operative pain killers was significantly less in the BPB versus LA group ($P = 0.0363$ and $P = 0.0318$, respectively). Moreover, time to postoperative pain initiation was significantly higher in the RA versus LA group. Thus, we conclude that RA provides better pain control intra- as well as post-operatively in dialysis AVF operations, enabling patients to feel more comfortable [5].

Study or Subgroup	BPB anesthesia Events	BPB anesthesia Total	Local anesthesia Events	Local anesthesia Total	Weight	Odds Ratio M-H, Fixed, 95% CI
Aitken 2016	53	63	39	63	18.2%	3.26 [1.40, 7.60]
Lo Monte 2011	20	20	18	20	1.3%	5.54 [0.25, 123.08]
Meena 2015	30	30	27	30	1.3%	7.76 [0.38, 157.14]
Mouquet 1989	9	9	9	9		Not estimable
Nofal 2017	58	70	49	70	24.7%	2.07 [0.93, 4.63]
Sahin 2011	28	30	25	30	4.9%	2.80 [0.50, 15.73]
Solomonson 1994	140	155	230	253	49.7%	0.93 [0.47, 1.85]
Total (95% CI)		**377**		**475**	**100.0%**	**1.88 [1.24, 2.84]**
Total events	338		397			

Heterogeneity: Chi² = 7.24, df = 5 (P = 0.20); I² = 31%
Test for overall effect: Z = 2.98 (P = 0.003)

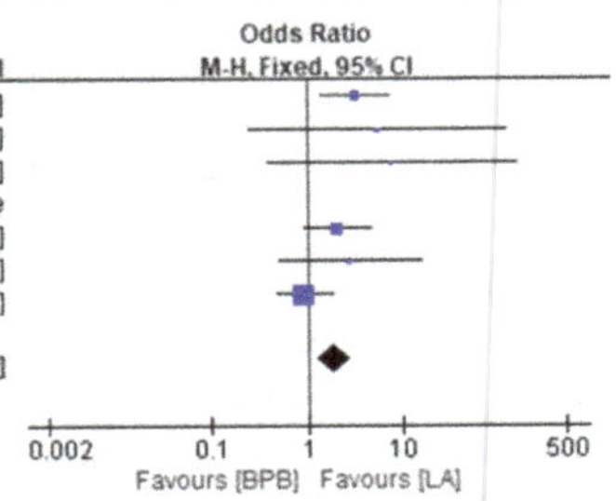

Fig. 3 Patency of brachial plexus block (regional anesthesia) versus local anesthesia

Table 3 Main clinical results

Outcome variable	Number of convective therapy study arms	Number of patients	Absolute mean net change [95% CI]	I^2
Duration of surgery	2	229	−29.63 [− 32.78, -26.48]	100%
Brachial artery diameter	3	284	0.83 [0.75, 0.92]	97%
Brachial artery blood flow rate	2	144	47.15 [35.18, 59.12]	83%
Complication of infection	3	594	0.68 [0.23, 2.02]	0%
Thrombosis	3	163	0.21 [0.03, 1.27]	0%
Hematoma	1	60	0.19 [0.01, 4.06]	–
Intraoperative analgesia	1	103	0.65 [0.30, 1.42]	–

CI confidence interval, I^2 inconsistency test

The results of our study are consistent with those of previous meta-analyses. In a systematic review of 6 randomized trials (462 patients) and 1 retrospective study (408 patients), Ismail et al [18] reported that RA improves the primary patency rate of AVF compared to LA. In conclusion, our meta-analysis suggests that RA is preferable to LA in patients with end-stage renal disease in guaranteeing AVF patency and increasing brachial artery diameter.

Limitations

Our study has several limitations. First, BPB can be performed with interscalene, supraclavicular, infraclavicular and axillar approaches. We included studies using different approaches for BPB, and did not consider the effects of these approaches in our comparison of LA versus RA. Future studies are thus required to explore the effect of different anesthetic approaches on the outcomes of BPB. Second, three of the studies included in this study were single-center trials with an inherent risk of bias. Moreover, there are relatively few primary studies available in the literature. Both factors restrict the generalizability of our findings. Third, only short-term data are reported in the literature; thus, future studies are required to explore longer-term outcomes. Finally, only one study explored patients' attitudes towards anesthesia and, thus, future trials are recommended to explore the differences between LA and RA in terms of patient-oriented outcomes.

Conclusions

In summary, our meta-analysis suggests that RA is advantageous over LA, providing sufficient branchial artery blood flow to guarantee AVF patency whilst increasing brachial artery diameter to avoid thrombosis and several other related complications. Nevertheless, large, head-to-head RCTs with longer follow-up periods are required to support the use of BPB and illustrate the safety differences between RA and LA.

Abbreviations

AVF: Arteriovenous fistulae; RA: Regional anesthesia; LA: Local anesthesia; GA: General anesthesia; BPB: Brachial plexus block; RCTs: Randomized controlled trials

Acknowledgements

Not applicable.

Authors' contributions

HCH and CG was involved in the study design, participated in drafting the manuscript and also helped to analyse the study data. CYW, QLY, JLX were participated in study design and drafting the manuscript. All authors have read and approved the manuscript.

Author details

[1]Department of Nephrology, The Hangzhou Fuyang Hospital of Traditional Chinese Medicine, Zhejiang, Hangzhou, China. [2]The First Clinical Medical of Zhejiang Chinese Medicine University, Zhejiang, Hangzhou, China. [3]Department of Internal Medicine, The Affiliated Hospital of Hangzhou Normal University, 126 Wenzhou Road, Zhejiang, Hangzhou, China.

References

1. Riella MC, Roy-Chaudhury P. Vascular access in haemodialysis: strengthening the Achilles' heel. Nat Rev Nephro. 2013;9:348–57.
2. Lo Monte AI, et al. Comparison between local and regional anesthesia in arteriovenous fistula creation. J Vasc Access. 2011;12:331–5. https://doi.org/10.5301/JVA.2011.8560.
3. Sahin L, et al. Ultrasound-guided infraclavicular brachial plexus block enhances postoperative blood flow in arteriovenous fistulas. J Vasc Surg. 2011;54(3):749–53.
4. Shoshiashvili V, et al. Evaluation of efficacy of regional and local anesthesia techniques in arteriovenous fistula criation for dialysis. Georg Med News. 2014;(236):7–12.
5. Meena S, et al. Ultrasound-guided supraclavicular brachial plexus anaesthesia improves arteriovenous fistula flow characteristics in end-stage renal disease patients. South Afr J Anaesth Anal. 2015;21(5):12–5.
6. Aitken E, et al. Effect of regional versus local anaesthesia on outcome after arteriovenous fistula creation: a randomised controlled trial. Lancet. 2016; 388(10049):1067–74.
7. Nofal WH, et al. Ultrasound-guided axillary brachial plexus block versus local infiltration anesthesia for arteriovenous fistula creation at the forearm for hemodialysis in patients with chronic renal failure. Saudi J Anaesth. 2017; 11(1):77–82.
8. Mouquet C, et al. Anesthesia for creation of a forearm fistula in patients with endstage renal failure. Anesthesiology. 1989;70(6):909–14.
9. Solomonson MD, Johnson ME, Ilstrup D. Risk factors in patients having surgery to create an arteriovenous fistula. Anesth Analg. 1994;79(4):694–700.
10. Malinzak EB, Gan TJ. Regional anesthesia for vascular access surgery. Anesth Analg. 2009;109:976–80.
11. Malovrh M. The role of sonography in the planning of arteriovenous fistulas for hemodialysis. Semin Dial. 2003;16:299–303.

12. Ebert B, Braunschweig R, Reill P. Quantification of variations in arm perfusion after plexus anesthesia with color Doppler sonography. Anaesthesist. 1995;44:859–62.
13. Brimble KS, Rabbat CG, Schiff D, Ingram AJ. The clinical utility of Doppler ultrasound prior to arteriovenous fistula creation. Semin Dial. 2001;14:314–7.
14. Abrahams MS, Aziz MF, Fu RF, Horn JL. Ultrasound guidance compared with electrical neurostimulation for peripheral nerve block: a systematic review and meta analysis of randomized controlled trials. Br J Anaesth. 2009;102:408–17.
15. Rang S, et al. Anaesthesia for chronic renal disease and renal transplantation. EAU-EBU Update Ser. 2006;4:246–56.
16. Capdevila X, Biboulet P, Morau D, et al. How and why to use ultrasound for regional blockade. Acta Anaesthesiol Belg. 2008;59:147–54.
17. Marhofer P, Schrögendorfer K, Koinig H, Kapral S, Weinstabl C, Mayer N. Ultrasound guidance improves sensory block and onset time of three-in-one blocks. Anesth Analg. 1997;85:854–7.
18. Ismail A. Abdelrahman Ibrahim Abushouk.: regional versus local anesthesia for arteriovenous fistula creation in end-stage renal disease: a systematic review and meta-analysis. J Vasc Access. 2017;18(3):177–84.

7

Electric vagal nerve stimulation inhibits inflammation and improves early postoperation cognitive dysfunction in aged rats

Jun Xiong[1], Huijun Wang[2], Yin Bao[2], Yuliang Guo[2] and Yongxing Sun[1*]

Abstract

Background: This study aimed to evaluate effects of electric vagal nerve stimulation on early postoperation cognitive dysfunction in aged rats.

Methods: A total of 33 male Sprague Dawley rats were selected and assigned randomly to three groups, control group (C, $n = 10$), splenectomy group (S, $n = 10$) and splenectomy+vagal nerve stimulation group (SV, $n = 13$). Behavior and memory of rats were evaluated by Open Field Test and Morris Water Maze. Levels of TNF-α, IL-6 and IL-10 in serum were measured by ELISA. The level of TNF-α protein in hippocampus was assessed by Western blotting. rt-PCR was used to detect mRNA expression of NF-κB in hippocampus.

Results: During anesthesia/operation, vital life signs of rats were stable. In SV group, vagal nerve stimulation decreased heart rate lower than 10% of basic level and kept it at a stable range by regulating stimulation intensity. After stimulation stop, heart rate returned to the basic level again. This indicated that the model of vagal nerve stimulation was successful. Serum levels of TNF-α and IL-6 increased by the operation/anesthesia, but they decreased with vagal nerve stimulation (all $P < 0.05$). TNF-α protein and mRNA expression of NF-κB in hippocampus were also eliminated by vagal nerve stimulation compared to S group ($P < 0.05$). Results of Morris Water Maze showed escape latency of postoperation in S group was significantly longer than C group ($P < 0.05$), and times of crossing platform in S group was lower than that of C group ($P < 0.05$). Although escape latency of postopration in SV group was shorter than that of S group, there was no significant difference between two groups. Meanwhile there were no significant differences of behavior test in Open Field test between three groups, although vagal nerve stimulation improved partly active explore behavior compared to S group.

Conclusion: The inflammation caused by operation and general anesthesia was an important reason of early postoperation cognitive dysfunction, and electric vagal nerve stimulation could inhibit the inflammation. Meanwhile, vagal nerve stimulation could ameliorate early postoperation cognitive dysfunction partly, but its protective effects were not enough and should be studied and improved in future.

Keywords: Vagus nerve stimulation, Cognitive dysfunction, Inflammation, General anesthesia

* Correspondence: B2008194@126.com
[1]Department of Anesthesiology, Sanbo Brain Hospital, Capital Medical University, No. 50 Yikesong, Xiangshan, Haidian District, Beijing 100093, China

Background

Postoperation cognitive dysfunction (POCD) is a severe complication of surgery and general anesthesia. Fourteen percent of patients have been found cognitive decline and confusion after surgery with anesthesia [1, 2]. POCD is frequent in patients older than 60-year undergoing major non-cardiac surgery, which increases both morbidity and mortality [3]. These cognitive impairments are related to language comprehension, attention, social integration and short term memory. Also, POCD may extent recovery process and hospital stay, and diminish quality of patients' life [4]. There are many risks developing postoperative cognitive decline in elderly patients, such as increased age, longer time in surgery, longer stay in an intensive care unit and mechanical ventilation time [2]. Although POCD is not rare, its underlying pathogenic mechanisms have not been known completely.

The systemic inflammation has been identified as an important process for occurrence and development of POCD [4, 5]. Not only surgical trauma, but also inhaled anesthetics could produce systemic inflammatory response, which leads to blood-brain barrier disruption, neuro-inflammation and cognitive dysfunction [6, 7]. So inhibiting this systemic inflammation might be a potential strategy preventing and/or treating cognitive dysfunction.

Vagal nerve has been identified to link to inflammatory response, its activity could suppress TNF-α and other pro-inflammatory cytokines. This anti-inflammation arc has been well-known as cholinergic anti-inflammation pathway [8]. Vagal nerve regulates inflammatory response through hypothalamic-pituitary-adrenal axis, release of cortisol and vagovagal reflex [9]. Anti-inflammatory effects of vagal nerve stimulation (VNS) were firstly researched by Borovikova and colleague [10]. They found not only acetylcholine, as vagal neurotransmitter, inhibited release of inflammatory cytokines in lipopolysaccharide stimulated human macrophage cultures, but also direct VNS could reduce systemic inflammatory response and prevent progress of infectious shock by attenuating inflammatory cytokines synthesis. Following their works, the anti-inflammation mechanisms of VNS have been researched systemically. Although the whole mechanisms and the signaling pathway have been unknown completely, wider range of inflammatory disorders might be ameliorated by VNS [11].

The aim of this study, firstly, was to demonstrate whether surgery and general anesthesia could induce systemic- and neuro-inflammatory response and impair cognitive function in elder rats. Secondly, it was to evaluate effects of VNS improving cognitive dysfunction by inhibiting the inflammatory response.

Methods

Experimental animals

A total of 33 male Sprague Dawley (SD) rats were obtained from Beijing Vital River Laboratory Animal Technology Co. Ltd. (Beijing, 100,012, China. \ (Jing)2012–0001.) and maintained in suitable rooms with controlled conditions of temperature at 22 ± 1 °C, 40 ± 10% relative humidity and light-dark cycles (12 h- 12 h, light onset at 7:00). Five rats were housed in one cage. During this experiment, standard food and drink water were available to the animals ad libitum. This study was approved by the institution ethical committee for animal care and use, Sanbo Brain Hospital, Capital Medical University. All efforts were made to minimize the number of animals used and their suffering. Experiments were performed during day, always at the same time, to avoid circadian variations. After finishing behavior tests, all animals were humanely euthanized using intraperitoneal injection of 3% sodium pentobarbital (50 mg/kg) and rapid decapitation. The process was as soon as possible to avoid interference on the results of experiment.

Experiment protocol

A random number generator was used to allocate the rats into different groups: control group ($n = 10$, C group, 577.00 ± 47.53 g) that received no surgery and anesthesia, splenectomy group ($n = 10$, S group, 577.60 ± 33.73 g) that was isolated cervical vagal nerve without stimulation, and splenectomy+VNS group ($n = 13$, SV group, 571.15 ± 50.63 g). Then all rats were conducted with Morris Water Maze (MWM) train (day 1–4) and test on day 7, Open Field Test (OFT) train on day 3 and test on day 7, splenectomy was carried on the day 4. Finishing behavior tests, all animals were decapitated for tissue preparation on day 7 (Fig. 1).

Electric vagal nerve stimulation

Rats were fixed in a cage and anesthetized with 1% propofol (Fresenius Kabi AB. Rapsgatan 7, 751 74 Uppsala. Sweden. Serial number: 10MC2871.) 80 mg/Kg intraperitoneally, after losing righting reflex, their tail vein was cathetered with 24-gauge catheter infusion set (Tuoren Medical Device Co., Ltd. Henan, 453,401, China.) for continuous propofol infusion [12]. During the experiment, rats were allowed to breathe pure oxygen through a tube filled with oxygen continuously, which fixed in front of their nose in order to prevent hypoxia. After 10 min stabilization, heart rate was recorded as basic line. Thus, neck hair shaving and skin cleaning, aseptic technique was used to make a ventral midline incision in neck skin. Then skin and muscles were retracted. Because right vagal nerve primarily innervates atria and sinoatrial node, and these stimulation may induce significant change in cardiac rhythm. At the same time, right VNS produce smaller cardiorespiratory response, so right vagal nerve was applied [13, 14]. Isolating right cervical vagal nerve and common carotid artery bundle, a 1.5 mm diameter silver bipolar cuff electrode was

Day 1	Day 2	Day 3	Day 4	Day 5	Day 6	Day 7
MWM	MWM	MWM	MWM	Rest	Rest	MWM
		OFT	Operation			OFT

Fig. 1 The experiment protocol. MWM: Morris water maze. OFT: Open field test

gently wrapped around the nerve bundle and fixed to the sternocleidomastoid muscle. Then the electrode was connected to stimulator (BL-820 Biological signal acquisition and processing system. Chengdu Techman Software Co. Ltd. Sichuan, Chengdu, 610,100, China). The basic stimulation parameters were adapted to the threshold of individual animal and included 2 V, 10 Hz and 1 ms, but these parameters were regulated constantly to preserve heart rate lower than 10% of basic line [14–17].

Splenectomy

After 30 min of VNS, splenectomy began with a small lateral peritoneal incision. Using 3.0 silk thread to dissociate and ligate spleen artery and vein at hilum of spleen, spleen was removed at the root of far end of spleen pedicle. The completely removed spleen was examined to ensure that no residual spleen was left. Then the incision was closed, covering it with sterile activated-iodine gauze, and securing it with adhesive tape. The operation time was within 60 min.

Behavioral tests

Open field test

OFT was applied in an apparatus, which was made of brown plywood, surface area was 50 × 50 cm, surrounded by 50 cm high walls. The floor was divided by black line into 25 rectangles. Rats were allowed to freely move in this apparatus for 5 min. The movement of individual animal in the arena was automatically tracked by AVTAS ver5.0 animal video analysis system (AniLab Software & Istruments Co., Ltd. Ningbo, China.) The number of crossing and rearing activities by each rat during 5 min was used to assess rats' active explore behavior. After every test, the apparatus was cleaned with 5% ethanol.

Morris water maze

MWM was used to evaluate spatial reference learning and memory. A circle pool (150 cm in diameter and 80 cm deep) was filled with water and divided into four quadrants. An escape platform, which 40 cm in height and 15 cm in diameter, was submerged by 2 cm under water surface and conserved to the center of northwest (NW) quadrant of this pool. Water was maintained at temperature of 23 ± 2 °C. The evaluation consisted of four training days of five consecutive trails per day, the last trail of each day was accepted. Rats were randomly introduced in this tank from different quadrants facing wall to find the escape platform in 60 s. If the rats did not find the platform within 60s in the first trial, they were gently guided to the platform to remain for 30s. Then the rats were removed from the tank. This procedure ensured animals to retain visual-spatial information during trail. The movement of individual rat was automatically tracked by AVTAS ver5.0 animal video analysis system (AniLab Software & Istruments Co., Ltd. Ningbo, China.) On the last day of the test after operation, rats were assessed in this tank without the platform. The time to find the platform, the times of passing through the platform location, and the duration of time in the quarter of platform were counted.

Assessment of TNF-α, IL-6, IL-10 in serum

Levels of serum TNF-α, IL-6, IL-10 were measured by Enzyme-Linked Immunosorbent Assay (ELISA). Aliquots containing 100ul of serum were placed into wells of ELISA plates and the plate was incubated at 37 °C for 2 h. Primary antibodies were rabbit monoclonal antibodies to TNF-α (Huamei, Wuhan. Number CSB-E11987r, 1:100 dilution), IL-6 (Huamei, Wuhan. Number CSB-E04640r, 1:100 dilution), IL-10 (Huamei, Wuhan. Number CSB-E04595r, 1:100 dilution). The primary antibodies were added to each wells and incubated at 37 °C for 1 h. After three washes with PBS-Tween 20 (0.1%), a horseradish-peroxidase-conjugated goat anti-rabbit IgG was added into the wells and incubated for 1 h at 37 °C. The antibody-antigen complex was revealed by addition of 100ul of 2,2′-azinobis (3-ethylbenzthiazoline-6-sulfonic acid) (ABTS) containing 0.3% H_2O_2 into each well. After 15 min, optical density (OD) was determined using Bio Tek Epoch (Bio Tek Instruments, Inc. China. Beijing, 100,025, China.) at 450 nm. All samples were processed under the same experimental conditions and time.

TNF-α protein in hippocampus

The proteins were extracted from hippocampus and their concentration was determined by Bicinchoninic Acid Kit (Catalog BCA02, Dingguo Changsheng Biology Technology LTD, Beijing, China). 30μg protein samples were separated by SDS-PAGE, followed by semi-dry transfer onto a PVDF membrane. The membrane was blocked in 5% non-fat dry milk. Further, membranes were incubated with rat monoclonal primary antibody, anti-TNF-α and anti-tubulin, for overnight at 4 °C. This was followed by triple washing with 0.1% TBST and incubation with HRP labeled secondary antibodies for 2 h at RT. Immunoreactive bands were detected by ECL and Western blot detection system using Quantity one (Bio-Rad Laboratories. Inc. Hercules, CA, USA). These steps were repeated triply in order to calculate mean value. Expressions of each interest protein were calculated after normalizing the interest protein with endogenous control tubulin in the same sample.

NF-κB in hippocampus expression

Total RNA was isolated from 100 mg of hippocampal cortex using 1 ml of TRIzol (Invitrogen Corporation; Carlsbad, CA, USA) and then RNA was treated with RNase-free DNase I and quantified using Q5000 Spectrophotometer (Quawell Technology, Inc. San Jose, CA, USA). cDNA was obtained from 5μg of total RNA using 2ul of ReverTra Ace reverse transcriptase kit (Catalog TRT-101, TOYOBO STC (Shanghai) CO., LTD, Shanghai, China), 2ul of Oligo dT 50um, 2ul of dNTP mix 10 mM, and water grade molecular biology to 20ul. Retrotranscription conditions were 30 °C for 10 min, followed 42 °C for 60 min and 99 °C for 5 min, then 4 °C for 5 min. Finally, the cDNA was stored at − 20 °C.

cDNA was used to amplify each gene using Sybr Green I (Catalog GG1301–50, Gen-View Scientific Inc. Florida, USA). The amplification reactions contained 1 ul of respective SybrGreen I, 12.5ul of Mix (Catalog PER012–1, Dingguo Changsheng Biology Technology LTD, Beijing, China), and 1ul of cDNA in a final volume of 25ul. The conditions were for qPCR were 3 min for pre-denaturation at 95 °C, followed by 35 cycles of amplification of 30s denaturation at 94 °C, 30s annealing at 60 °C and 30s extending at 72 °C. The last extending step was 10 min at 72 °C. Rat GAPDH was used as internal control gene for normalization. The amplification assays were made using ABI PRISM 7700 Sequence Detection System (ThermoFisher Scientific (China) LTD, Shanghai, China). Primer pairs for quantitative real-time PCR were as follows: NF-κB, 5′-AACCTGGGAATACTTCATGTGA CTAA-3′(sense) and 5′-GCACCAGAAGTCCAGGATTA TAGC-3′ (anti-sense), GADPH, 5′- GCTGAGTATGTCGT GGACTC-3′ (sense) and 5′- TTGGTGGTGCAGGATGCA TT-3′ (anti-sense). The steps were repeated triply in order to calculate mean value. The $2^{-\Delta\Delta Ct}$ analyses were applied to calculate the relative transcript levels expressed as fold change for gene expression [18].

Statistical analysis

SPSS 16.0 for Windows software package (SPSS, Inc., Chicago, IL, USA.) was used to perform statistical analysis. Quantitative data were expressed as mean ± standard deviation ($\bar{x} \pm s$). Normal distribution of data was check by Kolmogorov-Smirnov analysis. One-way ANOVA Post Hoc Multiple-Comparisons was used for multi-group comparisons of means. When homogeneity of variances occurred, L-S-D was used to compare between groups. When variances were heterogeneous, Dunnett T3 was used to compare between groups. Two-way repeated-measured ANOVA was use to analysis the data of escape latency. The mean difference was significant at 0.05 level.

Results

There were no significant different between three groups on body weight ($F = 0.073$, $P = 0.930$) and basic heart rate ($F = 1.163$, $P = 0.326$) (Table 1). Three minutes after beginning of VNS, heart rates of SV group (312.85 ± 27.52) was reduced significantly, compared to C group (373.90 ± 21.40) and S group (375.30 ± 16.26) ($F = 28.928$, $P < 0.01$). Three minutes after stopping VNS, heart rates of SV group (394.85 ± 32.19) rose up, compared to C group (369.60 ± 21.46) ($P = 0.021$). Till to ten minute after stopping VNS, heart rates were not significantly different between three groups ($F = 0.230$, $P = 0.796$), and recovered to the basic level (Fig. 2).

The level of inflammatory cytokines in serum

TNF-α level was increased by surgery and general anesthesia in S group (61.028 ± 8.642 pg/ml, $P < 0.001$, Dunnett T3) and SV group (41.609 ± 8.249 pg/ml, $P < 0.001$, Dunnett T3), compared to C group (27.180 ± 2.038 pg/ml). And it could be reduced by VNS, because TNF-α in SV group was significant lower than that in S group ($P < 0.001$, Dunnett T3). IL-6 level was similar to TNF-α. Compared to C group (1.278 ± 0.258 pg/ml), IL-6 in S group (6.789 ± 1.827 pg/ml) and SV group (3.623 ± 0.685 pg/ml) were increased significantly ($P < 0.001$, Dunnett T3). But VNS decreased IL-6 in SV group compared to that of S group ($P < 0.001$, Dunnett T3). Anti-

Table 1 The body weight and basic heart rate of three groups

Groups	Body weight	Basic heart rate
C group	577.00 ± 47.53	366.60 ± 15.12
S group	577.60 ± 33.73	375.10 ± 14.39
SV group	571.15 ± 50.63	365.38 ± 17.73
F	0.073	1.163
P	0.930	0.326

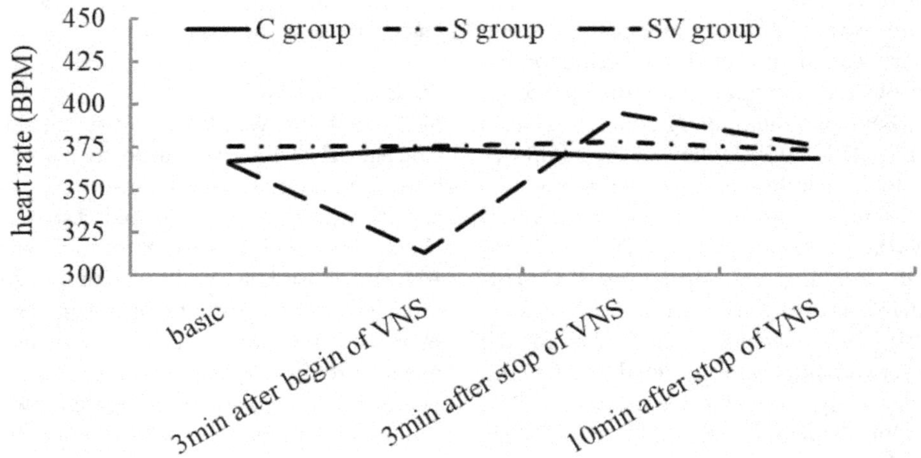

Fig. 2 The basic HR was no significant difference between three groups. At 3 min after begin of VNS, the HR in SV group was lower than the other groups. And at 3 min after stop of VNS, the HR of SV group was slightly increased, compared to the other groups. Ten min after stopping VNS, the HR of SV group return to the basic level, no difference of HR between three groups

inflammatory cytokine IL-10 was higher in S group (95.351 ± 6.236 pg/ml) and SV group (99.387 ± 5.236 pg/ml) caused by splenectomy and general anesthesia, compared to C group (38.587 ± 0.645 pg/ml, $P < 0.001$, Dunnett T3). However, there was no significant difference between IL-10 of S and SV group ($P = 0.302$, Dunnett T3) (Fig. 3).

The TNF-α level in the hippocampus

As internal reference protein, tubulin level in three groups was no significant difference ($F = 0.036$, $P = 0.965$). Normalization with tubulin, TNF-α of three groups was significant difference ($F = 10.018$, $P = 0.002$).TNF-α in S group (8.00 ± 1.99) was significantly higher than that in C group (4.78 ± 0.63, Dunnett T3, $P = 0.025$) and SV group (5.13 ± 1.11, Dunnett T3, $P = 0.043$). But TNF-α protein of C and SV groups was similar (Dunnett T3, $P = 0.872$) (Fig. 4).

The NF-κB gene expression in the hippocampus

After normalization with endogenous control GAPDH, NF-κB expression in three groups was significantly different ($F = 12.648$, $P = 0.001$, ANOVA). NF-κB gene of S group (1.839 ± 0.652) was increased significantly than

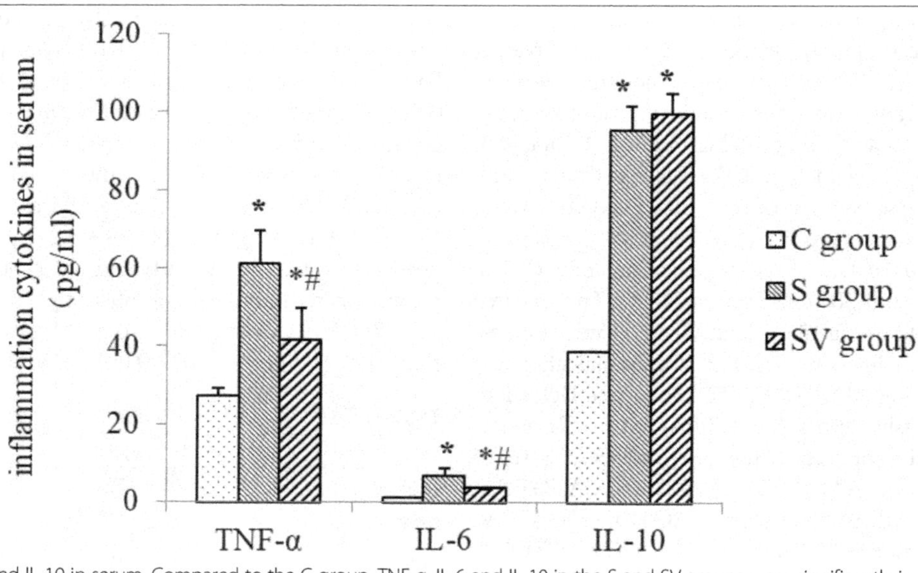

Fig. 3 TNF-α, IL-6 and IL-10 in serum. Compared to the C group, TNF-α, IL-6 and IL-10 in the S and SV groups were significantly increased, $P < 0.05$. VNS could reduce TNF-α and IL-6 in serum significantly, compared to the S group, $P < 0.05$. VNS did slightly raised IL-10 in serum, but there was no significant difference between both of them. *$P < 0.05$, comparing to the C group, #$P < 0.05$ comparing to the SV group

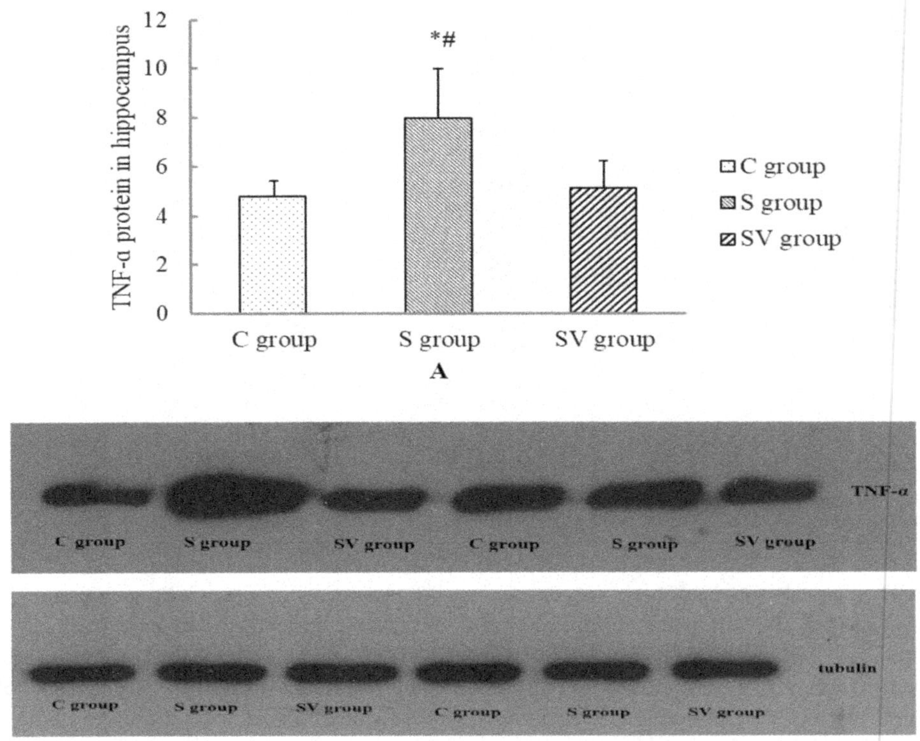

B

Fig. 4 The TNF-α protein in hippocampus. **a** TNF-α protein in hippocampus was higher than that of other groups, $P < 0.05$. But TNF-α of the C and SV group were similar. $^*P < 0.05$, comparing to the C group, $\#P < 0.05$ comparing to the SV group (**b**)

that of C group (0.685 ± 0.253, $P < 0.001$, LSD) and SV group (0.849 ± 0.258, $P = 0.001$, LSD). And there was no significant difference of NF-κB gene expression between C and SV group ($P = 0.518$, LSD) (Fig. 5).

Locomotor and exploratory activities

OPT was used to evaluate rat crossing and rearing activities, before and after splenecotmy respectively. Before the surgery, there were no significant different on the number of crossing ($F = 0$, $P = 0.995$) and rearing between three groups ($F = 0.003$, $P = 0.966$). After the operation, the number of crossing ($F = 0.302$, $P = 0.587$) and the number of rearing ($F = 2.040$, $P = 0.148$) were also similar in three groups, but the number of crossing (11.85 ± 15.44) and rearing (2.62 ± 3.30) in SV group were higher than the number of crossing (10.00 ± 13.19) and rearing (1.80 ± 2.82) in S group (Fig. 6).

Effects of VNS on the MWM test

As shown in (Fig. 7), two-way repeated-measures ANOVA revealed that escape latency of three groups reduced over the 4 days training period before the operation ($F = 103.062$, $P < 0.01$), and there was no interaction between days, splenecotmy and VNS ($F = 0.498$, $P = 0.807$). Also escape latency of each day was no significant difference between three groups during 4 days' training ($F = 1.715$, $P = 0.208$).

After the operation, S group had a longer escape latency (42.45 ± 13.23) than C group (25.07 ± 15.66, $P = 0.045$, Dunnett T3). And escape latency of C and SV group (34.37 ± 22.57, $P = 0.578$) was not significantly different. So escape latency was reduced by VNS compared to S group, but the difference was not significant. Results of times of crossing platform after the operation were similar to the results of escape latency. The rats of S group (1.6 ± 0.8) crossed few times than those of C group (2.9 ± 1.9, $P = 0.046$, LSD). And there was no significant difference between the times of crossing of C and SV groups (2.5 ± 1.3, $P = 0.543$, LSD). The times of crossing platform of SV group were more than that of S group, but the difference was not significant. After the operation, the duration of time spent in target quadrant was no significant difference between three groups ($F = 1.751$, $P = 0.191$). However, the time spending on the platform in S group (11.49 ± 2.58) was shorter than that of C group (15.54 ± 6.72) and SV group (15.73 ± 6.88).

Discussion

Our results showed that surgery and general anesthesia could produce damage to memory and study capability,

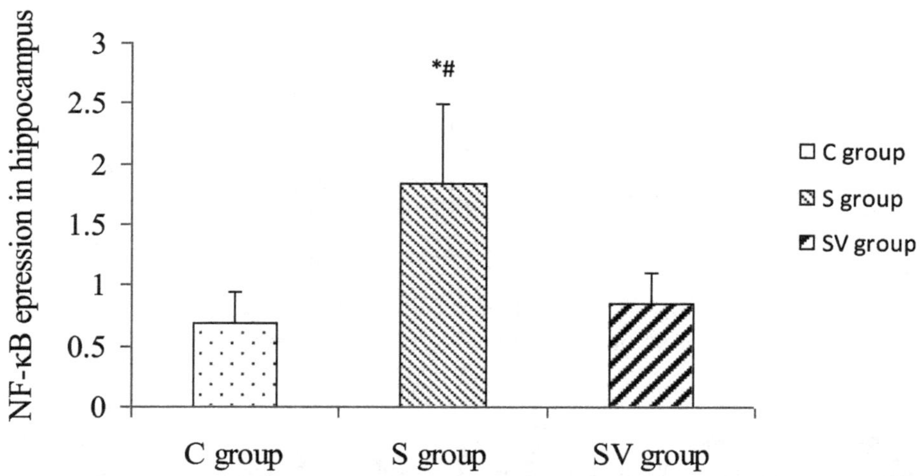

Fig. 5 The NF-κB gene expression in hippocampus. The NF-κB expression of the S group was increased significantly compared to the C and SV groups. There was similar expression between the C and SV groups

and aggravate POCD in elderly rats early after surgery and general anesthesia, because they induced systemic- and neuro-inflammation [19]. Although improvement of cognitive function was not significantly, electrical VNS did reduce POCD in some degree. The underlying mechanism might be related to inhibition of the inflammatory response caused by surgery and general anesthesia.

The inflammation caused by surgery and general anesthesia is one of most important reasons of POCD. There is strong evidence to suggest that acute inflammation affects and exacerbates cognitive function or cause delirium, one kind of clinical important postoperative complication. And ongoing inflammation might constantly impair cognitive function after surgery and anesthesia. Thus, inhibition or resolution of the inflammation is an important prerequisite for improvement of cognition [20]. In the present study, surgery and general anesthesia increased pro-inflammatory cytokines, TNF-α and IL-6. Meanwhile, IL-10, a kind of anti-inflammatory cytokine, was also upgraded. These changes demonstrated that acute systemic inflammation was induced via activation of innate immune system.

As an initiating medium of systemic inflammation, TNF-α activates and amplifies inflammation cascade. In addition, TNF-α can do damage directly to blood brain barrier and induce inflammatory cells infiltration in hippocampus [21]. Besides, NF-κB is an essential transcription factor to regulate inflammation and innate immunity genes expression. Its activation eventually increases level of pro-inflammatory cytokines in brain, such as TNF-α and IL-6, which subsequently cause cognitive impairment [22]. So NF-κB has been known as a potential therapeutic target, inhibition of NF-κB might improve cognitive dysfunction caused by sevoflurane anesthesia [23]. In our study, increase of pro-inflammation cytokines in serum and higher expression of TNF-α and NF-κB in hippocampus provided directly evidences that surgery and general anesthesia might induce acute inflammation, which took place systemically and locally, and lead to cognitive damage early after surgery and general anesthesia.

As to why right vagal nerve was stimulated in our study, this was because heart rate changed obviously when it was stimulated [13]. In other words, the change of heart rate is not only the evidence that VNS is successful, but also is the baseline for regulating stimulation parameters, such as stimulation intensity and frequency. In the present study, 3 min after onset of stimulation, heart rate reduced to about 85% of basic heart rate, and 10 min after stop of stimulation, heart rate increased to basic level. During the operation, continuous VNS kept heart rate at this level, till the operation was finished. In addition, right VNS might produce relatively slighter interruption to circulation and respiration than left VNS [14].

The more important is that vagal nerve plays key role in inflammation regulation, which is known as cholinergic anti-inflammation pathway. The vagal nerve efferent fibers release acetylcholine, which binding with special receptor on macrophages and inhibit production and release of TNF-α [24]. In our study, this effects of VNS were certified that VNS could decrease not only levels of pro-inflammatory cytokines in serum, such as TNF-α and IL-6, also TNF-α protein and transcription factor NF-κB in hippocampus were downgraded by VNS. As to the level of IL-10, although VNS could increase it slightly, there was no significant difference between S and SV groups. We inferred that anti-inflammation effects of vagal nerve focus on inhibition of pro-inflammatory cytokines, not upgrade of anti-inflammatory cytokines. So there was no significant change of IL-10.

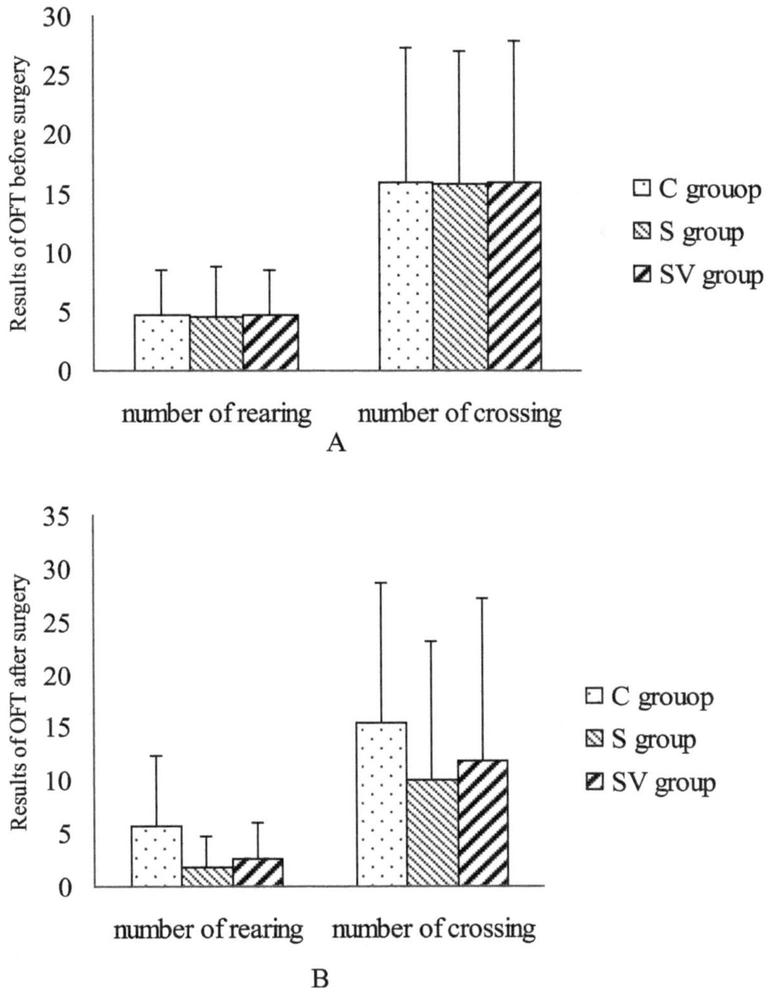

Fig. 6 The results of Open Field Test. **a** Before the surgery, the numbers of crossing and the number of rearing were similar in three groups. **b** After the surgery, both of crossing and rearing number were no significant difference between three groups. But comparing to the S group, the number of crossing and rearing in the SV group increased

Recently, Huffman and colleague reported that VNS could ameliorate cognitive response and decrease systemic and brain inflammation induced by lipopolysaccharide endotoxemia. In their study TNF-α was significantly inhibited by VNS [25], which was similar to results of our research. Besides effects of inhibiting inflammatory response, cholinergic system might regulate hippocampus function and memory, so it is not impossible to prevent or ameliorate POCD by VNS [26].

OFT is used to evaluate spontaneous activity and anxiety-like behaviors. In this study, results of OFT demonstrated that spontaneous movement in three groups were similar after the operation. Although VNS could ameliorate crossing and rearing movement, a kind of actively explore behaviors [27], there were no significant difference between three group. VNS was reported to increase score of OFT in depression model of rat and antagonized depressive status [28]. The results in the present study were not contradictory with the previous study, however these effects of VNS in our study was not significant statistically.

After the operation and general anesthesia, learning and memory function of rats were damaged, as indicated by increase of escape latency, and decrease of times of crossing platform and time spending on target region. VNS, as a kind of treatment, in our study, it did decrease escape latency, lengthen time spending on target quarter, and increase times of crossing platform, when compared to S group. These results were consistent with previous study which reported VNS ameliorated cognitive function [29]. However, in this study, these effects of VNS were not enough to produce protection against POCD completely.

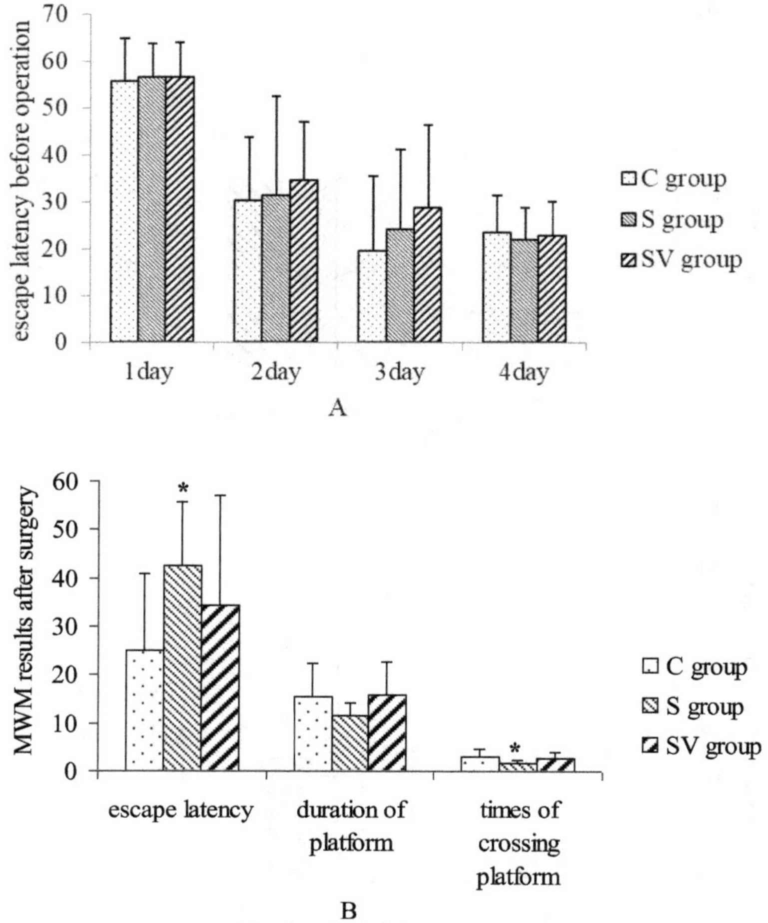

Fig. 7 a Before the surgery on the continuous training days, the escape latency of three groups decreased day by day. There was no interaction between time and different intervention. Each day, the escape latency were no significant difference between three groups. **b** After the surgery, the escape latency and times of crossing platform in the S group were significantly different with these of the C group. The escape latency, duration of platform and times of crossing platform were similar in the C and SV groups. Although these parameters relating to study and memory were ameliorated by VNS, the difference was not significant

Above results of OFT and MWM tests provided evidences that POCD could occur early after surgery, and inflammation caused by surgery and general anesthesia played more important role to induce POCD. These results were similar to recent studies [30, 31]. However, the detail mechanisms of POCD have not completely elucidated. For example, systemic inflammation, neuroinflammatin, cerebral microemboli and hypotension, all of these may cause POCD. In other words, any pathogenies could cause POCD as long as they interrupt central nerve system metabolic status and its homeostasis [32]. As well known, inflammation is one relatively important pathogeny for POCD, but it is not the only. Thus, we could explain the results of our study. Because VNS could inhibit the inflammation induced by surgery and general anesthesia, which demonstrated by lower level of pro-inflammation cytokines in serum and pro-inflammation protein and transcription factor NF-κB in hippocampus. However, there might be other pathogenies to promote the development of POCD. So VNS could ameliorate learning, memory function and actively explore movement in some degree, but its protection was not sufficient.

Our study indicated that surgery and general anesthesia could induce systemic and local inflammation. At the same time, cognitive function of rats was damaged. VNS might inhibit the inflammation to produce protective effect against POCD in some degree. However, this protection of VNS was insufficient. Maybe combination of VNS with other therapies might provide better clinical effects, this need to be researched in future.

The limitation of this study

There were some limitations in our study. NF-κB is a key transcription factor to modulate inflammatory responses via regulating expression of pro-inflammation mediators. It is regulated by its inhibitor, IκB. NF-κB will be released by degradation of IκB. Then it enters nucleus and activates transcription of multiple inflammatory response genes by interacting with κB elements in promoter region. Thus, increased NF-κB activation is considered as an important pathogenic factor in many inflammatory disorders. In our study, we only tested total NF-κB expression. If the expression of IκB in hippocampus was tested, the more information relative with central nerve systemic inflammatory response would be demonstrated.

Abbreviations

ELISA: Enzyme-linked immunosorbent assay; MWM: Morris water maze; OFT: Open field test; POCD: Postoperation cognitive dysfunction; VNS: Vagal nerve stimulation

Acknowledgements

Not applicable.

Authors' contributions

JX is the first author who was responsible for the experiment. HJW is responsible for data analysis. JX and HJW made the equal contribution to the article. YB and YLG took part in revising this article, they gave constructive advices to this study and English writing. YXS is the corresponding author. All authors have read and approved the manuscript, and ensure that this is the case.

Author details

[1]Department of Anesthesiology, Sanbo Brain Hospital, Capital Medical University, No. 50 Yikesong, Xiangshan, Haidian District, Beijing 100093, China. [2]Department of Anesthesiology, Tongren Hospital, Capital Medical University, No. 1 Dongjiao Minxiang, Dongcheng District, Beijing 100730, China.

References

1. Xiong B, Shi Q, Fang H. Dexmedetomidine alleviates postoperative cognitive dysfunction by inhibiting neuron excitation in aged rats. Am J Transl Res. 2016;8(1):70–80 PMID: 27069541.
2. Norkienė I, Samalavičius R, Misiūrienė I, Paulauskienė K, Budrys V, Ivaškevičius J. Incidence and risk factors for early postoperative cognitive decline after coronary artery bypass grafting. Medicina (Kaunas). 2010;46(7):460–4 PMID: 20966618.
3. Besch G, Vettoretti L, Claveau M, Boichut N, Mahr N, Bouhake Y, Liu N, Chazot T, Samain E, Pili-Floury S. Early post-operative cognitive dysfunction after closed-loop versus manual target controlled-infusion of propofol and remifentanil in patients undergoing elective major non-cardiac surgery: Protocol of the randomized controlled single-blind POCD-ELA trial. Medicine (Baltimore). 2018;97(40):e12558. https://doi.org/10.1097/MD.0000000000012558.
4. Zhu H, Liu W, Fang H. Inflammation caused by peripheral immune cells across into injured mouse blood brain barrier can worsen postoperative cognitive dysfunction induced by isoflurane. BMC Cell Biol. 2018;19(1):23. https://doi.org/10.1186/s12860-018-0172-1.
5. Zhang M, Zhang YH, Fu HQ, Zhang QM, Wang TL. Ulinastatin May Significantly Improve Postoperative Cognitive Function of Elderly Patients Undergoing Spinal Surgery by Reducing the Translocation of Lipopolysaccharide and Systemic Inflammation. Front Pharmacol. 2018;9:1007. https://doi.org/10.3389/fphar.2018.01007.
6. Cao Y, Li Z, Ma L, Ni C, Li L, Yang N, Shi C, Guo X. Isoflurane-induced postoperative cognitive dysfunction is mediated by hypoxia-inducible factor-1α-dependent neuroinflammation in aged rats. Mol Med Rep. 2018; 17(6):7730–6. https://doi.org/10.3892/mmr.2018.8850.
7. Danielson M, Reinsfelt B, Westerlind A, Zetterberg H, Blennow K, Ricksten SE. Effects of methylprednisolone on blood-brain barrier and cerebral inflammation in cardiac surgery-a randomized trial. J Neuroinflammation. 2018;15(1):283. https://doi.org/10.1186/s12974-018-1318-y.
8. Zila I, Mokra D, Kopincova J, Kolomaznik M, Javorka M, Calkovska A. Vagal-immune interactions involved in cholinergic anti-inflammatory pathway. Physiol Res. 2017;66(Supplementum 2):S139–45 PMID: 28937230.
9. Bonaz B, Sinniger V, Pellissier S. Vagus Nerve Stimulation at the Interface of Brain-Gut Interactions. Cold Spring Harb Perspect Med. 2018. https://doi.org/10.1101/cshperspect.a034199.
10. Borovikova LV, Ivanova S, Zhang M, Yang H, Botchkina GI, Watkins LR, Wang H, Abumrad N, Eaton JW, Tracey KJ. Vagus nerve stimulation attenuates the systemic inflammatory response to endotoxin. Nature. 2000;405(6785):458–62. https://doi.org/10.1038/35013070.
11. Johnson RL, Wilson CG. A review of vagus nerve stimulaton as a therapeutic intervention. J Inflamm Res. 2018;11:203–2123. https://doi.org/10.2147/JIR.S163248.
12. Li Z, Liu X, Zhang Y, Shi J, Zhang Y, Xie P, Yu T. Connection changes in somatosensory cortex induced by different doses of propofol. PLoS One. 2014;9(2):e87829. https://doi.org/10.1371/journal.pone.0087829.
13. Lee SW, Kulkarni K, Annoni EM, Libbus I, KenKnight BH, Tolkacheva EG. Stochastic vagus nerve stimulation affects acute heart rate dynamics in rats. PLoS One. 2018;13(3):e0194910. https://doi.org/10.1371/journal.pone.0194910.
14. Stauss HM. Differential hemodynamic and respiratory responses to right and left cervical vagal nerve stimulation in rats. Physiol Rep. 2017;5(7):e13244. https://doi.org/10.14814/phy2.13244.
15. Broncel A, Bocian R, Kłos-Wojtczak P, Konopacki J. Medial septal cholinergic mediation of hippocampal theta rhythm induced by vagal nerve stimulation. PLoS One. 2018;13(11):e0206532. https://doi.org/10.1371/journal.pone.0206532.
16. Stauss HM, Stangl H, Clark KC, Kwitek AE, Lira VA. Cervical vagal nerve stimulation impairs glucose tolerance and suppresses insulin release in conscious rats. Physiol Rep. 2018;6(24):e13953. https://doi.org/10.14814/phy2.13953.
17. Cao J, Lu KH, Powley TL, Liu Z. Vagal nerve stimulation triggers widespread responses and alters large-scale functional connectivity in the rat brain. PLoS One. 2017;12(12):e0189518. https://doi.org/10.1371/journal.pone.0189518.
18. Livak KJ, Schmittgen TD. Analysis of relative gene expression data using real-time quantitative PCR and the 2(-Delta Delta C(T)) Method. Methods. 2001;25(4):402–8. https://doi.org/10.1006/meth.2001.1262.
19. Xin X, Xin F, Chen X, Zhang Q, Li Y, Huo S, Chang C, Wang Q. Hypertonic saline for prevention of delirium in geriatric patients who underwent hip surgery. J Neuroinflammation. 2017;14(1):221. https://doi.org/10.1186/s12974-017-0999-y.
20. Nadelson MR, Sanders RD, Avidan MS. Perioperative cognitive trajectory in adults. Br J Anaesth. 2014;112(3):440–51. https://doi.org/10.1093/bja/aet420.
21. Kalliolias GD, Ivashkiv LB. TNF biology, pathogenic mechanisms and emerging therapeutic strategies. Nat Rev Rheumatol. 2016;12(1):49–62. https://doi.org/10.1038/nrrheum.2015.169.
22. Hua FZ, Ying J, Zhang J, Wang XF, Hu YH, Liang YP, Liu Q, Xu GH. Naringenin pre-treatment inhibits neuroapoptosis and ameliorates cognitive impairment in rats exposed to isoflurane anesthesia by regulating the PI3/Akt/PTEN signalling pathway and suppressing NF-κB-mediated inflammation. Int J Mol Med. 2016;38(4):1271–80. https://doi.org/10.3892/ijmm.2016.2715.
23. Zheng JW, Meng B, Li XY, Lu B, Wu GR, Chen JP. NF-κB/P65 signaling pathway: a potential therapeutic target in postoperative cognitive dysfunction after sevoflurane anesthesia. Eur Rev Med Pharmacol Sci. 2017; 21(2):394–407 PMID: 28165545.
24. Bonaz B, Sinniger V, Pellissier S. Anti-inflammatory properties of the vagus nerve: potential therapeutic implications of vagus nerve stimulation. J Physiol. 2016;594(20):5781–90. https://doi.org/10.1113/JP271539.
25. Huffman WJ, Subramaniyan S, Rodriguiz RM, Wetsel WC, Grill WM, Terrando N. Modulation of neuroinflammation and memory dysfunction using percutaneous vagus nerve stimulation in mice. Brain Stimul. 2019;12(1):19–29. https://doi.org/10.1016/j.brs.2018.10.005.
26. Maurer SV, Williams CL. The Cholinergic System Modulates Memory and Hippocampal Plasticity via Its Interactions with Non-Neuronal Cells. Front Immunol. 2017;8:1489. https://doi.org/10.3389/fimmu.2017.01489.
27. Zhou JP, Wang F, Li RL, Yuan BL, Guo YL. Effects of febrile seizure on motor, behavior, spatial learning and memory in rats. Zhonghua Er Ke Za Zhi. 2004; 42(1):49–53 PMID: 14990108. Chinese.
28. Liu RP, Fang JL, Rong PJ, Zhao Y, Meng H, Ben H, Li L, Huang ZX, Li X, Ma YG, Zhu B. Effects of electroacupuncture at auricular concha region on the

depressive status of unpredictable chronic mild stress rat models. Evid Based Complement Alternat Med. 2013;2013:789674. https://doi.org/10.1155/2013/789674.
29. Liu AF, Zhao FB, Wang J, Lu YF, Tian J, Zhao Y, Gao Y, Hu XJ, Liu XY, Tan J, Tian YL, Shi J. Effects of vagus nerve stimulation on cognitive functioning in rats with cerebral ischemia reperfusion. J Transl Med. 2016;14:101. https://doi.org/10.1186/s12967-016-0858-0.
30. Zhu YZ, Yao R, Zhang Z, Xu H, Wang LW. Parecoxib prevents early postoperative cognitive dysfunction in elderly patients undergoing total knee arthroplasty: A double-blind, randomized clinical consort study. Medicine (Baltimore). 2016;95(28):e4082. https://doi.org/10.1097/MD.0000000000004082.
31. Chen K, Wei P, Zheng Q, Zhou J, Li J. Neuroprotective effects of intravenous lidocaine on early postoperative cognitive dysfunction in elderly patients following spine surgery. Med Sci Monit. 2015;21:1402–7. https://doi.org/10.12659/MSM.894384.
32. Pappa M, Theodosiadis N, Tsounis A, Sarafis P. Pathogenesis and treatment of post-operative cognitive dysfunction. Electron Physician. 2017;9(2):3768–75. https://doi.org/10.19082/3768.

8

Dexmedetomidine suppresses sevoflurane anesthesia-induced neuroinflammation through activation of the PI3K/Akt/mTOR pathway

Nan Wang and Mingyu Wang*

Abstract

Background: Sevoflurane, an inhalational general anesthetic, has become one of the most widely used inhalational anesthetics in surgery. However, previous studies have found that sevoflurane anesthesia can trigger an inflammatory response, resulting in secondary damage. Dexmedetomidine (DEX), a highly-selective α adrenergic receptor agonist, is widely used as an anesthetic adjuvant in the clinic. In this study we investigated whether DEX was able to suppress sevoflurane-induced neuroinflammation.

Methods: The aim was to determine the mechanism of action of the suppressive effect of DEX using a rat model. Rats were randomly divided into a control group ($n = 10$), low-dose sevoflurane group (L-Sev; $n = 10$), high-dose sevoflurane group (H-Sev; n = 10), vehicle group (n = 10), DEX group (n = 10) and DEX + LY294002 (a specific inhibitor of PI3K) group (n = 10). The rats in vehicle, DEX and DEX + LY294002 groups were in the presence of high-dose sevoflurane exposure. Western blotting was used to measure the expression of proinflammatory cytokines (IL-6, IL-8, TNF-α) and the activity level of the phosphatidylinositol 3-hydroxy kinase/protein kinase B/mammalian target of rapamycin (PI3K/Akt/mTOR) pathway.

Results: We found that sevoflurane anesthesia induced an increase in the levels of pro-inflammatory cytokines, while decreasing activation of the PI3K/Akt/mTOR pathway in both the cortex and hippocampus of rats. Treatment with DEX reduced pro-inflammatory cytokine levels and prevented inactivation of the PI3K/Akt/mTOR pathway. Moreover, LY294002, an inhibitor of the PI3K/Akt/mTOR pathway, reduced the anti-inflammatory activity of DEX.

Conclusions: These data suggest that the PI3K/Akt/mTOR pathway contributes to sevoflurane-induced neuroinflammation and that activation of PI3K/Akt/mTOR signaling by DEX could help reduce the neuroinflammatory effects of sevoflurane.

Keywords: Dexmedetomidine, Sevoflurane, Neuroinflammation, PI3K/Akt/mTOR pathway

Background

In recent years the inhalational anesthetic sevoflurane has replaced other volatile anesthetics due to its quick induction, stable maintenance, rapid revival and because the irritation it causes is mild [1]. However, recent evidence has shown that sevoflurane can lead to pathophysiological alterations of the brain during the recovery period, such as neuronal apoptosis, tau aggresomes, abnormal discharge of neurons, and neuroinflammation, which cause neurodegenerative changes in the development of the mammalian brain [2–6]. Exposure to anesthesia in childhood may lead to adverse neurodevelopmental outcomes in children [7]. Despite evidence linking inhalational anesthesia to neurodegenerative effects, it is still considered safer than other methods of anesthesia, and more than 3 million children undergo inhaled anesthesia every year [8, 9]. Therefore, there is an urgent

* Correspondence: mingyuwang1211@163.com
Department of Anesthesiology, Cancer Hospital of China Medical University, Liaoning Cancer Hospital & Institute, Dalian Medical University Clinical Oncology College, Shenyang 110042, Liaoning, China

need to find anesthetic adjuvants that reduce the neurotoxicity of inhaled anesthetics.

Dexmedetomidine (DEX), a selective α2-adrenoceptor agonist, is used intravenously as a sedative or adjuvant of local anesthetics used in peripheral nerve blocks, where it prolongs the duration of sensory and motor blockades without causing toxicity [10–12].In addition, DEX is able to cross the blood brain barrier and stimulate α2-adrenoceptors centrally and has been shown to exert a neuroprotective effect [13]. Wang et al. found that treatment with DEX could inhibit the expression of inflammatory cytokines and their mediators, resulting in reduced focal cerebral ischemia-reperfusion injury in rats. These data suggest that inhibition of the nuclear factor-κB pathway (NF-κB) may be a mechanism underlying the neuroprotective action of DEX [14]. Treatment with DEX after subarachnoid haemorrhage (SAH) attenuated SAH-induced early brain injury, partially through suppression of the toll like receptor 4 (TLR4)/NF-κB pathway and the NLRP3 inflammasome [15]. Additionally, DEX has been shown to improve post-operative cognitive dysfunction in aging mice by inhibition of the hippocampal inflammatory response and reduction of neuronal apoptosis [16]. Taken together, these data suggest that DEX has anti-inflammatory properties in the central nervous system (CNS).

Given the inflammation induced by sevoflurane and the anti-inflammatory properties of DEX, we aimed to ascertain whether DEX could provide protection from sevoflurane anesthesia-induced inflammation in the CNS and ascertain whether these protective effects were closely associated with the phosphatidylinositol 3-hydroxy kinase/protein kinase B/mammalian target of rapamycin (PI3K/Akt/mTOR) pathway.

Methods

Animals

Fifty healthy Sprague-Dawley (SD) rats, weighing 150–200 g were purchased from the Animal Experiment Center of the Institute of Radiation Medicine of the Chinese Academy of Medical Sciences, China. The rats were fed food and water under specific pathogen-free conditions and housed in a 12 h light/dark cycle at 22–24 °C. All animal procedures were approved by the Institute of Radiation Medicine of the Chinese Academy of Medical Sciences and conducted in accordance with the ethical principles for Experiments on Animals, in addition to international standards.

Groups and treatments

Rats were randomly divided into six groups: control group ($n = 10$), low-dose sevoflurane group (L-Sev; n = 10), high-dose sevoflurane group (H-Sev; n = 10), vehicle group (n = 10), DEX group (n = 10) and DEX + LY294002 (a specific inhibitor of PI3K) group (n = 10). All rats were placed in an anesthesia induction chamber and received anesthesia using an inhalation machine. Oxygen concentration and anesthesia doses were continuously monitored. The control group was treated with 60% O_2 for 2 h, the L-Sev group with 1.5% sevoflurane inhalation for 2 h and the remaining groups (H-Sev group, vehicle group, DEX group and DEX + LY294002 group) were treated with 3% sevoflurane inhalation for 2 h [17]. One hour prior to sevoflurane treatment, the vehicle group received an intraperitoneal injection of saline, the DEX group received an intraperitoneal injection of 4 μg/kg DEX [18] and the DEX + LY294002 group received an intraperitoneal injection of 4 μg/kg DEX and intracerebroventricular injection of 25 μg/5 μl LY294002 (Sigma-Aldrich Chemical Company, USA) [19]. The time at which anesthesia commenced was when sevoflurane concentration had reached a maximum for each group. Gas flow in the anesthesia chamber was maintained at a rate of 4 L/min.

Tissue preparation

At the end of the experiment, rats were sacrificed under anesthesia using 50 mg/kg sodium pentobarbital by intraperitoneal injection. The brain tissue was removed and a subset of brain samples used to prepare 10 μm sections for use in immunofluorescence staining. The remaining brains were placed on Aluminum foil and the cortical and the hippocampal tissues separated then stored at − 80 °C for Western blot analysis.

Western blot analysis

Cortical and hippocampal tissue samples were lysed and total protein extracted using whole-cell protein extraction kits (Beyotime, China) in accordance with the manufacturer's protocols. A bicinchoninic acid (BCA) protein quantification kit (Beyotime, China) was used to measure protein concentration in the samples. Proteins were separated using 10% SDS-PAGE then transferred to polyvinylidene difluoride (PVDF) membranes. The membranes were blocked using 2% BSA in TBST at room temperature for 2 h. Membranes were then incubated with primary antibodies overnight at 4 °C. The primary antibodies used in our study included rabbit anti-IL-6 (1:1000, Abcam, USA), IL-8 (1:1000, Abcam, USA), TNFα (1: 1000, Abcam, USA), PI3K (1:1000, CST, USA), p-PI3K (1:1000, CST, USA), Akt (1:1000, CST, USA), p-Akt (1:1000, CST, USA), mTOR (1:1000, CST, USA), p-mTOR (1:1000, CST, USA) and GAPDH (1: 4000, Proteintech, USA). Following staining with a primary antibody, three TBST washes were preformed and the membranes were then incubated with a horseradish peroxidase-conjugated goat anti-rabbit IgG secondary antibody (1:4000, Proteintech, USA) for 2 h at room temperature. PVDF membranes were then washed three times with TBST and developed using an ECL Plus reagent. The optical density of each protein was analyzed using Image J software (National Institutes of Health, USA) and was standardized to GAPDH or corresponding total protein.

Statistical analysis

All values are presented as means ± SD. Comparisons between groups were conducted using t-tests and one-way ANOVA followed by a post hoc Tukey test. Differences were considered statistically significant at a level of $P < 0.05$.

Results

Sevoflurane induced neuroinflammation in rats

To determine the effect of sevoflurane on neuroinflammation, expression levels of the inflammatory markers IL-6, IL-8 and TNF-α were measured in the cortex and hippocampus of rats in the control, L-Sev and H-Sev groups by Western blotting. IL-6, IL-8 and TNF-α expression increased significantly in the cortex and hippocampus after low or high-dose sevoflurane anesthesia compared with that of the control group (Fig. 1, $p < 0.05$). Moreover, the high-dose sevoflurane group exhibited significantly higher levels of IL-6, IL-8 and TNF-α than the low-dose group, indicating that the induction of inflammation was dose-dependent (Fig. 1, $p < 0.05$).

Sevoflurane inhibited the PI3K/Akt/mTOR pathway in rats

The levels of PI3K, Akt and mTOR expression were assayed, in addition to their phosphorylation status, in the cortex and hippocampus of rats from the control, L-Sev, and H-Sev groups in order to assess the effect of sevoflurane anesthesia on PI3K/Akt/mTOR signaling. As shown in Fig. 2, both low and high-dose sevoflurane treatment groups exhibited significantly decreased levels of PI3K/Akt/

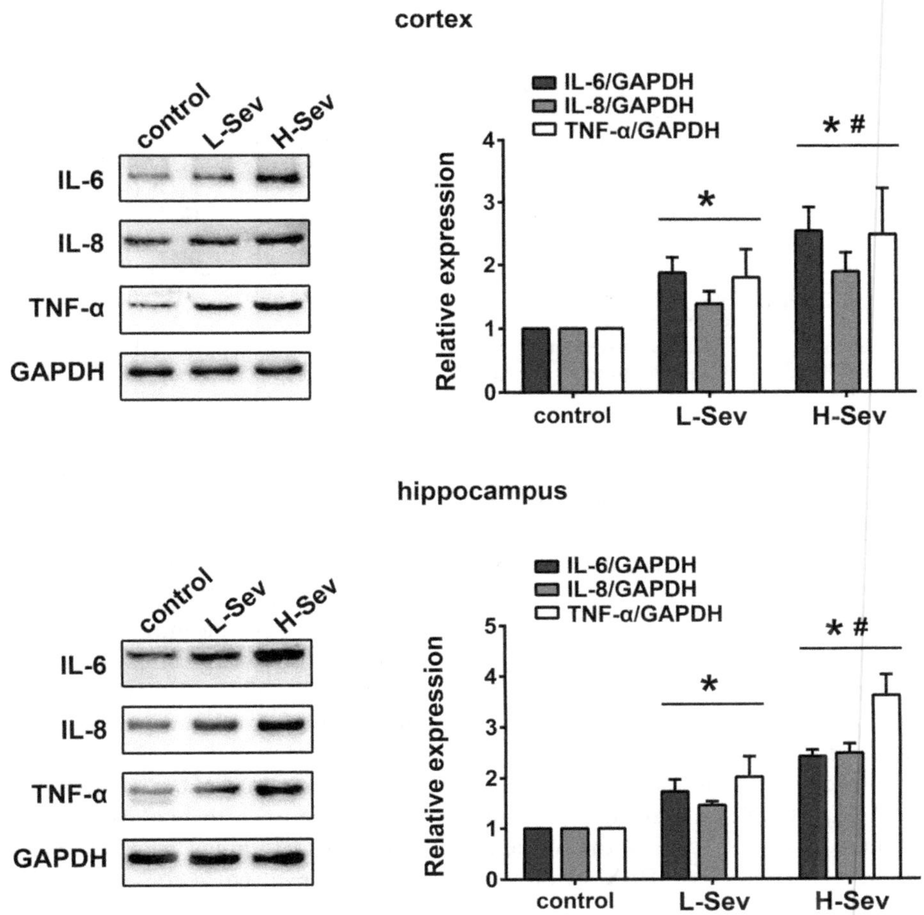

Fig. 1 Sevoflurane treatment increases inflammatory markers in the hippocampus. Expression levels of IL-6, IL-8 and TNF-α in the cortex and hippocampus of rats in the control, L-Sev and H-Sev groups were measured by Western blotting (mean ± SD, $n = 5$ per group, one-way ANOVA). *$p < 0.05$ vs control group, #p < 0.05 vs L-Sev group

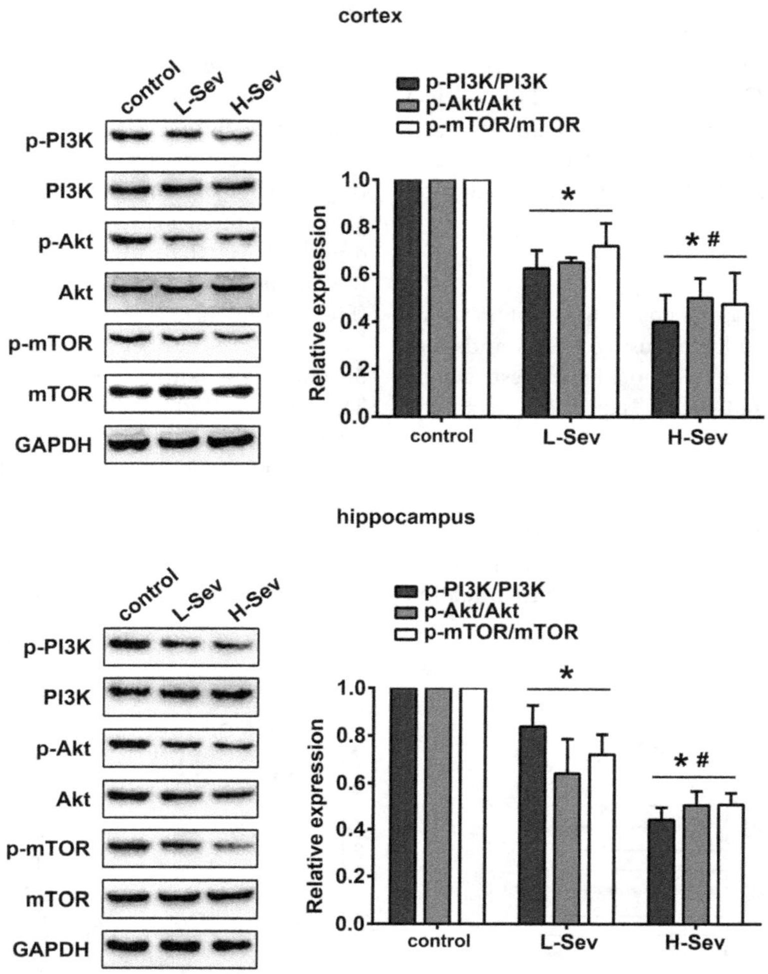

Fig. 2 Sevoflurane inhibited the PI3K/Akt/mTOR pathway in rats. Cortical and hippocampal levels of PI3K, p-PI3K, Akt, p-Akt, mTOR and p-mTOR of rats in the control, L-Sev and H-Sev groups were measured by Western blotting (mean ± SD, $n = 5$ per group, one-way ANOVA). *$p < 0.05$ vs control group, #$p < 0.05$ vs L-Sev group

mTOR pathway phosphorylation ($p < 0.05$). Moreover, the level of PI3K/AKT/mTOR pathway activity was significantly lower in the cortex and hippocampus after high-dose sevoflurane anesthesia compared with that in the L-Sev group (Fig. 2, $p < 0.05$).

Dexmedetomidine suppressed sevoflurane-induced neuroinflammation in rats

To determine if dexmedetomidine could reduce neuroinflammation induced by sevoflurane anesthesia, the levels of IL-6, IL-8 and TNF-α were measured in the cortex and hippocampus of rats in the vehicle and DEX groups. Rats treated with DEX exhibited decreased levels of IL-6, IL-8 and TNF-α compared with the vehicle control group, suggesting that DEX can inhibit sevoflurane anesthesia-induced neuroinflammation (Fig. 3, $p < 0.05$).

Dexmedetomidine activated the PI3K/Akt/mTOR pathway in sevoflurane-treated rats

Using Western blotting, we assayed the effects of DEX on PI3K/Akt/mTOR pathway activation. As shown in Fig. 4, the levels of PI3K, Akt and mTOR phosphorylation increased significantly in the cortex and hippocampus in the DEX group compared with the vehicle group, indicating that DEX could activate the PI3K/Akt/mTOR pathway under sevoflurane anesthesia ($p < 0.05$).

Blockade of the PI3K/Akt/mTOR pathway reduced the anti-inflammatory activity of dexmedetomidine

Finally, to determine whether the PI3K/Akt/mTOR pathway is involved in the anti-inflammatory effects of DEX, rats were treated with DEX in the presence or absence of LY294002 and the expression of IL-6, IL-8 and TNF-α in the cortex and hippocampus assessed by Western blot analysis. As shown in Fig. 5, the levels of

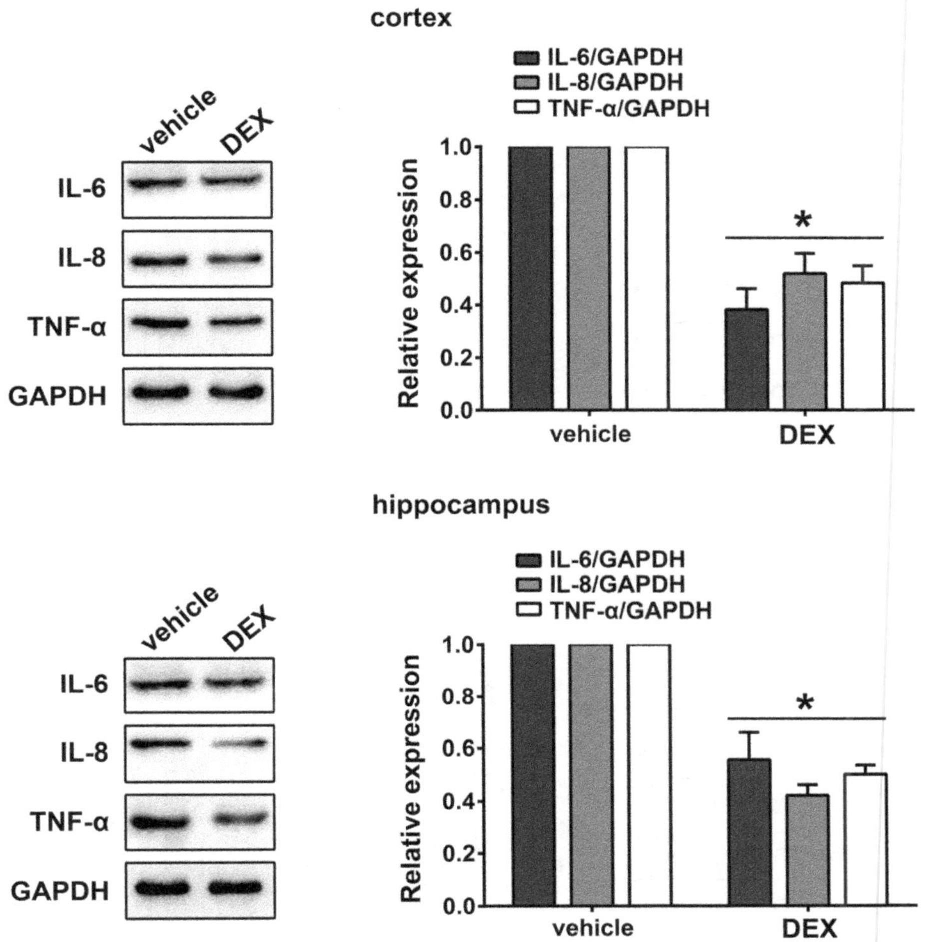

Fig. 3 Dexmedetomidine suppressed sevoflurane-induced neuroinflammation in rats Western blot measurements of IL-6, IL-8 and TNF- α from cortical and hippocampal samples of DEX and vehicle-treated rats (mean ± SD, $n = 5$ per group, t test). *$p < 0.05$ vs vehicle group

IL-6, IL-8 and TNF-α increased significantly in the cortex and hippocampus in the DEX+LY294002 group compared with the DEX group, indicating that LY294002 reduced the anti-inflammatory activity of DEX under sevoflurane anesthesia ($p < 0.05$).

Discussion

In the present study, we observed that sevoflurane anesthesia induced an increase in the expression of pro-inflammatory factors and a decrease in PI3K/Akt/mTOR pathway activity in both the cortex and hippocampus of rats. Additionally, we found that DEX treatment could restore PI3K/Akt/mTOR activity in rats treated with sevoflurane anesthesia and blockade of the PI3K/Akt/mTOR pathway reduced the anti-inflammatory activity of DEX. Thus, we propose that DEX can suppress sevoflurane anesthesia-induced neuroinflammation by modulating PI3K/Akt/mTOR pathway activity.

Postoperative neuroinflammation is a common pathological phenomenon in the CNS, which can lead to secondary damage, such as delirium, cognitive dysfunction, Alzheimer's disease and additional detrimental effects [20, 21]. A healthy immune response is crucial to ensure proper wound healing and repair of tissue damage, in addition to combating infection without harming the host's own cells or tissues. In contrast, an excessive inflammatory response is harmful and can result in severe tissue damage and even death [20, 22]. Inhalational anesthetics, such as isoflurane and sevoflurane, can trigger pathological inflammatory responses during surgery. Isoflurane, which has been used since the 1980s, is metabolized slowly leading to reduced induction of anesthesia during surgery and shorter recovery times [23]. The use of sevoflurane began a decade later. It has a lower blood-gas partition coefficient than other anesthetics, leading to rapid induction of anesthesia and faster recovery times after anesthesia [24, 25]. Several decades of research have been conducted on the toxicity and side effects of these volatile anesthetics. Here, we investigated the relationship

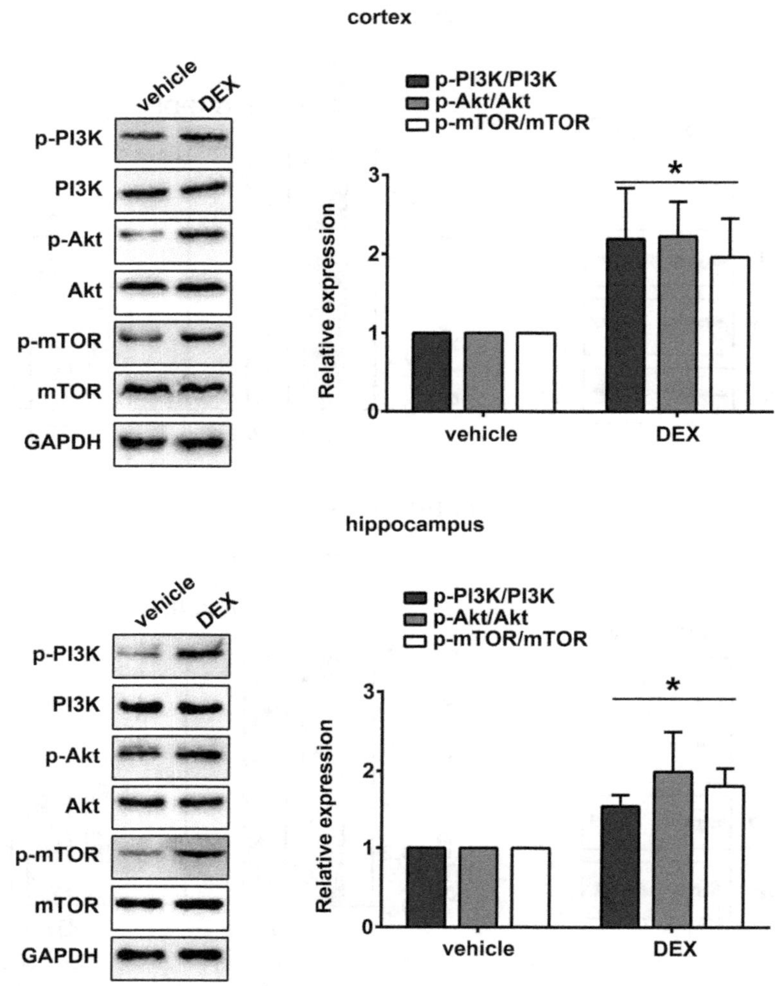

Fig. 4 Dexmedetomidine activated the PI3K/Akt/mTOR pathway in sevoflurane-treated rats Images and quantification of Western blot measurements of PI3K, p-PI3K, Akt, p-Akt, mTOR and p-mTOR in the cortex and hippocampus of rats in the vehicle and DEX groups (mean ± SD, $n = 5$ per group, t test). $^*p < 0.05$ vs vehicle group

between sevoflurane anesthesia and neuroinflammation. We used low- or high-dose sevoflurane in rats, then detected the expression of proinflammatory cytokines (IL-6, IL-8, TNF-α). We confirmed that sevoflurane could increase the levels of IL-6, IL-8 and TNF-α in the cortex and hippocampus of anesthetized rats, in agreement with previous research which indicated that both isoflurane and sevoflurane were able to increase IL-6 levels via activation of NF-κB signalling [26].

The PI3K/Akt/mTOR cascade is important in mediating the release of proinflammatory cytokines [27–29]. PI3K is a ubiquitous lipid kinase which plays a crucial role in signal transduction through receptor tyrosine kinases. PI3K phosphorylates phosphatidylinositol-4,5-bis-phosphate (PIP2) to form phosphatidylinositol-4,5-tri-phosphate (PIP3); PIP3 recruits other downstream molecules, such as serine-threonine kinases, including the major effector of PI3K activation, Akt [30]. Activated Akt can then in turn activate mTOR, leading to the phosphorylation of two downstream effectors, p70 ribosomal protein S6 kinase 1 (S6K1) and eIF4E binding protein (4E-BP1), which promotes translational initiation and elongation [31–34]. In addition to its role in protein synthesis, mTOR also regulates the ubiquitin-proteasome system (UPS) [34, 35]. The UPS is an important regulator of NF-κB signaling, as the inhibitory regulator of NF-κB must be degraded by the proteasome in order for NF-κB to become active. Harston et al. suggested that inhibition of mTOR by rapamycin could increase polyubiquitination and ubiquitin-mediated degradation of IκB-α, leading to NF-κB-induced transcriptional activation. This result suggests that activation of mTOR could prevent the occurrence of inflammation through suppression of NF-κB activation [27], as NF-κB activity promotes the expression of proinflammatory cytokines [28, 29]. We observed an

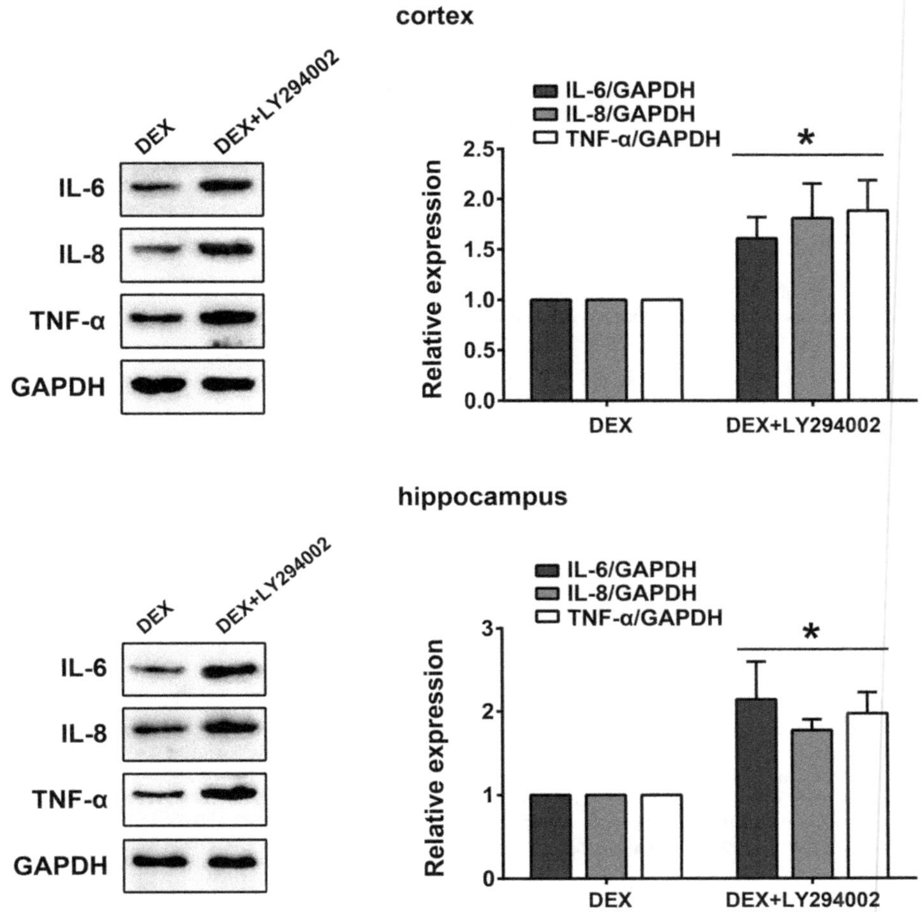

Fig. 5 Blockade of the PI3K/Akt/mTOR pathway reduced the anti-inflammatory activity of dexmedetomidine Western blot measurements of IL-6, IL-8 and TNF- α from cortical and hippocampal samples of rats in the DEX and DEX + LY294002 groups (mean ± SD, $n = 5$ per group, t test). $^{*}p < 0.05$ vs DEX group

increase in pro-inflammatory cytokine release after treatment with sevoflurane anesthesia, and this release was accompanied by the inactivation of the PI3K/Akt/mTOR pathway, suggesting that inactivation of the PI3K/Akt/mTOR pathway may be associated with sevoflurane anesthesia-induced neuroinflammation. Thus, increasing PI3K/Akt/mTOR pathway activity may be a promising and novel therapeutic strategy against postoperative neuroinflammation.

Recent studies have suggested that DEX has anti-inflammatory properties. Chen et al., for example, found that DEX treatment could suppress retinal ischemia/reperfusion injury, and showed effective anti-inflammatory effects through inhibition of toll-like receptor 4 (TLR4)/NF-κB expression [36]. Additionally, Huang et al. also suggested that DEX could inhibit the nuclear translocation and binding activity of activated NF-κB, thus reducing the release of inflammatory cytokines [37]. Given the anti-inflammatory properties of DEX and its effects on the PI3K/Akt/mTOR signaling pathway, we hypothesized that DEX could suppress sevoflurane anesthesia-induced neuroinflammation. We found that treatment with DEX down-regulated pro-inflammatory cytokines (IL-6, IL-8 and TNF-α) and up-regulated the phosphorylation levels of PI3K/Akt/mTOR. A previous study indicated that DEX exerts an anti-inflammatory effect via the activation of PI3K/Akt/mTOR signaling in rats with traumatic brain injury [19]. In addition, blockade of the PI3K/Akt/mTOR pathway reduced the anti-inflammatory activity of DEX. Thus, we propose that DEX can ameliorate sevoflurane-induced neuroinflammation through activation of the PI3K/Akt/mTOR signaling pathway.

Conclusions

Sevoflurane anesthesia induces neuroinflammation in the CNS and this inflammation may be the result of decreased signaling through the PI3K/Akt/mTOR pathway. The administration of DEX can reduce neuroinflammation caused by sevoflurane, providing an important reference basis for clinical anesthesia.

Abbreviations

DEX: Dexmedetomidine; NF-κB: Nuclear factor-κB pathway; PI3K/Akt/mTOR: Phosphatidylinositol 3-hydroxy kinase/protein kinase B/mammalian target of rapamycin; PIP2: Phosphatidylinositol-4,5-bis-phosphate; PIP3: Phosphatidylinositol-4,5-tri-phosphate; S6K1: S6 kinase 1; SAH: Subarachnoid haemorrhage; TLR4: Toll like receptor 4; UPS: Ubiquitin-proteasome system

Acknowledgments

We thank members of the laboratory for technical help.

Authors' contributions

The research idea and project design: MW. Data collection and dataset setup: NW. Data analysis: NW. All authors contributed to the development of the manuscript, and approved the final version.

References

1. Tang L, Liu H, Wu Y, Li M, Li W, Jiang M, Hou J, Jiang Y, Xia Z, Meng Q. Sevoflurane may be more beneficial than propofol in patients receiving endoscopic variceal ligation and endoscopic variceal sclerotherapy: a randomized, double-blind study. Exp Ther Med. 2017;14:3145–52.
2. Huang L, Huang K, Ning H. Autophagy induction by hispidulin provides protection against sevoflurane-induced neuronal apoptosis in aged rats. Biomed Pharmacother. 2018;98:460–8.
3. Wang L, Zheng M, Wu S, Niu Z. MicroRNA-188-3p is involved in sevoflurane anesthesia-induced neuroapoptosis by targeting MDM2. Mol Med Rep. 2018;17:4229–36.
4. Tao G, Zhang J, Zhang L, Dong Y, Yu B, Crosby G, Culley DJ, Zhang Y, Xie Z. Sevoflurane induces tau phosphorylation and glycogen synthase kinase 3β activation in young mice. Anesthesiology. 2014;121:510–27.
5. Liang P, Li F, Liu J, Liao D, Huang H, Zhou C. Sevoflurane activates hippocampal CA3 kainate receptors (Gluk2) to induce hyperactivity during induction and recovery in a mouse model. Br J Anaesth. 2017;119:1047–54.
6. Li D, Liu L, Li L, Li X, Huang B, Zhou C, Zhang Z, Wang C, Dong P, Zhang X, Yang B, Zhang L. Sevoflurane induces exaggerated and persistent cognitive decline in a type II diabetic rat model by aggregating hippocampal inflammation. Front Pharmacol. 2017;8:886.
7. Poor Zamany Nejat Kermany M, Roodneshin F, Ahmadi Dizgah N, Gerami E, Riahi E. Early childhood exposure to short periods of sevoflurane is not associated with later, lasting cognitive deficits. Paediatr Anaesth. 2016;26:1018–25.
8. Sun LS, Li G, Dimaggio C, Byrne M, Rauh V, Brooks-Gunn J, Kakavouli A, Wood A. Anesthesia and neurodevelopment in children: time for an answer. Anesthesiology. 2008;109:757–61.
9. Bo LJ, Yu PX, Zhang FZ, Dong ZM. Dexmedetomidine mitigates sevoflurane-induced cell cycle arrest in hippocampus. J Anesth. 2018; 32:717–24.
10. Kim BS, Choi JH, Baek SH, Lee DH. Effects of Intraneural injection of Dexmedetomidine in combination with Ropivacaine in rat sciatic nerve block. Reg Anesth Pain Med. 2018;43:378–84.
11. Brummett CM, Norat MA, Palmisano JM, Lydic R. Perineural administration of dexmedetomidine in combination with bupivacaine enhances sensory and motor blockade in sciatic nerve block without inducing neurotoxicity in rat. Anesthesiology. 2008;109:502–11.
12. Tan JA, Ho KM. Use of dexmedetomidine as a sedative and analgesic agent in critically ill adult patients: a meta-analysis. Intensive Care Med. 2010;36:926–39.
13. Alam A, Suen KC, Hana Z, Sanders RD, Maze M, Ma D. Neuroprotection and neurotoxicity in the developing brain: an update on the effects of dexmedetomidine and xenon. Neurotoxicol Teratol. 2017;60:102–16.
14. Wang L, Liu H, Zhang L, Wang G, Zhang M, Yu Y. Neuroprotection of Dexmedetomidine against cerebral ischemia-reperfusion injury in rats: involved in inhibition of NF-κB and inflammation response. Biomol Ther (Seoul). 2017;25:383–9.
15. Yin D, Zhou S, Xu X, Gao W, Li F, Ma Y, Sun D, Wu Y, Guo Q, Liu H, Han L, Wang Z, Wang Y, Zhang J. Dexmedetomidine attenuated early brain injury in rats with subarachnoid haemorrhage by suppressing the inflammatory response: the TLR4/NF-κB pathway and the NLRP3 inflammasome may be involved in the mechanism. Brain Res. 2018;1698:1–10.
16. Qian XL, Zhang W, Liu MZ, Zhou YB, Zhang JM, Han L, Peng YM, Jiang JH, Wang QD. Dexmedetomidine improves early postoperative cognitive dysfunction in aged mice. Eur J Pharmacol. 2015;746:206–12.
17. Cui RS, Wang K, Wang ZL. Sevoflurane anesthesia alters cognitive function by activating inflammation and cell death in rats. Exp Ther Med. 2018;15:4127–30.
18. Yi C, Fu Z, Luo X. Dexmedetomidine on autophagy of hippocampal neurons in aged rats under sevoflurane anesthesia. Exp Ther Med. 2018;16:837–41.
19. Shen M, Wang S, Wen X, Han XR, Wang YJ, Zhou XM, Zhang MH, Wu DM, Lu J, Zheng YL. Dexmedetomidine exerts neuroprotective effect via the activation of the PI3K/Akt/mTOR signaling pathway in rats with traumatic brain injury. Biomed Pharmacother. 2017;95:885–93.
20. Umholtz M, Nader ND. Anesthetic immunomodulation of the Neuroinflammation in postoperative cognitive dysfunction. Immunol Investig. 2017;46:805–15.
21. Cortese GP, Burger C. Neuroinflammatory challenges compromise neuronal function in the aging brain: postoperative cognitive delirium and Alzheimer's disease. Behav Brain Res. 2017;322:269–79.
22. Pol RA, van Leeuwen BL, Izaks GJ, Reijnen MM, Visser L, Tielliu IF, Zeebregts CJ. C-reactive protein predicts postoperative delirium following vascular surgery. Ann Vasc Surg. 2014;28:1923–30.
23. Eger EI. New inhaled anesthetics. Anesthesiology. 1994;80:906–22.
24. Esper T, Wehner M, Meinecke CD, Rueffert H. Blood/gas partition coefficients for isoflurane, sevoflurane, and desflurane in a clinically relevant patient population. Anesth Analg. 2015;120:45–50.
25. Lee YM, Song BC, Yeum KJ. Impact of volatile anesthetics on oxidative stress and inflammation. Biomed Res Int. 2015;2015:242709.
26. Zhang L, Zhang J, Yang L, Dong Y, Zhang Y, Xie Z. Isoflurane and sevoflurane increase interleukin-6 levels through the nuclear factor-kappa B pathway in neuroglioma cells. Br J Anaesth. 2013;110(Suppl 1):i82–91.
27. Harston RK, McKillop JC, Moschella PC, Van Laer A, Quinones LS, Baicu CF, Balasubramanian S, Zile MR, Kuppuswamy D. Rapamycin treatment augments both protein ubiquitination and Akt activation in pressure-overloaded rat myocardium. Am J Physiol Heart Circ Physiol. 2011;300: H1696–706.
28. Tak PP, Firestein GS. NF-kappaB: a key role in inflammatory diseases. J Clin Invest. 2001;107:7–11.
29. Yang J, Li S, Wang L, Du F, Zhou X, Song Q, Zhao J, Fang R. Ginsenoside Rg3 attenuates lipopolysaccharide-induced acute lung injury via MerTK-dependent activation of the PI3K/AKT/mTOR pathway. Front Pharmacol. 2018;9:850.
30. Ko JK, Auyeung KK. Target-oriented mechanisms of novel herbal therapeutics in the chemotherapy of gastrointestinal cancer and inflammation. Curr Pharm Des. 2013;19:48–66.
31. Ma XM, Blenis J. Molecular mechanisms of mTOR-mediated translational control. Nat Rev Mol Cell Biol. 2009;10:307–18.
32. Iadevaia V, Huo Y, Zhang Z, Foster LJ, Proud CG. Roles of the mammalian target of rapamycin, mTOR, in controlling ribosome biogenesis and protein synthesis. Biochem Soc Trans. 2012;40:168–72.
33. Albert V, Hall MN. mTOR signaling in cellular and organismal energetics. Curr Opin Cell Biol. 2015;33:55–66.
34. Xu L, Brink M. mTOR, cardiomyocytes and inflammation in cardiac hypertrophy. Biochim Biophys Acta. 1863;2016:1894–903.
35. Zhang Y, Nicholatos J, Dreier JR, Ricoult SJ, Widenmaier SB, Hotamisligil GS, Kwiatkowski DJ, Manning BD. Coordinated regulation of protein synthesis and degradation by mTORC1. Nature. 2014;513:440–3.
36. Chen Z, Qiu PY, Ma CG. Dexmedetomidine preconditioning protects against retinal ischemia/reperfusion injury and inhibits inflammation response via toll-like receptor 4 (TLR4) pathway. Biomed Pharmacother. 2017;93:1018–24.
37. Huang Y, Lu Y, Zhang L, Yan J, Jiang J, Jiang H. Perineural dexmedetomidine attenuates inflammation in rat sciatic nerve via the NF-κB pathway. Int J Mol Sci. 2014;15:4049–59.

9

Maternal sciatic nerve administered bupivacaine induces hippocampal cell apoptosis in offspring

Alireza Mirkheshti[1], Alireza Shakeri[1], Elham Memary[1], Mansoureh Baniasadi[2], Jalal Zaringhalam[2*], Ardeshir Tajbakhsh[1], Marzieh Mirzaei[3] and Elena Lak[4]

Abstract

Background: Bupivacaine, an amid-type local anesthetic, is widely used for clinical patients especially in pregnant women. In addition to neurotoxicity effect of bupivacaine, it can cross the placenta, accumulates in this tissue and retained in fetal tissues. Nevertheless, whether bupivacaine can cause neurotoxicity in fetus remains unclear. Hence, this study was design to investigate the effects of maternal bupivacaine use on fetus hippocampal cell apoptosis and the possible related mechanism.

Methods: On day 15 of pregnancy, sciatic nerve of pregnant wistar rat (180–200 g) were exposed by lateral incision of the right thigh and 0.2 ml of bupivacaine was injected. After their delivery, we randomly selected one male offspring of every mother. On day 30 after of their birth, the rat's hippocampi were isolated for molecular studies. Western blotting was used to examine the expression of cleaved caspase-3, caspase-8 and p-Akt in fetal hippocampus.

Results: Our results showed that maternal bupivacaine use caused a significant increment of cleaved caspase-3 and caspase-8 expression in fetal hippocampus compared with the sham group. In addition, maternally administered bupivacaine could significantly decrease hippocampal P.Akt/T.Akt ratio which was concurrent with an increment of cleaved caspase-3 and caspase-8 expression.

Conclusion: Our data suggest that maternal bupivacaine use increases fetal hippocampal cell apoptosis markers such as caspase 8 and cleaved caspase 3, at least in part, via inhibiting the Akt activation.

Keywords: Bupivacaine, Apoptosis, Akt, Pregnancy

Background

Bupivacaine, an amid-type local anesthetic, is widely used for spinal and epidural anesthesia, peripheral nerve blockade, sympathetic nerve block and postoperative analgesia in clinical patients, especially in pregnant patients by providing excellent sensory anesthesia [1, 2]. However, local anesthetics may have potential neurotoxicity and induce nonreversible neurological complications [1, 3–5]. In this regard, a growing body of data indicates that bupivacaine triggers a complex cascade response leading to neuronal apoptosis [6–9]. It has been reported that disruption of calcium homeostasis, reduced mitochondrial membrane potential, ROS generation and DNA damage in the neuronal population are implicated in the pathogenesis of bupivacaine-induced neurotoxicity [3, 10, 11]. The exact mechanisms by which bupivacaine induces apoptosis have not been elucidated entirely. However, different studies have reported that several

* Correspondence: jzaringhalam@yahoo.com
[2]Department of Physiology, School of Medicine, Shahid Beheshti University of Medical Sciences, Tehran, Iran

signaling pathways such as the PERK [12, 13], IRE1 [3], glycogen synthase kinase-3 (GSK3) [14], MAPK [15, 16] and Akt [4, 12] might be responsible for bupivacaine- induced apoptosis.

Although the placenta is proposed as a protective barrier, there are mechanisms of drug transport across this tissue that expose the fetus to drugs taken by pregnant women [17–19]. It has been a general finding that the placenta does not limit the fetal transfer of local anesthetics [20–22]. By using a human placental model in rats, it is revealed that bupivacaine accumulates in the placenta and is retained in fetal tissues [22, 23]. Some animal studies have shown that bupivacaine has an adverse effect on the fetus so, according to the US FDA, bupivacaine is a pregnancy category C drug. While, based on the Australian categorization system for prescribing medicines in pregnancy, bupivacaine is a category A drug that is widely used in pregnant women and has no reported direct or indirect harmful effects on the fetus [2, 22]. Because of controversial reports, further research is required to determine the possible neurotoxic potency of maternal bupivacaine use on the fetus and newborn. Therefore, our main purpose in the present study was to investigate the effects of maternal bupivacaine use on fetus hippocampal apoptosis and the possible related mechanism.

Methods

Laboratory animals and experimental procedures

All procedures were approved by the ethics committee of Shahid Beheshti University of Medical Sciences (IR.SBMU.RETECH.REC.1398.031) which followed Guidelines of ethical standards for the care and use of laboratory animals for animal research [24]. The animals were obtained from Laboratory Animal Center, Shahid Beheshti University of Medical Sciences. They were housed in polypropylene cages under standard environmental conditions (22 ± 2 °C, humidity 60–70%, and 12 h light/dark cycle) and allowed standard water and food intake. Adult female Wistar rat weighting 180–200 g was used for mating. Pregnant rats on day 15 of pregnancy randomly divided into three groups as follows (a) Control group (sciatic nerve was exposed but no drug was administered), (b) Sham+ vehicle group (sciatic nerve was exposed and saline was injected) and (c) Bupivacaine group (sciatic nerve was exposed and blocked with bupivacaine administration) ($n = 6$ / each group).

Surgery and drug administration

On day 15 of pregnancy, the pregnant rats became anesthetized with intraperitoneal injection of Ketamine 100 mg/kg and Xylazine 10 mg/kg mixture. Then, the sciatic nerve of the rat's right thigh was isolated and based on previous studies [25, 26], 0.2 ml of Bupivacaine 0.5% (Astra Zeneca, Austria), in Bupivacaine group, and 0.2 ml of Normal Saline 0.9%, in the Sham+vehicle group, was injected beneath the clear fascia surrounding the sciatic nerve but outside the perineurium. After performing nerve block, we sutured the muscles and skin by Vicryl 6–0 and Nylon 4–0 sutures. After recovery, all rats were returned to their places and were cared at the time of their delivery. Then, we randomly selected one male offspring of every mother and kept under standard condition until the 30th day after of their birth. All offspring in control, sham and bupivacaine group have no significant difference in birth weight and weight gain during the study. In day 30, the rats ($n =$ 6 per each group) were anaesthetized by CO_2 inhalation then decapitated. The hippocampi were immediately isolated on the ice and kept in liquid nitrogen for 24 h and then stored in − 80 °C until molecular analysis. All animals used in the present study, finally were anaesthetized by CO2 inhalation then scarified by decapitation.

Western blotting

The hippocampi were homogenized in the cold RIPA lysis buffer (50 mM Tris-HCl, pH 8.0; 150 mM NaCl; 1% Triton X-100; 0.5% Na-Deoxycholate; 0.1% SDS (sodium dodecyl sulfate)) supplemented with protease and phosphatase inhibitors cocktail (was purchased from Pierce). Bradford method was used to quantify the protein content of each sample. Then, the equal amounts of proteins (40 μg) were separated using 12% polyacrylamide gel electrophoresis, transferred to a activated PVDF membrane (Roche Diagnostics, Indianapolis, IN, USA), blocked with blocking buffer (5% BSA) 1 h in room temperature and incubated at 4 °C overnight with primary anti-rabbit antibodies against phospho-Akt (Ser473) (1:3000, cell signaling #4060), Akt (1:3000, cell signaling #4685), caspase-3 (1;3000, ab184787), caspase-8 (1;3000, cell signaling #4790) and β-actin (1:15000, cell signaling #4970). After washing with TBST, the membranes incubated for 1:30 h with secondary HRP-conjugated anti-rabbit antibody (1:20000, cell signaling #7074) at room temperature, visualized by Amersham ECL select Western Blotting Detection Kit (RPN2235), and exposed to radiography films (Kodak). All membranes were stripped and incubated with primary antibody against β-actin. Finally, the radiographic films were scanned and blot quantification of protein bands density was calculated by Image-J software.

Statistical analysis

Statistical analyses of data and drawing charts were performed using the GraphPad Prism 7.01. For comparison of variables between the groups, one-way analysis of variance (ANOVA) followed by Post hoc Tukey's test was used. All data have been shown as means ± S.E.M. In all statistical comparisons, $P < 0.05$ is considered as a significant difference.

Results

Maternal bupivacaine administration increases the level of fetal hippocampal cleaved caspase-3

Activation of caspase-dependent apoptosis was assessed through western blot analysis of cleaved caspase-3. Caspase-3 play a main role in apoptosis and its cleavage represents its activation [27]. There was no significant difference in caspase-3 activity between the control and sham group while, maternal bupivacaine use caused a significant increase in cleaved caspase-3 expression in the fetal hippocampus compared with the sham group ($P < 0.001$) (Fig. 1).

Overexpression of fetal hippocampal caspase-8 after maternal bupivacaine use

To test the role of maternal bupivacaine use on fetal hippocampal cell apoptosis, caspase-8 expression was also assessed by western blotting. The data showed that there was no significant difference in caspase-8 expression between the control and sham groups. One- way ANOVA followed by Tukey's test showed that maternal bupivacaine use could increase hippocampal caspase-8 expression in the bupivacaine group compared with the sham group ($P < 0.001$) (Fig. 2).

Phosphorylation of Akt decreases after maternal bupivacaine use

PI3K/Akt pathway plays a regulatory role in different biological processes such as proliferation and cell survival [28–30]. Western blot was done to investigate the effect of maternal bupivacaine use on fetal hippocampal P.Akt/T.Akt ratios. Our results revealed that maternal bupivacaine use significantly decreased hippocampal P.Akt/T.Akt ration in the bupivacaine group compared with sham group ($P < 0.001$) (Fig. 3).

Discussion

Pregnancy is a unique experience in the lifetime of women. The mother's health is directly connected to the fetus's health. Therefore, it is essential to maintain the health of pregnant women. Since, local anesthetics are commonly used for surgical procedures in the pregnant women [31–33], it is necessary to understand the effects of maternally administered local anesthetics on the fetus. For this purpose, this study aimed to elucidate the adverse effects of maternal bupivacaine use on fetus hippocampal cell apoptosis and the possible related mechanism. To assess the activation of caspase-dependent apoptosis pathways in fetal hippocampal following maternally administered bupivacaine, we measured activation of caspase-3 and caspase-8. It is revealed that

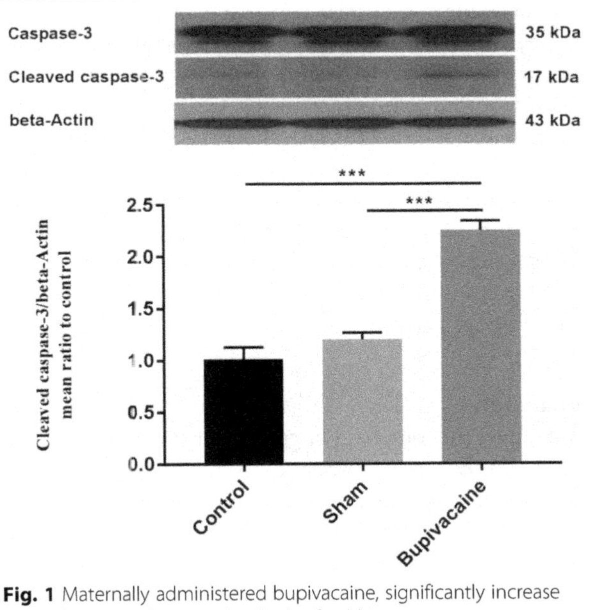

Fig. 1 Maternally administered bupivacaine, significantly increase cleaved caspase-3 expression in the fetal hippocampus. Representative cropped western blot of cleaved caspase-3 (19 kDa) which is normalized to beta-Actin. Data are represented as mean ± SEM ($n = 6$ rats/group). ***$P < 0.001$: comparison of cleaved caspase-3 protein band intensity between different groups. Full-length blots are presented in Supplementary Fig. 1

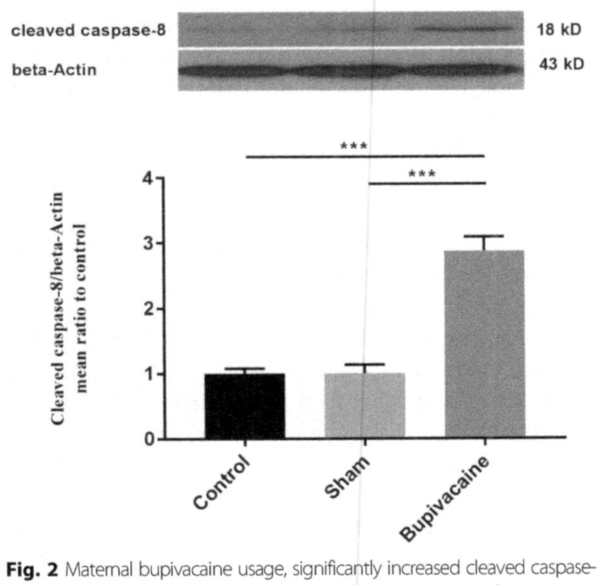

Fig. 2 Maternal bupivacaine usage, significantly increased cleaved caspase-8 expression in the fetal hippocampus. Representative cropped western blot of cleaved caspase-8 (18 kDa) which is normalized to beta-Actin. Data are represented as mean ± SEM ($n = 6$ rats/group). ***$P < 0.001$: comparison of cleaved caspase-8 protein band intensity between different groups. Full-length blots are presented in Supplementary Fig. 2

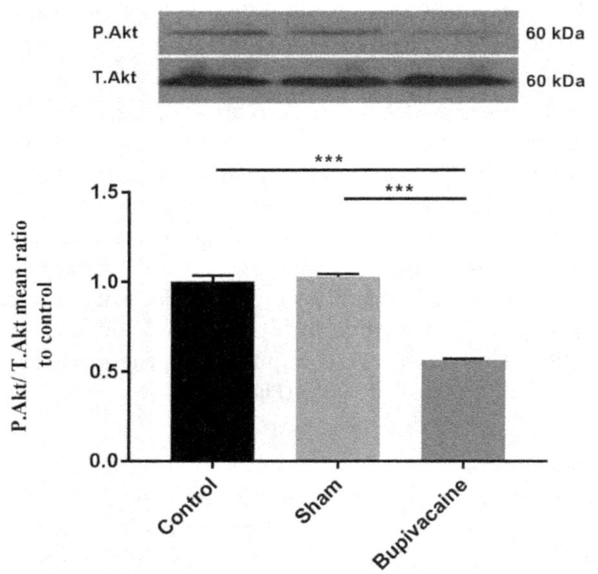

Fig. 3 Maternal administration of bupivacaine significantly decreased Akt activity in fetal hippocampus. Representative cropped western blot of P. Akt (60 kDa) which is normalized to T.Akt. Data are represented as mean ± SEM ($n = 6$ rats/group). ***$P < 0.001$: comparison of P. Akt protein band intensity between different groups. Full-length blots are presented in Supplementary Fig. 3

caspase-3 play a key role in apoptosis and its cleavage represents its activation [27, 34]. Caspase-3 is activated during both extrinsic and intrinsic apoptosis pathways [27, 35]. Also, caspase-8 is the initiator caspase that play a critical role in the extrinsic apoptotic signaling pathway. Our result revealed that maternal bupivacaine use could increase apoptosis-related proteins, cleaved caspase-3 and caspase- 8 expressions in the hippocampal of the fetus compared with the sham group.

A growing body of researches in the last years, both laboratory and clinical settings, reported that, although happened in rare-event situations, local anesthetic reagents, like bupivacaine, ropivacaine, lidocaine and mepivacaine, might induce severe neurological injury in both animal and humans [14, 36–38]. In this regard, Yu et al. (2017) shown that in neuronal population, bupivacaine could significantly increase apoptosis and induce much severe neurotoxicity than other local anesthetics, such as mepivacaine or procaine [10]. In addition, another study showed that bupivacaine could induce neural apoptosis and neurite degeneration in DRG neurons [11]. Available evidences shows that local anesthetics have systemic absorption, and placenta does not limit the fetal transfer of maternally administered amide-linked local anesthetics, such as bupivacaine [19, 20, 39]. It is revealed that bupivacaine crosses the placenta, accumulates in this tissue and is retained in fetal tissues [18, 21, 22]. Bupivacaine enters in the fetal liver through umbilical venous blood perfused in this organ. The 3-hydroxybupivacaine can remain detectable in the fetus liver up to 4 h. This suggesting that bupivacaine can metabolize in the fetal liver [22]. The fetus eliminates the bupivacaine by diffusing it into the maternal compartment through the placental membrane. Although the majority of the bupivacaine metabolites are more polar, and it is unlikely that the placental membrane crosses these metabolites back into the maternal compartment, possibly resulting in the accumulation of metabolites in various fetal tissues. The half of the fetal circulation directly reaches the heart and brain, thus it is possible that reduced fetal ability to remove drugs can cause prolonged adverse effects on these tissues [40, 41]. Although there are no adequate and well-controlled studies about the adverse effect of maternal bupivacaine on the fetus, our results for the first time suggest that, maternally administered bupivacaine, could have an adverse effect on fetal brain and induce hippocampal cell apoptosis.

The exact mechanism by which bupivacaine induces apoptosis have not been elucidated entirely. However different studies have reported that several signaling pathways, such as PERK [12, 13], IRE1 [3], GSK3 [14], MAPK [15, 16] and Akt [4, 12], might be responsible for bupivacaine- induced apoptosis. In exploring the signaling mechanism; we focused on Akt, which is a well-known anti-apoptosis molecule. Our results showed that maternal bupivacaine use markedly decreases the phosphorylation levels of Akt. A number of studies have demonstrated that Akt, a key kinase downstream of the PI3-kinase, plays a crucial role in cell survival and death pathway of neurons [12, 29, 42, 43]. Recent studies have confirmed that Akt-signaling pathway involves in the bupivacaine-induced apoptosis in adults [44, 45]. In this regard, Fan et al. (2016) reported that bupivacaine-induced neurotoxicity in SH-SY5Y cells is mediated thorough inactivating Akt signaling pathway [1]. In consistent with previous studies, we observed that bupivacaine decreased the phosphorylation levels of Akt in the fetal hippocampus, which was concurrent with an increment of apoptotic markers.

Conclusions

Taken together, our data suggest that maternally administered bupivacaine increases fetal hippocampal cell apoptosis markers such as caspase 8 and cleaved caspase 3, at least in concurrent with inhibition of the Akt activation.

Abbreviations

Akt: Protein kinase B; P.Akt: Phosphorylated Akt; PI3K: Phosphatidylinositol 3-kinases; T.Akt: Total Akt

Acknowledgements

Not applicable.

Authors' contributions

AM and JZ designed the study and made the conception of the work, AS made data acquisition and wrote the manuscript. MB performed western blot technique and made data analysis. EL provided statistical advice. EM made data interpretation. MM substantively revised the work. All authors read and approved the final manuscript.

Author details

[1]Department of Anesthesiology, Shahid Beheshti University of Medical Sciences, Tehran 1985717443, Iran. [2]Department of Physiology, School of Medicine, Shahid Beheshti University of Medical Sciences, Tehran, Iran. [3]Department of Gynecology, Tehran Azad University, Tehran, Iran. [4]Department of Gastroenterology, Shahid Beheshti University of Medical Sciences, Tehran, Iran.

References

1. Fan Y-L, Li H-C, Zhao W, Peng H-H, Huang F, Jiang W-H, Xu S-Y. Curcumin attenuated bupivacaine-induced neurotoxicity in SH-SY5Y cells via activation of the Akt signaling pathway. Neurochem Res. 2016;41(9):2425–32.
2. Rudolph AM. Pharmacodynamics in the maternal-fetal-placental unit. NIDA Res Monogr. 1995;154:163–74.
3. Liu Y, Sun L, Ma Y, Wei B, Gao M, Shang L. High glucose and bupivacaine-induced cytotoxicity is mediated by enhanced apoptosis and impaired autophagy via the PERK-ATF4-CHOP and IRE1-TRAF2 signaling pathways. Mol Med Rep. 2019;20(3):2832–42.
4. Zhang H, Wang W, Du Q. Andrographolide attenuates bupivacaine-induced cytotoxicity in SH-SY5Y cells through preserving Akt/mTOR activity. Drug Des Devel Ther. 2019;13:1659.
5. Zheng Q, Peng X, Zhang Y. Cytotoxicity of amide-linked local anesthetics on melanoma cells via inhibition of Ras and RhoA signaling independent of sodium channel blockade. BMC Anesthesiol. 2020;20(1):1–9.
6. Li L, Zhang Q-g, Lai L-y, Wen X-j, Zheng T, Cheung C-w, Zhou S-q, Xu S-y. Neuroprotective effect of ginkgolide B on bupivacaine-induced apoptosis in SH-SY5Y cells. Oxidative Med Cell Longev. 2013;2013.
7. Lu J, Xu SY, Zhang QG, Lei HY. Bupivacaine induces reactive oxygen species production via activation of the AMP-activated protein kinase-dependent pathway. Pharmacology. 2011;87(3–4):121–9.
8. Zhang H, Wang K. Downregulation of MicroRNA-33-5p protected bupivacaine-induced apoptosis in murine dorsal root ganglion neurons through GDNF. Neurotox Res. 2019;35(4):860–6.
9. Wang S, Xia B, Qiao Z, Duan L, Wang G, Meng W, Liu Z, Wang Y, Zhang M. Tetramethylpyrazine attenuated bupivacaine-induced neurotoxicity in SH-SY5Y cells through regulating apoptosis, autophagy and oxidative damage. Drug Des Devel Ther. 2019;13:1187.
10. Yu X-j, Zhao W, Li Y-j, Li F-x, Liu Z-j, Xu H-l, Lai L-y, Xu R, Xu S-y. Neurotoxicity comparison of two types of local anaesthetics: amide-bupivacaine versus ester-procaine. Sci Rep. 2017;7:45316.
11. Radwan IA, Saito S, Goto F. The neurotoxicity of local anesthetics on growing neurons: a comparative study of lidocaine, bupivacaine, mepivacaine, and ropivacaine. Anesth Analg. 2002;94(2):319–24.
12. Maurice JM, Gan Y, Chang Y-c, Hibner M, Huang Y. Bupivacaine causes cytotoxicity in mouse C2C12 myoblast cells: involvement of ERK and Akt signaling pathways. Acta Pharmacol Sin. 2010;31(4):493.
13. Antonio AM, Druse MJ. Antioxidants prevent ethanol-associated apoptosis in fetal rhombencephalic neurons. Brain Res. 2008;1204:16–23.
14. Yu T, Lin W. Small-molecule GSK-3 inhibitor rescued apoptosis and neurodegeneration in anesthetics-injured dorsal root ganglion neurons. Biomed Pharmacother. 2016;84:395–402.
15. Tan Z, Dohi S, Chen J, Banno Y, Nozawa Y. Involvement of the mitogen-activated protein kinase family in tetracaine-induced PC12 cell death. Anesthesiology. 2002;96(5):1191–201.
16. Lirk P, Haller I, Peter H, Lang L, Tomaselli B, Klimaschewski L, Gerner P. In vitro, inhibition of mitogen-activated protein kinase pathways protects against bupivacaine-and ropivacaine-induced neurotoxicity. Anesth Analg. 2008;106(5):1456–64.
17. Al-Enazy S, Ali S, Albekairi N, El-Tawil M, Rytting E. Placental control of drug delivery. Adv Drug Deliv Rev. 2017;116:63–72.
18. Morishima HO, Heymann MA, Rudolph AM, Barrett CT, James LS. Transfer of lidocaine across the sheep placenta to the fetus: hemodynamic and acid-base responses of the fetal lamb. Am J Obstet Gynecol. 1975;122(5):581–8.
19. Santos AC, Arthur GR, Lehning EJ, Finster M. Comparative pharmacokinetics of ropivacaine and bupivacaine in nonpregnant and pregnant ewes. Anesth Analg. 1997;85(1):87–93.
20. Kennedy R, Miller R, Bell J, Doshi D, deSousa H, Kennedy M, Heald D, David Y. Uptake and distribution of bupivacaine in fetal lambs. Anesthesiology. 1986;65(3):247–53.
21. Gordon HR. Fetal bradycardia after paracervical block: correlation with fetal and maternal blood levels of local anesthetic (mepivacaine). N Engl J Med. 1968;279(17):910–4.
22. Morishima HO, Ishizaki A, Zhang Y, Whittington RA, Suckow RF, Cooper TB. Disposition of bupivacaine and its metabolites in the maternal, placental, and fetal compartments in rats. Anesthesiology. 2000;93(4):1069–74.
23. Eslamian L, KABIRI NM, AGHA HM, Azimaraghi O, Barzin G, Movafegh A. Adding sufentanil to TAP block hyperbaric bupivacaine decreases post-cesarean delivery morphine consumption; 2016.
24. Council NR. Guide for the care and use of laboratory animals: eighth edition. Washington, DC: The National Academies Press; 2011.
25. Kau Y-C, Hung Y-C, Zizza AM, Zurakowski D, Greco WR, Wang GK, Gerner P. Efficacy of lidocaine or bupivacaine combined with ephedrine in rat sciatic nerve block. Reg Anesth Pain Med. 2006;31(1):14–8 14-18.
26. Memari E, Hosseinian M-A, Mirkheshti A, Arhami-Dolatabadi A, Mirabotalebi M, Khandaghy M, Daneshbod Y, Alizadeh L, Shirian S. Comparison of histopathological effects of perineural administration of bupivacaine and bupivacaine-dexmedetomidine in rat sciatic nerve. Exp Toxicol Pathol. 2016; 68(10):559–64.
27. Ni J, Hou X, Wang X, Shi Y, Xu L, Zheng X, Liu N, Qiu A, Zhuang S. 3-deazaneplanocin a protects against cisplatin-induced renal tubular cell apoptosis and acute kidney injury by restoration of E-cadherin expression. Cell Death Dis. 2019;10(5):355.
28. Knight Z, Shokat K. Chemically targeting the PI3K family. In: Portland Press Limited; 2007.
29. Chung H, Seo S, Moon M, Park S. Phosphatidylinositol-3-kinase/Akt/glycogen synthase kinase-3b and ERK1/2 pathways mediate protective effects of acylated and unacylated ghrelin against oxygen-glucose deprivation-induced apoptosis in primary rat cortical neuronal cells. J Endocrinol. 2008;198(3):511–22.
30. Ma R, Wang X, Lu C, Li C, Cheng Y, Ding G, Liu L, Ding Z. Dexamethasone attenuated bupivacaine-induced neuron injury in vitro through a threonine–serine protein kinase B-dependent mechanism. Neuroscience. 2010;167(2):329–42.
31. Gündüz Ş, Yalçın SE, Karakoç G, Akkurt MÖ, Yalçın Y. Comparison of bupivacaine and ropivacaine in combination with fentanyl used for walking epidural anesthesia in labor. Turkish J Obstet Gynecol. 2017;14(3):170.
32. B-s L, Wang W, Wang Z-q, Wang X-w, Wang J-h, Fang F, Mi W-d. Efficacy and safety of local anesthetics bupivacaine, ropivacaine and levobupivacaine in combination with sufentanil in epidural anesthesia for labor and delivery: a meta-analysis. Curr Med Res Opin. 2014;30(11):2279–89.
33. Lee JM, Shin TJ. Use of local anesthetics for dental treatment during pregnancy; safety for parturient. J Dent Anesth Pain Med. 2017;17(2):81–90.
34. Elmore S. Apoptosis: a review of programmed cell death. Toxicol Pathol. 2007;35(4):495–516.
35. Baniasadi M, Manaheji H, Maghsoudi N, Danyali S, Zakeri Z, Maghsoudi A, Zaringhalam J. Microglial-induced apoptosis is potentially responsible for hyperalgesia variations during CFA-induced inflammation. Inflammopharmacology. 2019:1–11.
36. Brull R, McCartney CJ, Chan VW, El-Beheiry H. Neurological complications after regional anesthesia: contemporary estimates of risk. Anesth Analg. 2007;104(4):965–74.
37. Graham MR. Clinical update regarding general anesthesia-associated neurotoxicity in infants and children. Curr Opin Anaesthesiol. 2017;30(6): 682–7.
38. Vutskits L, Davidson A. Update on developmental anesthesia neurotoxicity. Curr Opin Anesthesiol. 2017;30(3):337–42.
39. Santos AC, Pedersen H, Sallusto JA, Johnson HV, Morishima HO, Finster M, Arthur GR, Covino BG. Pharmacokinetics of ropivacaine in nonpregnant and pregnant ewes. Anesth Analg. 1990;70(3):262–6.
40. Pacifici GM, Nottoli R. Placental transfer of drugs administered to the mother. Clin Pharmacokinet. 1995;28(3):235–69.
41. Guillén-Dolores Y. Bupivacaine pharmacokinetics in pregnant women. In: Local Anesthetics edn: IntechOpen; 2019.
42. Manning BD, Cantley LC. AKT/PKB signaling: navigating downstream. Cell.

2007;129(7):1261–74.

43. Nair VD, Olanow CW. Differential modulation of Akt/glycogen synthase kinase-3β pathway regulates apoptotic and cytoprotective signaling responses. J Biol Chem. 2008;283(22):15469–78.
44. Zhao W, Liu Z, Yu X, Lai L, Li H, Liu Z, Li L, Jiang S, Xia Z, Sy X. iTRAQ proteomics analysis reveals that PI3K is highly associated with bupivacaine-induced neurotoxicity pathways. Proteomics. 2016;16(4):564–75.
45. Wang Z, Shen J, Wang J, Lu T, Li C, Zhang X, Liu L, Ding Z. Lithium attenuates bupivacaine-induced neurotoxicity in vitro through phosphatidylinositol-3-kinase/threonine-serine protein kinase B-and extracellular signal-regulated kinase-dependent mechanisms. Neuroscience. 2012;206:190–200.

10

Variation of bispectral index in children aged 1–12 years under propofol anesthesia

Fang Wang[1], Jianmin Zhang[1], Jie Yu[1], Muyang Tian[1], Xiaohuan Cui[1] and Anshi Wu[2*]

Abstract

Background: The use of the bispectral index (BIS) is widespread in pediatric anesthesia, but few studies have attempted to perform a detailed evaluation of how BIS varies according to age in children under propofol anesthesia. This prospective study aimed to explore the exact relationship between BIS value and the age of 1- to 12-year-old children under propofol anesthesia.

Methods: This study enrolled 165 children (1 < yr. ≤ 12), scheduled for surgery under anesthesia, and divided them into 11 age groups. Of the 165 participants, 157 completed the study protocol. All patients were anesthetized with propofol for over 30 s. An observation period of 4 min followed. BIS values were recorded at 0 (immediately after propofol injection), 30, 40, 50, 60, 90, 120, 180, and 240 s after the injection. BIS values at each time point corresponding to the 11 age groups were compared using repeated measures ANOVA.

Results: BIS values significantly differed among the nine time points ($p < 0.01$) as well as among the different age groups ($p < 0.01$) after propofol administration. Post-hoc Bonferroni tests showed a difference in BIS values between groups 1–4 (1 < yr. ≤ 5) and groups 5–11(5 < yr. ≤ 12). BIS values were lower in the latter than in the former, from 50 to 240 s. The minimum BIS values in group 1 < yr. ≤ 5 and in group 5 < yr. ≤ 12 were recorded at 60 s as 49 ± 17 and 35 ± 14, respectively.

Conclusions: During propofol anesthesia, the BIS values were closely related to age, which can be divided into two groups: 1 < yr. ≤ 5 and 5 < yr. ≤ 12. BIS values of the older age group were lower than those of the younger age group at the same time points.

Keywords: Propofol, Anesthesia: intravenous, Bispectral index, Children

Background

Since the implementation of the bispectral index (BIS) as the only means of monitoring the depth of sedation by the American Food and Drug Administration, its application has become increasingly widespread in pediatric anesthesia. Although the reliability of BIS is similar among adults and children over the age of 1 year [1], whether BIS can accurately monitor the depth of sedation in children remains controversial. The BIS algorithm was initially derived from electroencephalography data obtained from adults under various anesthetic conditions [2]. However, the child's brain is different from that of an adult and is characterized by rapid development. Moreover, the Electroencephalogram (EEG) of children has different manifestations at different ages; thus, whether the BIS value can accurately reflect these changes across growth is directly related to its accuracy for monitoring sedation depth. Recent studies using various volatile and intravenous anesthetic agents have shown that BIS values are linked to the age of children [3–6]. However, most of these studies have involved children over the age of 3 years or traditional age groups; infants (1–12 months of age), toddlers (13–36 months), and

* Correspondence: wuanshi012@sina.com
[2]Department of Anesthesiology, Beijing Chaoyang Hospital, Capital Medical University, No. 8 Gongti South Road, Chaoyang District, Beijing 100020, China

children (37–144 months), and only indicated that a given BIS value was relevant for a specified age. Few studies have attempted to evaluate the details of BIS variation with age under propofol anesthesia in a pediatric population.

This prospective observational study explored the exact relationship between BIS values and children aged 1–12 years, grouped with one-year intervals, under propofol anesthesia to provide a reliable basis for clinical monitoring.

Methods

Ethical approval

This study (Chictr.org.cn identifier: chictr-roc-16,008, 630) was approved by the Ethical Committee of Beijing Children's Hospital, Capital Medical University, Beijing, China (Ethical Committee No 2016–67, Chairperson Prof Tianyou Wang) on 16 May 2016. Written informed consent for participation was obtained from the parents or guardians of all patients.

Study population

In total, 165 pediatric patients requiring elective surgery, including urological, orthopedic, thoracic, and general surgery, under general anesthesia via intubation or a laryngeal mask, were initially selected. The inclusion criteria were as follows: 1<yr. ≤ 12, an American Society of Anesthesiologists (ASA) score of I or II, the intraoperative use of total intravenous anesthesia, and the provision of written informed consent by a parent or guardian. The exclusion criteria were as follows: concomitant severe systemic disease; requirement of cranial surgery; long-term use of sedative, hypnotic, or antipsychotic drugs; history of epilepsy; concomitant mental development disorders; and concomitant cardiovascular disease. We divided the included patients into 11 age groups with 15 patients in each group: group 1 (1 < yr. ≤ 2), group 2 (2 < yr. ≤ 3), group 3 (3 < yr. ≤ 4), group 4 (4 < yr. ≤ 5), group 5 (5 < yr. ≤ 6), group 6 (6 < yr. ≤ 7), group 7 (7 < yr. ≤ 8), group 8 (8 < yr. ≤ 9), group 9 (9 < yr. ≤ 10), group 10 (10 < yr. ≤ 11), and group 11 (11 < yr. ≤ 12).

Anesthesia protocol

No children were pre-medicated. Children routinely fasted from food for ≥6 h and from drink for ≥4 h before surgery. Peripheral intravenous access was established for all patients in the hospital ward. In the operating room, a continuous monitor (S/5TM monitor; GE Healthcare, Germany) was used for noninvasive blood pressure (NIBP), pulse oxygen saturation (SpO_2), heart rate (HR), and electrocardiogram (ECG) monitoring. After oxygen inhalation via a facemask was initiated, general anesthesia was induced by the continuous intravenous injection of 3 mg/kg of propofol (1% propofol in a medium-chain/long-chain triglyceride emulsion; Fresenius Kabi Deutschland Gmbh, Germany) for over 30 s, followed by an observation period of 4 min. Routine oxygen inhalation via the facemask was continued during propofol administration, and the lower jaw was gently raised as needed to assist airway management and maintain a blood oxygen saturation of ≥97%. At the end of the observation period, 2 mg/kg of propofol (Fresenius Kabi Deutschland Gmbh, Germany), 2 μg/kg of fentanyl (Yichang Humanwell Pharmaceutical Co., Ltd., Hubei Province, China), and 0.5 mg/kg of rocuronium (Hameln Pharmaceuticals Gmbh, Germany) were administered for routine induction. The patient was intubated or received a laryngeal mask after a sufficient depth of anesthesia was achieved.

Data acquisition

BIS (Aspect Medical System, USA) was simultaneously monitored for all patients. The skin over the forehead was cleaned, and the BIS electrode was then placed according to the manufacturers instructions by the anesthesiologist. The BIS monitor requires a self-test before it begins to function. Propofol was injected after signal stabilization, which indicated the BIS value in the absence of anesthesia. The baseline values were recorded immediately after propofol injection was initiated (0 s). Subsequently, values were recorded at 30, 40, 50, 60, 90, 120, 180, and 240 s after the injection.

For all patients, the same anesthesiologist placed all electrodes and administered propofol. Moreover, data for all patients were recorded by the same individual.

Statistical analysis and data handling

The sample size of 15 cases per group in the present study was generally similar, but not identical, to that of previously published reports [7, 8].

BIS values were measured at nine time points in the 11 age groups. IBM SPSS 21.0 (SPSS Inc., Chicago, IL, USA) was used for data analysis. Normally distributed numerical data are expressed as means ± standard deviations (SDs;$\bar{x} \pm s$). Repeated measures ANOVA was used to analyze BIS values at multiple time points in groups. A post-hoc Bonferroni test was used to compare differences at same time points in different age groups and at different time points in same groups. A p-value of < 0.05 was considered statistically significant. Data analysis was independently performed by two data scientists.

Results

From the 165 initially recruited patients, eight were excluded because the electrodes fell off during the observation period; 157 patients were thus included in the analyses. The patient data are presented in Table 1.

Table 1 Patient characteristics of 11 groups

Groups	1	2	3	4	5	6	7	8	9	10	11	Total
Number of patients	15	15	15	15	13	15	15	15	13	12	14	157
Male/Female	13/2	14/1	13/2	10/5	7/6	10/5	12/3	13/2	6/7	9/3	9/5	116/41
Type of surgery												
Urology	11	10	6	7	9	5	5	1		3	5	62
Orthopaedics	1	3	9	6	3	7	10	9	9	9	7	73
Other	3	2		2	1	3		5	4		2	22

group 1 (1 < yr. ≤ 2), group 2 (2 < yr. ≤ 3), group 3 (3 < yr. ≤ 4), group 4 (4 < yr. ≤ 5), group 5 (5 < yr. ≤ 6), group 6 (6 < yr. ≤ 7), group 7 (7 < yr. ≤ 8), group 8 (8 < yr. ≤ 9), group 9 (9 < yr. ≤ 10), group 10 (10 < yr. ≤ 11), and group 11 (11 < yr. ≤ 12)

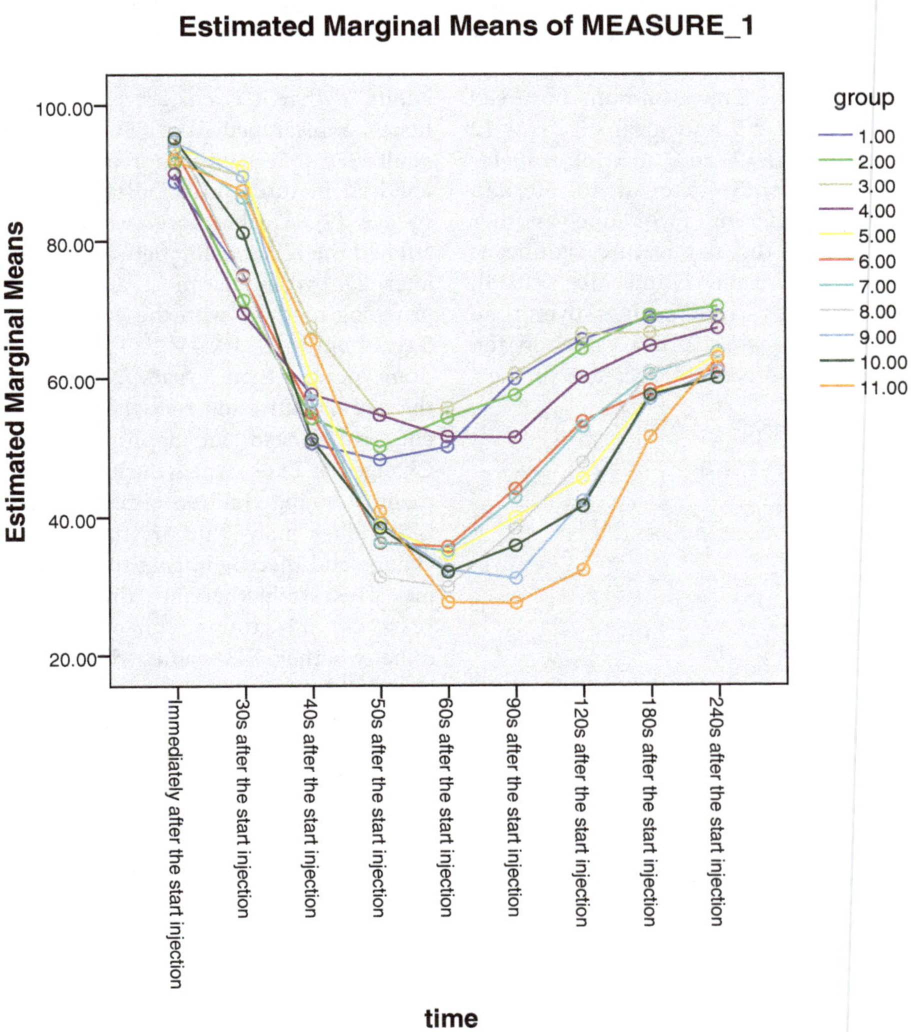

Fig. 1 Bispectral index (BIS) values according to the patient age and time point of measurement after propofol injection in children. Age groups:group 1 (1 < yr. ≤ 2), group 2 (2 < yr. ≤ 3), group 3 (3 < yr. ≤ 4), group 4 (4 < yr. ≤ 5), group 5 (5 < yr. ≤ 6), group 6 (6 < yr. ≤ 7), group 7 (7 < yr. ≤ 8), group 8 (8 < yr. ≤ 9), group 9 (9 < yr. ≤ 10), group 10 (10 < yr. ≤ 11), and group 11 (11 < yr. ≤ 12)

Repeated measures ANOVA showed that BIS values significantly differed among the nine time points ($P < 0.01$) as well as the different age groups ($P < 0.01$) after propofol administration. The post-hoc Bonferroni test showed a difference in BIS values between groups 1–4 (1 < yr. ≤ 5) and groups 5–11(5 < yr. ≤ 12) (Fig. 1).

The patients were reclassified for further analysis: group 1 < yr. ≤ 5, which included the 60 patients in groups 1–4, and group 5 < yr. ≤ 12, which included the 97 patients in groups 5–11. Table 2 presents the BIS values at each time point for group 1 < yr. ≤ 5 and group 5 < yr. ≤ 12. In both groups, the baseline BIS values (immediately after the start of injection; 0 s) differed significantly from the values at the subsequent eight time points, from 30 to 240 s ($p < 0.01$). The BIS values between the two groups were significantly different at each of the following time points: 50, 60, 90, 120, 180, and 240 s ($p < 0.05$). The BIS values in group 5 < yr. ≤ 12 were significantly lower than those in group 1 < yr. ≤ 5 at each time point from 50 to 250 s ($p < 0.05$). The minimum observed BIS values for group 1 < yr. ≤ 5 and group 5 < yr. ≤ 12 were recorded at 60 s: 49 ± 17 and 35 ± 14, respectively. In group 5 < yr. ≤ 12, BIS values at 40, 50, and 60 s were significantly different from one another ($p < 0.01$); group 1 < yr. ≤ 5 did not feature significant differences among these time points ($p > 0.05$). Figure 2 shows the changes in BIS values over time in groups 1 < yr. ≤ 5 and 5 < yr. ≤ 12. BIS values in the two patient groups exhibited a rapid decrease to their minimum values from 0 to 60 s, followed by an obvious trend towards an increase. Changes in BIS values were more obvious in group 5 < yr. ≤ 12 than in group 1 < yr. ≤ 5, with the former demonstrating a precipitous decrease between 40 and 60 s.

Table 2 BIS values at each time point in Group 1 < yr. ≤ 5 and Group 5 < yr. ≤ 12 ($\bar{x} \pm s$)

time/ s	BIS	
	Group 1 < yr. ≤ 5	Group 5 < yr. ≤ 12
0	91 ± 7	94 ± 5
30	75 ± 20*	82 ± 21*
40	57 ± 21*cd	58 ± 25*e
50	52 ± 18*ac	37 ± 16*af
60	49 ± 17*ac	35 ± 14*af
90	55 ± 13*acd	37 ± 11*af
120	63 ± 8*ad	46 ± 14*a
180	66 ± 5*ad	57 ± 8*ae
240	67 ± 5*ad	62 ± 5*ae

[a] $P < 0.05$, values of BIS were compared between the group 1 < yr. ≤ 5 and the group 1 < yr. ≤ 2 at the same time point
*$P < 0.01$, BIS values with superscript * compared with BIS values at 0 s time point
[c] $P < 0.05$, BIS values with superscript c compared with BIS values at the other time point of group 1 < yr. ≤ 5
[d] $P < 0.05$, BIS values with superscript d compared with BIS values at the other time point of group 1 < yr. ≤ 5
[e] $P < 0.05$, BIS values with superscript e compared with BIS values at the other time point of group 5 < yr. ≤ 12
[f] $P < 0.05$, BIS values with superscript d compared with BIS values at the other time point of group 5 < yr. ≤ 12

Time points

0: immediately after the start of injection.

30, 40, 50, 60, 90, 120, 180, and 240 s after the start of propofol injection.

Discussion

In this study, BIS value changes were studied in children aged 1–12 years, who were grouped according to age, under propofol anesthesia. We found that BIS values showed a similar trend at each time point after propofol injection in the 11 groups, but BIS values differed according to age groups. Our findings differed from those reported previously.

The pediatric nervous system differs from that of adults in that it is characterized by rapid development; hence, typical pediatric EEGs are more variable than adult EEGs. It has been reported that EEG signals of children mature and stabilize at approximately 12 years of age [9]. Furthermore, while previous reports have studied the relationship between BIS values and propofol after age grouping, most adopted the traditional age grouping method, with the youngest patients being over 3 years old [4, 8, 10, 11]. While relevant studies on children younger than 3 years of age have been conducted, the age classification that they employed was inconsistent and lacked an appropriate justification [1, 7]. Changes in EEG signals during the growth and development of young children occur in a short period of time; BIS values may thus feature a similarly significant change and thereby impact the accuracy of BIS monitoring. This study therefore divided children aged 1–12 years into 11 groups with one-year intervals to determine whether BIS values differed among the groups stratified by age.

As the utility of BIS for monitoring the sedative depth of propofol anesthesia in children has been established, propofol is widely used for both sedation and general anesthesia in children [12]. However, BIS monitoring is easily disrupted by the administration of other drugs, especially muscle relaxants. Because BIS features frontal electromyography (EMG) as a weighted parameter, the frontal EMG overlaps with the EEG at a frequency of 30–50 Hz, and the interference of frontal EMG can thus be excluded at frequencies lower than 47 Hz. However, after the application of muscle relaxants, BIS may decrease due to the drop in the components of the frontal EMG, and the monitoring of sedation depth may be disrupted. The BIS value can reportedly reduce to 33 when muscle relaxants are administered

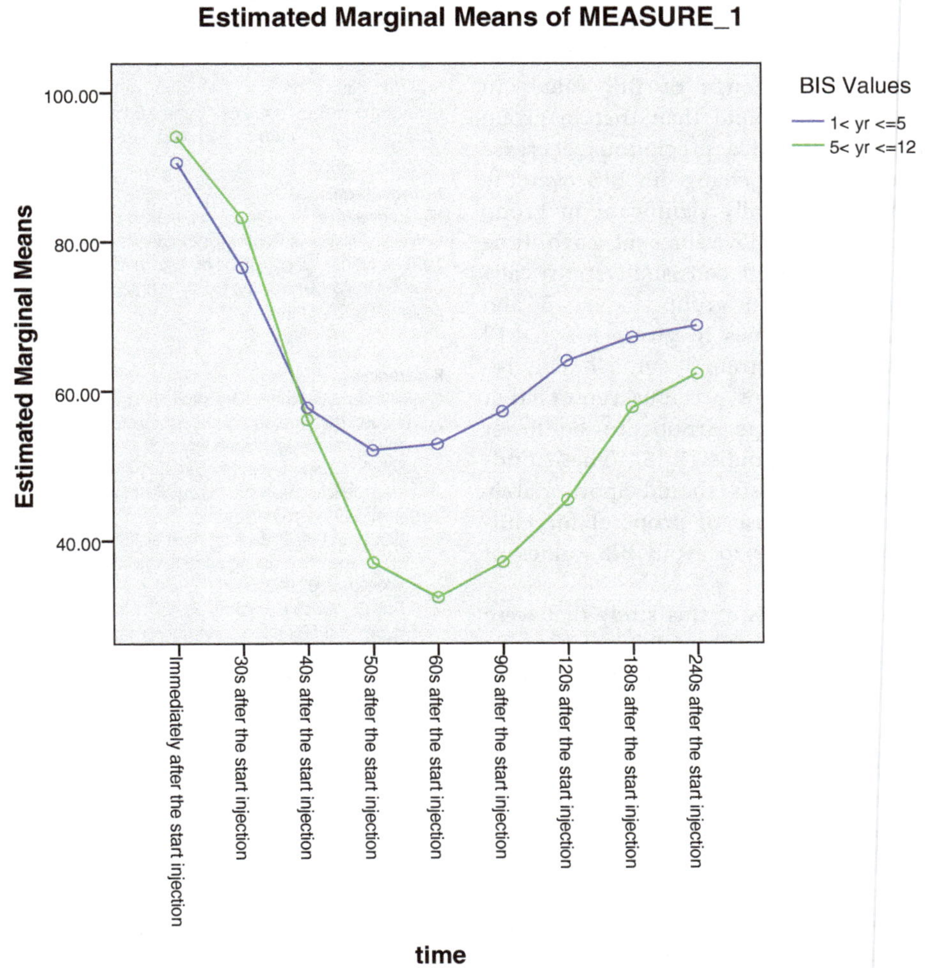

Fig. 2 Changes in bispectral index (BIS) values over time in group 1 < yr. ≤ 5 and group 5 < yr. ≤ 12. Group 1 < yr. ≤ 5: the 60 paediatric patients in groups 1–4 (group 1: 1 < yr. ≤ 2; group 2: 2 < yr. ≤ 3; group 3: 3 < yr. ≤ 4; group 4: 4 < yr. ≤ 5), who were combined because of the lack of significant differences in BIS values. Group 5<yr. ≤ 12: the 97 paediatric patients in groups 5–11 (group 5: 5 < yr. ≤ 6; group 6: 6 < yr. ≤ 7; group 7: 7 < yr. ≤ 8; group 8: 8 < yr. ≤ 9; group 9: 9 < yr. ≤ 10; group 10: 10 < yr. ≤ 11; group 11: 11 < yr. ≤ 12), who were combined because of the lack of significant differences in BIS values

to patients who are fully awake [13]. Whether opioids have an impact on the BIS value remains controversial: although many studies have reported that opioids do not affect BIS values [14, 15], Minto and colleagues [16] have described age-dependent EEG modification when remifentanil was administered to adults and found that changes in BIS values with an attendant loss of verbal command or eyelash reflex were more common in patients who received remifentanil combined with propofol than propofol alone [17, 18]. Therefore, this study administered a single propofol to eliminate the effect of the combined drugs on BIS value and improve the accuracy of the research results.

Previous literature has shown that BIS values for children under propofol anesthesia are significantly associated with age [1]; however, prior studies have only shown that BIS accuracy is better in children over the age of 1 year. In this study, the results of detailed age grouping indicated that BIS values in the 11 groups showed a similar trend in BIS: an initial decrease followed by an increase. However, the changes of BIS values at the same time points differed significantly across age. Moreover, we identified that such significant differences could be identified between two composite groups: 1–4 and 5–11. The results suggest that age persists as an important factor, affecting BIS in children over 1 year of age, and anesthesiologists must pay attention to this difference when monitoring sedation depth.

The minimum BIS values of 49 ± 17 and 35 ± 14 in group 1 < yr. ≤ 5 and group 5 < yr. ≤ 12, respectively, were observed at 60 s. Generally consistent with reports of the peak effect time being at 1.6 min (1–2.4 min) after the single-bolus intravenous injection of propofol [19]. From this finding we presume that BIS is sensitive to changes in blood propofol concentration and similar result had been reported in the previous literature [20]. The change of BIS values in group 5 < yr. ≤ 12 was more rapid than that in group 1 < yr. ≤ 5; the former featured a precipitous decrease between 40 and 60 s, and the change in BIS over the same period was not statistically significant in group 1 < yr. ≤ 5. In addition, the BIS values at each time point from 50 to 240 s showed consistent statistically significant differences between group 1 < yr. ≤ 5 and group 5 < yr. ≤ 12; the BIS values in group 5 < yr. ≤ 12 were all lower than those in group 1 < yr. ≤ 5. This result is consistent with those of previous reports that found BIS values in older age groups to be lower than those in younger age groups [7, 8]. These findings imply that anesthesiologists should appropriately reduce the single injection dose of propofol for children over 5 years old in order to avoid BIS values of less than 40.

There were several limitations of this study that were important to note. First, this study did not provide hemodynamics data at each time point. The current study was designed to observe the change of BIS value after single dose of propofol injection and the 10-s interval between each observation time point was narrow, it may be difficult to measure non-invasive blood pressure at each time points and we also considered that even if we did measure it, Moreover, cuff blood pressure measurement may be considered as one of stimulations during the observation period which may interfere with the sedative state of the child. But heart rate and pulse oxygen saturation were continuously monitored during the whole procedure. Secondly, the current study did not provide information of clinical parameters at each time points, the correlation between BIS value and clinical consciousness was therefore not evaluated in this study. This was the initial observational study for BIS value and propofol injection in different age groups and the correlation BIS values and clinical signs of sedative should be assessed in our future studies.

Conclusions

Our study indicates that BIS values showed a close relationship to two age groups: 1 < yr. ≤ 5 and 5 < yr. ≤ 12 during the administration of propofol anesthesia. BIS values of the older age group were lower than those of the younger age group at the same time points. This study suggests that attention should be paid to changes in children younger and older than 5 years when BIS monitoring is applied to children aged 1–12 years.

Abbreviations

BIS: Bispectral index; EEG: Electroencephalogram

Authors' contributions

All authors have read and approved the final version of this manuscript. AW contributed to the overall study design, data analysis, and revised the paper. FW helped design the study, performed the experiments, collected and analyzed data, and wrote the manuscript. JZ helped design the study and revised the manuscript. JY, MT and XC had performed the experiments, collected data. All authors had read and approved the final manuscript.

Author details

[1]Department of Anesthesiology, Beijing Children's Hospital, Capital Medical University, National Center for Children's Health, No. 56 Nanlishi Road, Beijing 100045, China. [2]Department of Anesthesiology, Beijing Chaoyang Hospital, Capital Medical University, No. 8 Gongti South Road, Chaoyang District, Beijing 100020, China.

References

1. Jeleazcov C, Schmidt J, Schmitz B, et al. EEG variables as measures of arousal during propofol anaesthesia for general surgery in children: rational selection and age dependence. Br J Anaesth. 2007;99:845–54.
2. Sebel PS, Lang E, Rampil IJ, et al. A multicenter study of bispectral electroencephalogram analysis for monitoring anesthetic effect. Anesth Analg. 1997;84:891–9.
3. Wodey E, Tirel O, Bansard JY, et al. Impact of age on both BIS values and EEG bispectrum during anaesthesia with sevoflurane in children. Br J Anaesth. 2005;94:810–20.
4. Tirel O, Wodey E, Harris R, et al. The impact of age on bispectral index values and EEG bispectrum during anaesthesia with desflurane and halothane in children. Br J Anaesth. 2006;96:480–5.
5. Wallenborn J, Kluba K, Olthoff D. Comparative evaluation of bispectral index and Narcotrend index in children below 5 years of age. Paediatr Anaesth. 2007;17:140–7.
6. Tirel O, Wodey E, Harris R, et al. Variation of bispectral index under TIVA with propofol in a paediatric population. Br J Anaesth. 2008;100:82–7.
7. Zhang JM, Wang F, Xin Z, et al. Treatment of different-aged children under bispectral index monitoring with intravenous anesthesia with propofol and remifentanil. Eur Rev Med Pharmacol Sci. 2015;19:64–9.
8. Liu JS, Zhang JM, Yun Y. Variation of bispectral index monitoring in pediatric patients undergoing propofol-remifentanil anesthesia. Eur J Anaesthesiol. 2008;25:821–5.
9. Eisermann M, Kaminska A, Moutard ML, et al. Normal EEG in childhood: from neonates to adolescents. Neurophysiol Clin. 2013;43:35–65.
10. Louvet N, Rigouzzo A, Sabourdin N, et al. Bispectral index under propofol anesthesia in children: a comparative randomized study between TIVA and TCI. Paediatr Anaesth. 2016 Sep;26(9):899–908.
11. Fuentes R, Cortínez I, Ibacache M, et al. Propofol concentration to induce general anesthesia in children aged 3-11 years with the Kataria effect-site model. Paediatr Anaesth. 2015 Jun;25(6):554–9.
12. Powers KS, Nazarian EB, Tapyrik SA, et al. Bispectral index as a guide for titration of propofol during procedural sedation among children. Pediatrics. 2005 Jun;115(6):1666–74.
13. Messner M, Beese U, Romstock J, et al. The bispectral index declines during neuromuscular block in fully awake persons. Anesth Analg. 2003;97:488–91.
14. Schmidt GN, Bischoff P, Standl T, et al. Narcotrend, bispectral index, and classical electroencephalogram variables during emergence from propofol/remifentanil anesthesia. Anesth Analg. 2002;95:1324–30.
15. Wang LP, McLoughlin P, Paech MJ, et al. Low and moderate remifentanil infusion rates do not alter targetcontrolled infusion propofol concentrations necessary to maintain anesthesia as assessed by bispectral index monitoring. Anesth Analg. 2007;104:325–31.
16. Minto CF, Schnider TW, Egan TD, et al. Influence of age and gender on the pharmacokinetics and pharmacodynamics of remifentanil. I. Model development. Anesthesiol. 1997;86:10–23.
17. Struys MM, Vereecke H, Moerman A, et al. Ability of the bispectral index, autoregressive modelling with exogenous inputderived auditory evoked potentials, and predicted propofol concentrations to measure patient responsiveness during anesthesia with propofol and remifentanil. Anesthesiology. 2003;99:802–12.
18. Lysakowski C, Dumont L, Pelle'grini M, et al. Effects of fentanyl, alfentanil, remifentanil and sufentanil on loss of consciousness and bispectral index during propofol induction of anaesthesia. Br J Anaesth. 2001;86:523–7.

19. Sepulveda PO, Mora X. Reevaluation of the time course of the effect of propoful described with the Schnider pharmacokinetic model. Rev Esp Anestsiol Reanim. 2012;59:542–8.
20. Doi M, Gajraj RJ, Mantzaridis H, et al. Relationship between calculated blood concentration of propoful and electrophysiological variables during emergence from anaesthesia: comparision of bispectral index , spectral edge frequency, median frequency and auditory evoked potential index. Br J Anaesth. 1997;78:180–4.

11

Differential effects and mechanisms of local anesthetics on esophageal carcinoma cell migration, growth, survival and chemosensitivity

Guanhua Zhu[1†], Ling Zhang[1†], Jiapeng Dan[1] and Qiong Zhu[2*]

Abstract

Background: Retrospective analysis and pre-clinical studies suggest that local anesthetics have anti-tumoral effects. However, the association between cancer recurrence and the use of local anesthesia is inconclusive and most reports are based on single local anesthetic results.

Methods: The biological effects (growth, migration and survival) of four common local anesthetics on esophageal carcinoma cells were compared. Biochemical assays on molecules involved in cell migration and proliferation were analyzed.

Results: Ropivacaine and bupivacaine significantly inhibited esophageal carcinoma cell migration, at clinically relevant micromolar concentrations. Mepivacaine and lidocaine showed less potent cell migration inhibition than ropivacaine or bupivacaine. All four local anesthetics inhibited cell proliferation. Of note, the effective concentration of anti-proliferative activities requires higher doses. At millimolar concentrations of these local anesthetics, cell apoptosis was moderately affected. Drug combination analysis demonstrated that two of four local anesthetics augmented chemotherapeutic drugs in inhibiting migration. However, all four local anesthetics significantly augmented chemotherapeutic drugs in inhibiting growth and inducing apoptosis. The anti-growth and anti-survival effects of four local anesthetics were attributed to mitochondrial dysfunction and oxidative damage. The anti-migratory effect of local anesthetics is likely through decreasing Rac1 activity.

Conclusions: Our work demonstrates the differential effects and proposes the mechanisms of local anesthetics on esophageal carcinoma cell migration, growth, survival and chemosensitivity.

Keywords: Local anesthetics, Esophageal carcinoma, Mitochondria, Rac1

* Correspondence: honeyzhujing@163.com
†Guanhua Zhu and Ling Zhang are equal contributors and co-first authors.
[2]Department of Anesthesiology, The First Affiliated Hospital of Yangtze University, Hangkong Road 8, Jingzhou 434020, Hubei Province, China

Background

Esophageal cancer is the sixth leading cause of cancer-related mortality and the eighth most common cancer worldwide. Despite advances in diagnostics and therapeutics, the five year survival rate in esophageal carcinoma remains poor [1]. Surgery remains the main curative option for advance local esophageal cancer to improve patient survival. However, local-regional disease recurrences and distant organ metastases are found in a significant proportion of patients after surgical procedures [2]. Studies suggest that anesthetics used in the perioperative period can potentially influence cancer recurrence [3, 4]. Certain local anaesthesia reduce cancer recurrence in a number of retrospective studies. However, these studies have small sizes and are subjected to selection bias [4–7].

Mepivacaine, bupivacaine, ropivacaine and lidocaine are amide-linked local anesthetics and often used during the perioperative period in cancer patients [8, 9]. Amide local anesthetics act on nerve cells through blocking voltage-gate sodium-channels, resulting in the decreased rate of depolarization and repolarization of excitable nerve cell membrane [10]. Substantial preclinical studies suggest that local anesthetics have direct inhibitory effects on the biological activities of cancer cells, including cell proliferation, migration, invasion and survival [11–15]. The mechanisms of the action of the local anesthetics in cancer cells are via targeting multiple signaling or related molecules, and furthermore are sodium-channel-independent [16, 17]. Ropivacaine has been recently reported to inhibit esophageal cancer cell migration via prenylation-dependent inhibition of Rac1/JNK/paxillin [16]. However, systematic evaluation and comparison of these commonly used local anesthetics in esophageal carcinoma biological functions are lacking.

In this work, we investigated the effects of four local anaesthetics on esophageal carcinoma cell growth, survival and migration, as well as their combinatory effects with chemotherapeutic drugs. We show that the four local anesthetics 1) have differential inhibitory effects on esophageal carcinoma cells in aspects of effective doses, cell lines and cellular activities; 2) acts differently with chemotherapeutic drugs; 3) acts on esophageal carcinoma cells via varying mechanisms.

Methods

Cell culture

Esophageal carcinoma cell lines OE19 and SK-GT-4 (Sigma, USA) were cultured in 75 ml flasks at 37 °C with 5% CO_2, using Dulbecco's Modified Eagle Medium supplemented with penicillin at 100/ml, streptomycin at 100 μg/ml and10% heat-inactivated fetal bovine serum (FBS) (Invitrogen, USA). The cell lines used in our study are validated with short tandem repeat (STR) profile analysis.

Drugs

Local anesthetics including lidocaine, mepivacaine, bupivacaine and ropivacaine were obtained from the Department of Pharmacy, Jingzhou Central Hospital. 5-Fluorouracil (5-FU) and paclitaxel were purchased from Sigma, USA.

Measurement of proliferation

Cells were seeded onto a 96-well plate with up to 50% confluency. Different agents were added to the culture plate the next day. These included different local anaesthetics at varying concentrations, single chemotherapeutic drug, or their combinations. After 72 h incubation, cell proliferation activity was determined by the BrdU Cell Proliferation Assay Kit (Cell Signaling, USA).

Measurement of apoptosis

Cells were seeded onto a 6-well plate with up to 50% confluency. Different agents were added to the culture plate the next day. These included different local anaesthetics at varying concentrations, single chemotherapeutic drug, or their combinations. After 72 h incubation, cells were harvested using trypsin for apoptosis analysis using Annexin V/7-AAD kit. The Annexin V-positive cells were determined by analysing cells on Beckman Coulter FC500 Flow Cytometer (Beckman Coulter, USA).

Boyden chamber migration assay

Migration assay was performed using the same method as described in our previous studies [13]. Briefly, pre-treated cells suspended in 2% FBS medium were seeded onto the cell culture inserts and 10% FBS medium as attractant was placed onto the lower chamber. Migration was captured for 8 h. The migrated cells were stained with 0.4% crystal violet and counted under microscope. Cell number of five random fields were quantified.

Measurement of oxygen consumption rate (OCR)

OCR was measured using a Seahorse XF24 extracellular flux analyser (Seahorse Bioscience, USA) as described in our previous studies [13]. Briefly, after 24 h drug treatment on XF24 tissue culture plates, cells were equilibrated to the un-buffered medium in a CO_2-free incubator. OCR was then measured on Seahorse Analyzer at basal condition.

ELISA assays

Cells were incubated with drug for 24 h and were then harvested and homogenized using a standard protocol. Cell lysates were adjusted to the same concentration using PBS. Cellular RhoA and Rac1 activity were assessed using total cell lysates and were determined using RhoA G-LISA Activation Assay Kit and Rac1 G-LISA Activation Assay Kit (Cytoskeleton, Inc. USA). Active RhoA and Rac1 level were measured on absorbance at 490 nm. The level of 8-hydroxydeoxyguanosine (8-OHdG) which is a ubiquitous marker of oxidative DNA damage was measured on absorbance at 450 nm as per protocol and reagents provided by OxiSelect™ Oxidative DNA Damage ELISA Kit (Cell Biolabs Inc., USA).

Measurement of reactive oxygen species (ROS)

Cells were incubated with drug for 24 h and were then harvested and homogenized using a standard protocol. ROS level was measured by using DCFDA/H2DCFDA - Cellular ROS Assay Kit (Abcam, USA) as per manufacture's protocol. The absorbance was measured on a fluorescence plate reader at ex/em of 495/525 nm.

Statistical analyses

The data are expressed as mean and standard deviation (SD). For comparison between groups of two categorical variables, these were analysed by the Student's t test. Across multiple groups, one-way analysis of variance (ANOVA) with post-hoc Tukey was performed. A p-value < 0.05 was considered statistically significant.

Results

The differential effects of local anesthetics on esophageal carcinoma cell migration

To establish the effects of local anesthetics on esophageal carcinoma metastasis, we conducted the Boyden Chamber migration assay using OE19 and SK-GT-4 cells in the presence of local anesthetics: mepivacaine, bupivacaine, lidocaine and ropivacaine. OE-19 was derived from an adenocarcinoma of a gastric/esophageal junction and SK-GT-4 was derived from a well-differentiated adenocarcinoma of the distal esophagus. Both are used as representatives of esophageal adenocarcinoma. We exposed esophageal carcinoma cells to local anesthetics at micromolar concentrations. Ropivacaine and bupivacaine were observed to significantly inhibit migration of both OE19 and SK-GT-4 cells in a dose-dependent manner, starting from 10 μM (Fig. 1). Of note, both ropivacaine and bupivacaine at 100 μM resulted in ~ 80% inhibition of migration. In contrast, lidocaine significantly inhibited migration of both OE19 and SK-GT-4 cells starting from 50 μM and lidocaine at 100 μM. These resulted in ~ 30% inhibition. Interestingly, mepivacaine inhibited migration of SK-GT-4 but not OE19 cells. Mepivacaine at 100 μM resulted in only ~ 20% inhibition. These results demonstrated that ropivacaine and bupivacaine were much more potent than lidocaine and mepivacaine in inhibiting migration of esophageal carcinoma cells. In addition, OE19 and SK-GT-4 cells responded to mepivacaine for cell migration inhibition in a different manner.

The differential effects of local anesthetics on esophageal carcinoma cell growth and survival

We next employed the BrdU incorporation assay and Annexin V labeling method to assess the proliferation and apoptosis of esophageal carcinoma cells exposed to local anesthetics. Based on our previous findings on the varying effective concentrations of bupivacaine on gastric cancer cell migration, growth and survival [13], we treated cells with local anesthetics at millimolar concentrations. We found that all tested local anesthetics significantly inhibited both OE19 and SK-GT-4 cell proliferation in a dose-dependent manner (Fig. 2a). In addition, OE19 was more sensitive to mepivacaine and bupivacaine than SK-GT-4 cells whereas OE19 and SK-GT-4 responded similarly to lidocaine and ropivacaine. Of note, mepivacaine and bupivacaine at 12.5 mM achieved ~ 100% growth inhibition whereas lidocaine and ropivacaine at 12.5 mM achieved ~ 50% growth inhibition in OE19 cells.

In contrast to growth inhibition, we observed a slight to modest apoptosis induction by all tested local anesthetics. Mepivacaine at 12.5 mM induced ~ 20% and ~ 40% apoptosis in OE19 and SK-GT-4 cells (Fig. 2b). Ropivacaine at 12.5 mM induced ~ 20% apoptosis in SK-GT-4 cells and did not affect OE19 survival. Bupivacaine at 12.5 mM induced ~ 40% and ~ 50% apoptosis in OE19 and SK-GT-4 cells. Lidocaine at 12.5 mM induced ~ 20% and ~ 30% apoptosis in OE19 and SK-GT-4 cells. We noted that ropivacaine at 2.5 mM and bupivacaine at 0.5 mM significantly decreased proliferation while sparing apoptosis (Fig. 2). Cell cycle analysis indicated that ropivacaine at 2.5 mM and bupivacaine at 0.5 mM increased G2/M percentage, suggesting that the cell cycle was arrested in G2/M phase by these two local anaesthetics (Fig. S1). Altogether, three of four tested local anesthetics up to 2.5 mM did not induce apoptosis in esophageal carcinoma cells.

The differential combinatory effects of local anaesthetics with chemotherapy drugs on esophageal carcinoma cell migration, growth and survival

To investigate whether local anaesthetics influence the efficacy of chemotherapy in esophageal carcinoma cells, we performed combination studies using local anaesthetics and commonly used chemotherapeutic drugs: 5-FU and paclitaxel. The concentration of anaesthetics and chemotherapeutic agent in earlier analyses that led to around 50% inhibition on cell proliferation, survival and migration as a single drug alone was chosen for the combination studies. We found that the combination of ropivacaine or bupivacaine with 5-FU or paclitaxel were significantly more effective in inhibiting migration of esophageal carcinoma cells than 5-FU or paclitaxel alone (Fig. 3a).

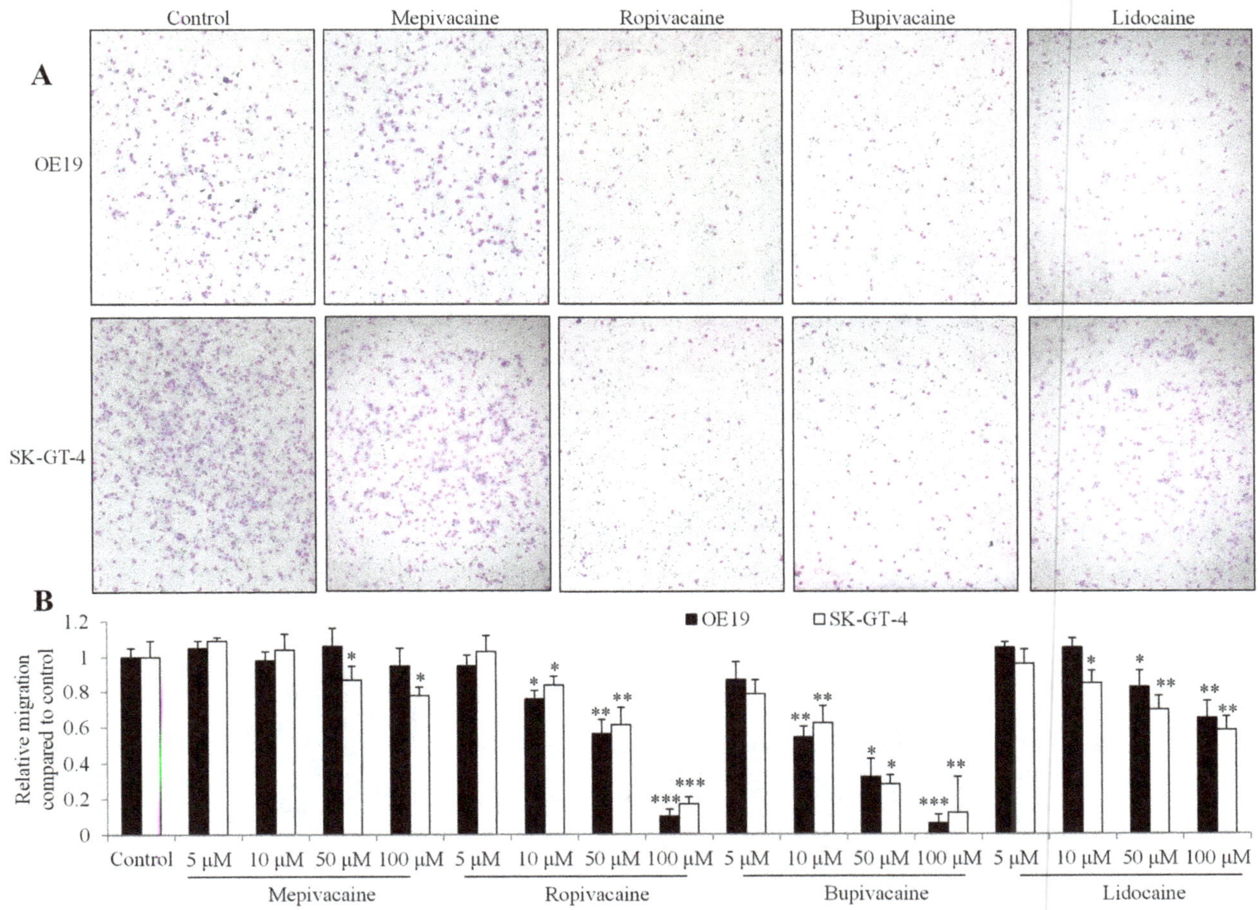

Fig. 1 The differential effects of local anesthetics on esophageal carcinoma cell migration. **a** Representative photos of cell migration assay. OE19 and SK-GT-4 were treated with control or four local anesthetics at 100 μM: mepivacaine, bupivacaine, ropivacaine and lidocaine. **b** Quantification of cell migration using the Image J software shows the differential degree of inhibition on esophageal carcinoma cells among four local anesthetics at concentration range from 5 to 100 μM. Cell number of five random fields were quantified. $*P < 0.05$, $**P < 0.01$, $***P < 0.001$, compared to control. All experiments were independently performed at least three times

However, combination of lidocaine or mepivacaine with 5-FU or paclitaxel inhibited cell migration in a similar manner as the chemotherapeutic drugs alone. These suggest that some but not all local anesthetics displays synergism with chemotherapeutic agents in inhibiting esophageal carcinoma cell migration.

We further observed that all tested local anaesthetics significantly augmented the anti-proliferative and pro-apoptotic effects of 5-FU or paclitaxel in esophageal carcinoma cells (Fig. 3b and c). It was noted that the combination of local anaesthetics with chemotherapeutic drugs resulted in ~ 90% growth inhibition and ~ 80% apoptosis induction in SK-GT-4 cells, suggesting the remarkably enhanced effects between local anesthetics and chemotherapy. In addition, we observed that ropivacaine failed to augment the pro-apoptotic effect of 5-FU and paclitaxel in OE19 cells.

The differential mechanisms of local anaesthetics' action in esophageal carcinoma cells

To investigate the mechanisms of local anesthetics' action in esophageal carcinoma cells, we examined the activities of essential molecules involved in cell migration, such as RhoA and Rac1 [18, 19]. We found that all tested local anesthetics did not affect RhoA activity in SK-GT-4 cells (Fig. 4a). Ropivacaine and bupivacaine but not mepivacaine or lidocaine at both 0.1 mM and 12.5 mM significantly decreased Rac1 activities (Fig. 4b). Time course analysis indicated that ropivacaine and bupivacaine decreased Rac1 activity as early as 2-h drug treatment (Fig. 4c).

Local anesthetics have been shown to interact with mitochondria and affect mitochondrial respiratory chain with compromised mitochondrial functions [20, 21]. We found that bupivacaine, mepivacaine, ropivacaine and

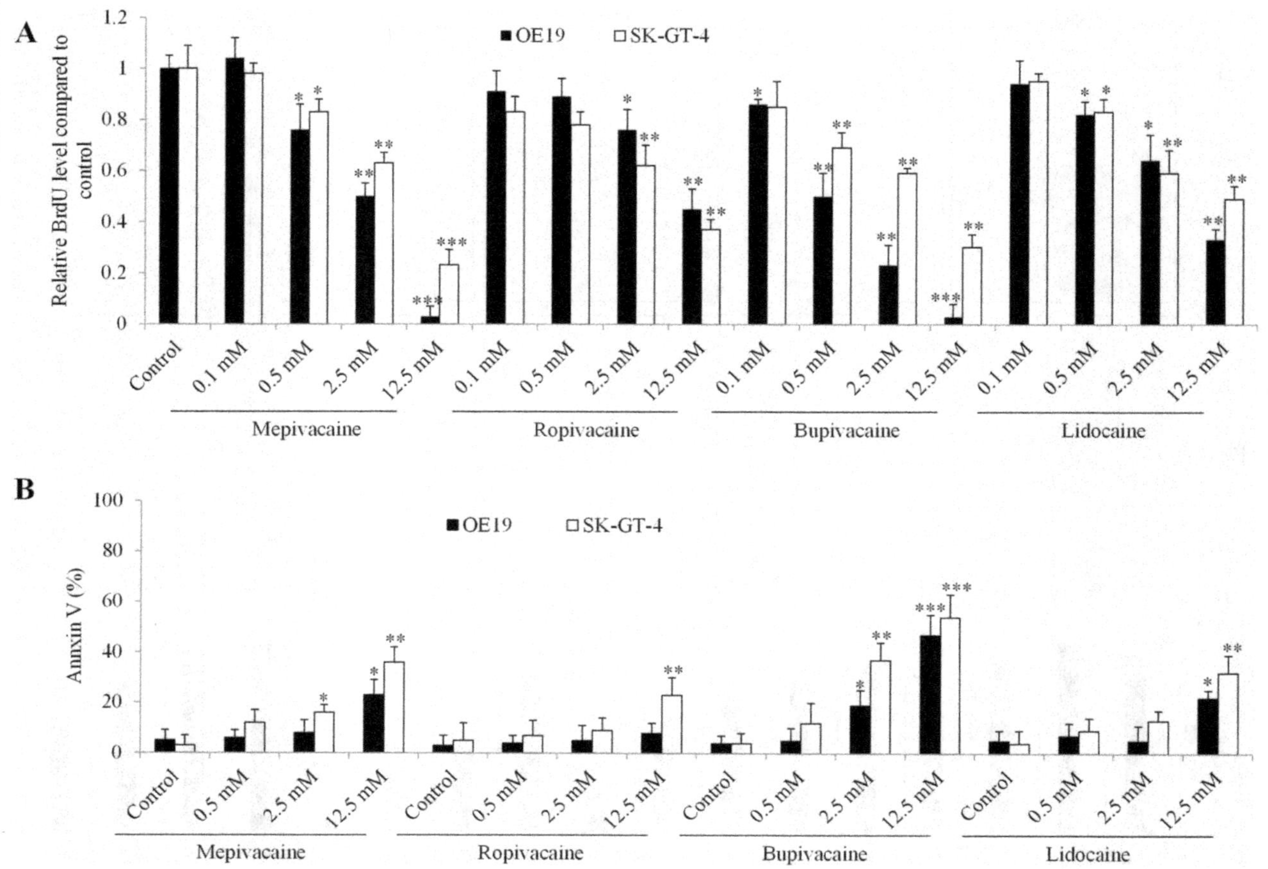

Fig. 2 The differential effects of local anesthetics on esophageal carcinoma cell growth and survival. The differential degree of growth inhibition (**a**) and apoptosis induction (**b**) among four local anesthetics at concentration range from 0.1 to 12.5 mM in esophageal carcinoma cell. **P* < 0.05, ***P* < 0.01, ****P* < 0.001, compared to control. All experiments were independently performed at least three times

lidocaine at 2.5 mM and 12.5 mM but not 0.1 mM significantly decreased OCR level, increased intercellular ROS and 8-OHdG levels (Fig. 4d-f and Fig. S2 to S4). Of note, all local anesthetics at concentrations that decreased proliferation significantly inhibited mitochondrial respiration, increased ROS and 8-OHdG levels (Fig. S2 to S4), suggesting that proliferation inhibition by local anesthetics might be due to their ability in inducing mitochondrial dysfunction, oxidative stress and damage in esophageal carcinoma cells.

Discussion

Although earlier small retrospective clinical trials suggest the beneficial roles of local anaesthetics in cancer patients with reduced tumor metastases and recurrence [22–24], prospective, large and randomized clinical trials on the effects of regional anaesthesia on long-term outcome after cancer surgery are required. This will provide confirmation of anaesthetics' implication in cancer patients to guide clinical practice. Our study complements the efforts to drive better understanding of its mechanisms using preclinical studies to evaluate the direct effects of local anaesthetics on representative cancer cells. Local anaesthetics can reach the circulatory system via absorption from the injection site or direct intravenous injection (eg, lidocaine) to affect circulating tumour cells released from the primary tumour during surgery. The anti-cancer activities of common amide-linked local anaesthetics have been identified in various cancers, such as lung cancer, hepatocellular carcinoma and thyroid cancer [25–27]. We previously revealed the anti-breast cancer activity of ropivacaine [20] and anti-migratory effect of bupivacaine in gastric cancer [13]. Given the fact that little is known on the effects of local anaesthetics on esophageal carcinoma cells, the present study comprehensively evaluated and compared the effects of four local anaesthetics on two well-characterized esophageal carcinoma cell lines: OE19 and SK-GT-4. We found that four local aesthetics had differential effects and mechanisms on esophageal carcinoma cell migration, growth, survival and chemosensitivity.

Metastatic disease is the most important cause of cancer-related death in patients after surgery. Using

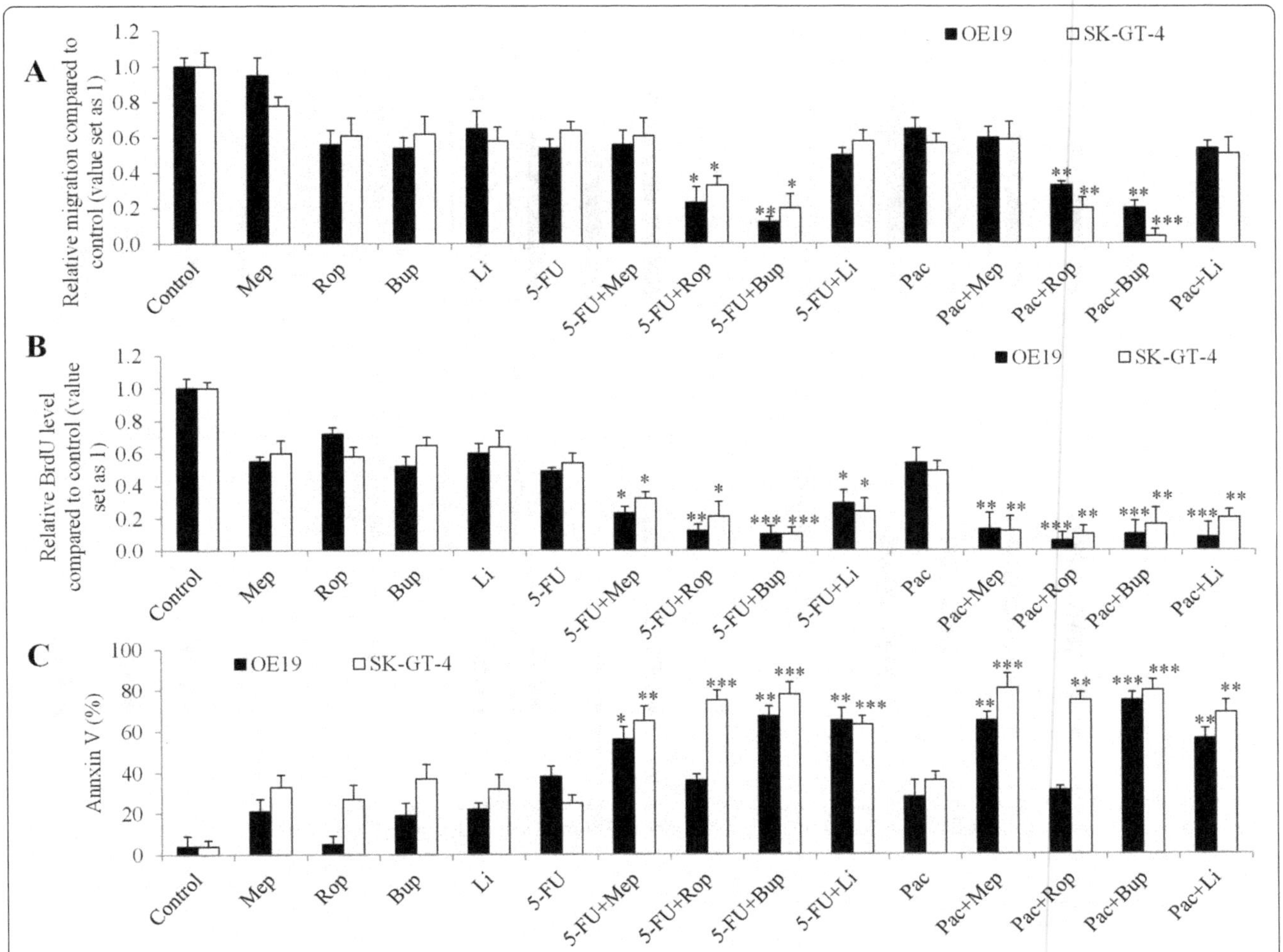

Fig. 3 The differential combinatory effects of local anesthetics on esophageal carcinoma cell migration, growth and survival. **a** Bupivacaine (Bup) and ropivacaine (Rop) but not mepivacaine (Mep) or lidocaine (Li) significantly augment the effects of 5-FU and paclitaxel in decreasing esophageal carcinoma cell migration. 100 μM of mepivacaine and lidocaine, 50 μM of ropivacaine and 10 μM of bupivacaine were used. All four local anesthetics significantly augment the effects of 5-FU and paclitaxel in decreasing esophageal carcinoma cell in inhibiting proliferation (**b**) and inducing apoptosis (**c**). 2.5 mM of mepivacaine, ropivacaine and lidocaine, and 0.5 mM of bupivacaine were used in proliferation assay. 12.5 mM of mepivacaine, ropivacaine and lidocaine, and 2.5 mM of bupivacaine were used in apoptosis assay. 5-FU at 100 nM and paclitaxel at 50 nM were used for the combination studies in migration, proliferation and apoptosis assays. *$P < 0.05$, **$P < 0.01$, ***$P < 0.001$, compared to paclitaxel or 5-FU alone. All experiments were independently performed at least three times

Boyden Chamber migration assay, we showed that bupivacaine and ropivacaine were more potent than lidocaine and mepivacaine in inhibiting migration (Fig. 1). The estimated IC50 of anti-migratory effect of bupivacaine, ropivacaine, lidocaine and mepivacaine in esophageal carcinoma cells are ~ 10 μM, ~ 50 μM, > 100 μM and > 100 μM. Plasma concentrations of these four local anesthetics ranged from 2.8 to 10 μM [15]. Our results suggest that bupivacaine is the only local anesthetics among the four, at clinically achievable concentration, to inhibit migration in esophageal carcinoma. In contrast, all four local anesthetics inhibited proliferation in a similar manner (Fig. 2a). Compared to anti-migratory activity, the effective concentration of anti-proliferative activity requires up to 250-time higher doses, with IC50 at ~ 2.5 mM in esophageal carcinoma cells (Fig. 2a). Although the plasma concentration of local anesthetics is at low micromolar range, local infiltration concentration of bupivacaine, ropivacaine, lidocaine and mepivacaine might reach sub-millimolar level [15]. Our results suggest that none of local anesthetics at plasma achievable concentration affects esophageal carcinoma cell proliferation. The varying effective doses of anti-migratory and anti-proliferative effects of local anesthetics observed in our study are consistent with the previous reports [28–30]. We further showed that the four local anesthetics at

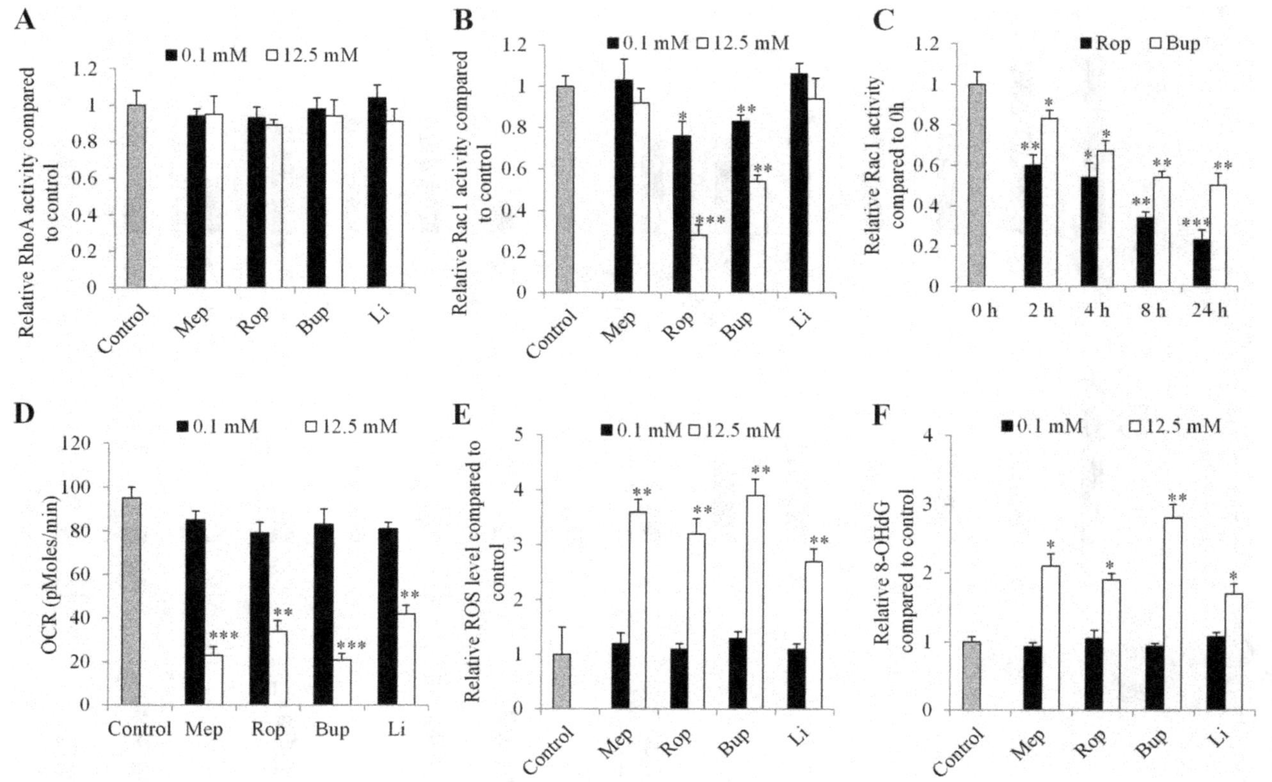

Fig. 4 The differential mechanisms of local anesthetics' action in esophageal carcinoma cells. **a** Local anesthetics up to 12.5 mM do not affect RhoA activity in SK-GT-4 cells. Ropivacaine and bupivacaine but not lidocaine or mepivacaine significantly decreases Rac1 activity (**b**) in SK-GT-4 cells. **c** Ropivacaine and bupivacaine decreased Rac1 activity in a time-dependent manner. Local anesthetics at 12.5 mM but not 0.1 mM significantly decreases OCR level (**d**) and increases ROS level (**e**) and 8-OHdG level (**f**) in SK-GT-4 cells. *$P < 0.05$, **$P < 0.01$, ***$P < 0.001$, compared to control. All experiments were independently performed at least three times

millimolar concentration had slight or modest pro-apoptotic effects (Fig. 2c), suggesting that local anesthetics are less likely to affect esophageal carcinoma cell survival.

Chemotherapeutic agents, such as 5-FU, cisplatin and paclitaxel, are the most frequently used chemotherapy for esophageal carcinoma [31]. Apart from the identification of local anaesthetics' effect as single drug alone, we further revealed that local anaesthetics significantly augmented the inhibitory effects of 5-FU and paclitaxel (Fig. 3). Our results are supported by the previous work on the combinatory effects of lidocaine and bupivacaine with chemotherapy agents on cancer cells [13, 32]. This finding provides pre-clinical evidence that local anaesthetics can be considered for pain management in patient with advanced esophageal carcinoma, especially in those who are concurrently receiving chemotherapy. Of note, our work showed the differential combinatory effects of local anaesthetics with chemotherapeutic agents in different aspects of tumour cell biological functions. Additionally, two esophageal cell lines displayed differential response to the drug combination (Fig. 3). Our results also highlight that there is no common mechanism to account for the anti-esophageal carcinoma activity for all four local anaesthetics. Generally, bupivacaine and ropivacaine but not lidocaine or bupivacaine inhibited migration through decreasing activity of Rac1 (Fig. 4a-c). Rac1 exerts an important regulatory role in cell motility by formation of lamellipodia [33]. Our findings on the inhibitory effects of ropivacaine on Rac1 activity is consistent with the previous report that ropivacaine inhibits Rac1/JNK/paxillin in cancer cells [16]. Our study demonstrates the well correlated effective concentrations of local anaesthetics between proliferation and mitochondrial respiration (Fig. 2a and Fig. S2). Taken together, these suggest that local anaesthetics are likely to inhibit cell migration via inhibiting Rac1, and inhibit cell proliferation via inhibiting mitochondrial respiration. The exact molecular targets which are responsible for local anaesthetics' differential action in esophageal carcinoma cells are worthy of further investigations.

Conclusion

In conclusion, our findings demonstrate the direct inhibitory effects of four local anesthetics in esophageal carcinoma cells with different effective concentrations. The mechanisms of the action of local anesthetics on esophageal carcinoma cells are likely due to their ability in inhibiting Rac1, inducing mitochondrial dysfunctions, and increasing oxidative stress and damage.

Supplementary information

Additional file 1: Fig. S1. Ropivacaine and bupivacaine arrest cell cycle via increasing G2/M percentage in esophageal carcinoma cells. After 24-h drug treatment, the cell cycle was assessed by staining cells with Propidium iodide (PI) and followed by flow cytometry. $*P < 0.05$, $**P < 0.01$, $***P < 0.001$, compared to control. **Fig. S2.** All local anesthetics decrease OCR level in esophageal carcinoma cells. $*P < 0.05$, $**P < 0.01$, $***P < 0.001$, compared to control. **Fig. S3.** All local anesthetics increase ROS level in esophageal carcinoma cells. $*P < 0.05$, $**P < 0.01$, $***P < 0.001$, compared to control. **Fig. S4.** All local anesthetics increase 8-OHdG level in esophageal carcinoma cells. $*P < 0.05$, $**P < 0.01$, $***P < 0.001$, compared to control.

Abbreviations

JNK: c-Jun N-terminal kinase; FBS: Fetal bovine serum; STR: Short tandem repeat; 5-FU: 5-Fluorouracil; ANOVA: One-way analysis of variance; 8-OHdG: 8-hydroxydeoxyguanosine; OCR: Oxygen consumption rate

Acknowledgements

No applicable.

Authors' contributions

QZ and GHZ designed the experiments. GHZ, JPD and LZ performed each of the tests and collated the data. All analysed the results and prepared the manuscript.

Author details

[1]Department of Anesthesiology, Jingzhou Central Hospital, Jingzhou, Hubei Province, China. [2]Department of Anesthesiology, The First Affiliated Hospital of Yangtze University, Hangkong Road 8, Jingzhou 434020, Hubei Province, China.

References

1. Pennathur A, Gibson MK, Jobe BA, Luketich JD. Oesophageal carcinoma. Lancet. 2013;381(9864):400–12.
2. Su XD, Zhang DK, Zhang X, Lin P, Long H, Rong TH. Prognostic factors in patients with recurrence after complete resection of esophageal squamous cell carcinoma. J Thorac Dis. 2014;6(7):949–57.
3. Gottschalk A, Sharma S, Ford J, Durieux ME, Tiouririne M. Review article: the role of the perioperative period in recurrence after cancer surgery. Anesth Analg. 2010;110(6):1636–43.
4. Tedore T: Regional anaesthesia and analgesia: relationship to cancer recurrence and survival. British journal of anaesthesia 2015, 115 Suppl 2:ii34–45.
5. Chen WK, Miao CH. The effect of anesthetic technique on survival in human cancers: a meta-analysis of retrospective and prospective studies. PLoS One. 2013;8(2):e56540.
6. Exadaktylos AK, Buggy DJ, Moriarty DC, Mascha E, Sessler DI. Can anesthetic technique for primary breast cancer surgery affect recurrence or metastasis? Anesthesiology. 2006;105(4):660–4.
7. Biki B, Mascha E, Moriarty DC, Fitzpatrick JM, Sessler DI, Buggy DJ. Anesthetic technique for radical prostatectomy surgery affects cancer recurrence: a retrospective analysis. Anesthesiology. 2008;109(2):180–7.
8. Kim B, Lee H, Chung H, Park JC, Shin SK, Lee SK, Lee YC. The efficacy of topical bupivacaine and triamcinolone acetonide injection in the relief of pain after endoscopic submucosal dissection for gastric neoplasia: a randomized double-blind, placebo-controlled trial. Surg Endosc. 2015;29(3):714–22.
9. Chamaraux-Tran TN, Piegeler T. The amide local anesthetic Lidocaine in Cancer surgery-potential Antimetastatic effects and preservation of immune cell function? A narrative review. Front Med (Lausanne). 2017;4:235.
10. Heavner JE. Local anesthetics. Curr Opin Anaesthesiol. 2007;20(4):336–42.
11. Zheng Q, Peng X, Yu H. Local anesthetic drug inhibits growth and survival in chronic myeloid leukemia through suppressing PI3K/Akt/mTOR. Am J Med Sci. 2013;355(3):266–73.
12. Ni J, Xie T, Xiao M, Xiang W, Wang L. Amide-linked local anesthetics preferentially target leukemia stem cell through inhibition of Wnt/beta-catenin. Biochem Biophys Res Commun. 2018;503(2):956–62.
13. Dan J, Gong X, Li D, Zhu G, Wang L, Li F: Inhibition of gastric cancer by local anesthetic bupivacaine through multiple mechanisms independent of sodium channel blockade. Biomedicine & pharmacotherapy = Biomedecine & pharmacotherapie 2018, 103:823–828.
14. Zhang L, Hu R, Cheng Y, Wu X, Xi S, Sun Y, Jiang H: Lidocaine inhibits the proliferation of lung cancer by regulating the expression of GOLT1A. Cell Prolif 2017, 50(5).
15. Li R, Xiao C, Liu H, Huang Y, Dilger JP, Lin J. Effects of local anesthetics on breast cancer cell viability and migration. BMC Cancer. 2018;18(1):666.
16. Zhang Y, Peng X, Zheng Q. Ropivacaine inhibits the migration of esophageal cancer cells via sodium-channel-independent but prenylation-dependent inhibition of Rac1/JNK/paxillin/FAK. Biochem Biophys Res Commun. 2018;501(4):1074–9.
17. Piegeler T, Votta-Velis EG, Liu G, Place AT, Schwartz DE, Beck-Schimmer B, Minshall RD, Borgeat A. Antimetastatic potential of amide-linked local anesthetics: inhibition of lung adenocarcinoma cell migration and inflammatory Src signaling independent of sodium channel blockade. Anesthesiology. 2012;117(3):548–59.
18. Ridley AJ. Rho GTPase signalling in cell migration. Curr Opin Cell Biol. 2015; 36:103–12.
19. Nabeshima K, Inoue T, Shimao Y, Sameshima T. Matrix metalloproteinases in tumor invasion: role for cell migration. Pathol Int. 2002;52(4):255–64.
20. Gong X, Dan J, Li F, Wang L. Suppression of mitochondrial respiration with local anesthetic ropivacaine targets breast cancer cells. J Thorac Dis. 2018; 10(5):2804–12.
21. La Monaca E, Fodale V. Effects of anesthetics on mitochondrial signaling and function. Curr Drug Saf. 2012;7(2):126–39.
22. Snyder GL, Greenberg S. Effect of anaesthetic technique and other perioperative factors on cancer recurrence. Br J Anaesth. 2010;105(2):106–15.
23. Tavare AN, Perry NJ, Benzonana LL, Takata M, Ma D. Cancer recurrence after surgery: direct and indirect effects of anesthetic agents. Int J Cancer. 2012; 130(6):1237–50.
24. Mao L, Lin S, Lin J. The effects of anesthetics on tumor progression. International journal of physiology, pathophysiology and pharmacology. 2013;5(1):1–10.
25. Le Gac G, Angenard G, Clement B, Laviolle B, Coulouarn C, Beloeil H. Local anesthetics inhibit the growth of human hepatocellular carcinoma cells. Anesth Analg. 2017;125(5):1600–9.
26. Wang HW, Wang LY, Jiang L, Tian SM, Zhong TD, Fang XM. Amide-linked local anesthetics induce apoptosis in human non-small cell lung cancer. J Thorac Dis. 2016;8(10):2748–57.
27. Chang YC, Hsu YC, Liu CL, Huang SY, Hu MC, Cheng SP. Local anesthetics induce apoptosis in human thyroid cancer cells through the mitogen-activated protein kinase pathway. PLoS One. 2014;9(2):e89563.
28. Chang YC, Liu CL, Chen MJ, Hsu YW, Chen SN, Lin CH, Chen CM, Yang FM, Hu MC. Local anesthetics induce apoptosis in human breast tumor cells. Anesth Analg. 2014;118(1):116–24.
29. Xuan W, Zhao H, Hankin J, Chen L, Yao S, Ma D. Local anesthetic bupivacaine induced ovarian and prostate cancer apoptotic cell death and underlying mechanisms in vitro. Sci Rep. 2016;6:26277.
30. Baptista-Hon DT, Robertson FM, Robertson GB, Owen SJ, Rogers GW, Lydon EL, Lee NH, Hales TG: Potent inhibition by ropivacaine of metastatic colon cancer SW620 cell invasion and NaV1.5 channel function. British journal of anaesthesia 2014, 113 Suppl 1:i39-i48.
31. Hirano H, Kato K. Systemic treatment of advanced esophageal squamous cell carcinoma: chemotherapy, molecular-targeting therapy and immunotherapy. Jpn J Clin Oncol. 2019;49(5):412–20.
32. Yang X, Zhao L, Li M, Yan L, Zhang S, Mi Z, Ren L, Xu J. Lidocaine enhances the effects of chemotherapeutic drugs against bladder cancer. Sci Rep. 2018;8(1):598.
33. Parri M, Chiarugi P. Rac and rho GTPases in cancer cell motility control. Cell Commun Signal. 2010;8:23.

12

Comparison of general anesthesia with endotracheal intubation, combined spinal-epidural anesthesia, and general anesthesia with laryngeal mask airway and nerve block for intertrochanteric fracture surgeries in elderly patients

Yang Liu[1], Mang Su[2], Wei Li[1], Hao Yuan[1] and Cheng Yang[1*]

Abstract

Background: There is no consensus on the optimal anesthesia method for intertrochanteric fracture surgeries in elderly patients. Our study aimed to compare the hemodynamics and perioperative outcomes of general anesthesia with endotracheal intubation, combined spinal-epidural anesthesia, and general anesthesia with laryngeal mask airway (LMA) and nerve block for intertrochanteric fracture surgeries in elderly patients.

Methods: This is a retrospective study of 75 patients aged > 60 years scheduled for intertrochanteric fracture surgeries with general anesthesia with intubation ($n = 25$), combined spinal-epidural anesthesia ($n = 25$), and general anesthesia with LMA and nerve block ($n = 25$). The intraoperative hemodynamics were recorded, and the maximum variation rate was calculated. Postoperative analgesic effect was evaluated using the visual analog scale (VAS). Postoperative cognitive status was assessed using the Mini-Mental State Exam (MMSE).

Results: The maximum variation rate of intraoperative heart rate, systolic blood pressure, diastolic blood pressure differed significantly between the three groups (general anesthesia with intubation > combined spinal-epidural anesthesia > general anesthesia with LMA and nerve block). The VAS scores postoperative 2 h, 4 h, 6 h, and 8 h also differed significantly between the three groups (general anesthesia with intubation > combined spinal-epidural anesthesia > general anesthesia with LMA and nerve block). The VAS scores postoperative 24 h were significantly lower in the general anesthesia with LMA/nerve block group than the general anesthesia with intubation group and the combined spinal-epidural anesthesia group. The MMSE scores postoperative 15 min and 45 min differed significantly between the three groups (general anesthesia with intubation < combined spinal-epidural anesthesia < general anesthesia with LMA and nerve block). The MMSE scores postoperative 120 min in the general anesthesia with intubation group were the lowest among the three groups. There was no significant difference in the incidence of respiratory infection postoperative 24 h, 48 h, and 72 h between the three groups.

(Continued on next page)

* Correspondence: 358353224@qq.com
[1]Department of Orthopedics, Chengdu Aerospace Hospital, Chengdu 610100, China

(Continued from previous page)

Conclusion: Compared to general anesthesia with intubation and combined spinal-epidural anesthesia, general anesthesia with LMA and nerve block had better postoperative analgesic effect and less disturbances on intraoperative hemodynamics and postoperative cognition for elderly patients undergoing intertrochanteric fracture surgeries.

Keywords: Anesthesia, elderly patient, intertrochanteric fracture, laryngeal mask airway,

Background

The global population aging has led to increasingly more elderly patients with hip fractures. Aging is associated with decreased hemodynamic stability, hypertension, poor physical status, risk of cognitive impairment, and osteoporosis [1–3]. Providing anesthesia for hip fracture surgeries in elderly patients can be challenging.

It has been shown that regional anesthesia is comparable to general anesthesia for hip fractures in adults [4]. However, it is not known whether regional anesthesia is superior to general anesthesia in terms of hemodynamic stability and postoperative cognitive impairment in elderly patients undergoing hip surgeries. A previous study found that general anesthesia with endotracheal intubation was associated with intraoperative hypotension and hemodynamic instability in elderly patients undergoing hip surgeries compared to general anesthesia with laryngeal mask airway (LMA) and nerve block [5]. The effect of these two anesthetic methods on postoperative cognitive function in elderly patients is still not clear.

Our study aimed to compare intraoperative hemodynamics, postoperative pain, postoperative cognitive function, and respiratory infection between general anesthesia with endotracheal intubation, combined spinal-epidural anesthesia, and general anesthesia with LMA and nerve block for elderly patients undergoing intertrochanteric fracture surgeries.

Methods

Patients

A total of 75 patients scheduled for closed reduction or open reduction with internal fixation for intertrochanteric fracture between January 2017 and November 2018 were included in this retrospective study. The inclusion criteria were age > 60 years and < 90 years, intertrochanteric fracture diagnosed by radiology, and American Society of Anesthesiologists (ASA) physical status I–III. Patients with the following conditions were excluded: cognitive impairment, allergy to anesthetic agents, operation time > 4 h, conversion to general anesthesia with intubation.

Anesthesia protocols

The patients were matched by sex, age, and weight and received general anesthesia with intubation (n = 25), combined spinal-epidural anesthesia (n = 25), and general anesthesia with LMA and nerve block (n = 25). All patients fasted preoperatively for 8 h. Hypertension and diabetes mellitus were controlled before the surgery. All anesthesia procedures were performed by one anesthesiologist.

For the general anesthesia with intubation, anesthesia was induced by infusing midazolam 0.05 mg/kg, lidocaine 0.5 mg/kg, fentanyl 3 μg/kg, propofol 1.5–2.0 mg/kg, and cisatracurium 0.2 mg/kg. Then the patients were intubated for mechanical ventilation.

For the combined spinal-epidural anesthesia, the patient was in the lateral decubitus position. Ropivacaine 0.5% 4 ml was injected into the subarachnoid space through the L2-L3 intervertebral space. An epidural catheter was positioned. The upper level of anesthesia was controlled bellow the T8 vertebra. Ropivacaine 0.5% 3–5 ml was administered epidurally if the surgery lasted over 2 h.

For the general anesthesia with LMA and nerve block, lumbar plexus-sciatic nerve block was first performed. A 100-mm stimulation needle (D22G, Stimuplex, B. Braun, Germany) was used to deliver electric stimulations at 2 Hz, with a starting current of 1 mA and a pulse time of 0.1 ms. Contraction of the quadriceps femoris and the gastrocnemius in response to a current < 0.3 mA indicated that the injection site had been reached. After confirming no aspiration of blood or cerebrospinal fluid, ropivacaine 0.5% 30 ml was injected respectively for lumbar plexus block and sciatic nerve block. Anesthesia was induced using etomidate 0.1–0.3 mg/kg, vecuronium bromide 0.1 mg/kg, and fentanyl 2–4 μg/kg. Then an LMA was inserted. General anesthesia was maintained using propofol 3–5 mg/h·kg. No postoperative analgesics were used.

Collection of patient data

Patient data was from a previous clinical trial in which intraoperative heart rate, systolic blood pressure, and diastolic blood pressure were recorded using a ventilator. Hemodynamic changes were evaluated using the maximum variation rate, which was calculated using the formula:

maximum variation rate = (maximum − minimum)/pre − anesthesia value.

Postoperative pain was evaluated at 2 h, 4 h, 6 h, 8 h, and 24 h using the visual analog scale (VAS). The VAS

Table 1 Patient general information

	General anesthesia with intubation (n = 25)	Combined spinal-epidural anesthesia (n = 25)	General anesthesia with LMA/nerve block (n = 25)	P
Male, n (%)	12 (48)	10 (40)	11 (44)	0.850
Age, year	74.7 ± 6.8	75.4 ± 6.1	75.5 ± 6.0	0.893
Weight, kg	62.1 ± 7.6	62.3 ± 6.4	64.8 ± 6.6	0.320
ASA physical status, n (%)				0.796
I	3 (12)	3 (12)	2 (8)	
II	21 (84)	20 (80)	21 (84)	
III	1 (4)	2 (8)	2 (8)	
Operation time (min)	61.1 ± 6.7	62.3 ± 6.7	63.8 ± 7.1	0.782
Anesthesia time (time)	85.7 ± 6.8	86.4 ± 7.0	86.6 ± 7.0	0.842
Hospital stay (day)	15.7 ± 2.2	16.4 ± 2.0	14.56 ± 2.02	0.860

LMA laryngeal mask airway, *ASA* American Society of Anesthesiologists

scores range from 0 to 10, with 0 indicating painless and 10 indicating the worst pain imaginable.

Patient cognitive function was assessed preoperatively, postoperative 15 min, 45 min, and 120 min using the Mini-Mental State Examination (MMSE). The MMSE assesses orientation to place and time, calculation, memory, language, reading, writing, and drawing. A reduction of 3 points in the postoperative MMSE score suggested postoperative cognitive dysfunction [6].

Postoperative respiratory infection was tested by bacteria culture using the respiratory secretions collected postoperative 24 h, 48 h, and 72 h.

Statistical analysis

Continuous data were presented as means and standard deviations. Categorical data were presented as percentages or frequencies. Comparisons were made using the one-way analysis of variance analysis followed by post-hoc analysis or the chi-square test. Ordinal data was compared using the Kruskal-Wallis test. All statistical analyses were performed using the SPSS 18.0 software (SPSS, Chicago, USA). A P-value < 0.05 was considered statistically significant.

Results

A total of 91 patients were eligible for inclusion and 16 patients were excluded for cognitive impairment (n = 7), allergy to anesthetic agents (n = 4), operation time > 4 h (n = 2), conversion to general anesthesia with intubation (n = 3). The patients included 33 men and 42 women (age range, 60–90 years). There was no significant difference in sex, age, weight, and ASA physical status between the three groups (Table 1).

The maximum variation rate of heart rate, systolic blood pressure, and diastolic blood pressure differed significantly between the three groups (general anesthesia with intubation > combined spinal-epidural anesthesia > general anesthesia with LMA and nerve block, all P < 0.001, Table 2).

The three groups showed no significant difference in preoperative VAS scores. The VAS scores postoperative 2 h, 4 h, 6 h, and 8 h differed significantly between the three groups (general anesthesia with intubation > combined spinal-epidural anesthesia > general anesthesia with LMA and nerve block, all P < 0.001, Table 3). The VAS scores at rest and during ambulation postoperative 24 h were significantly lower in the general anesthesia with LMA/nerve block group than the general anesthesia

Table 2 Comparison of intraoperative hemodynamics

Maximum variation rate	General anesthesia with intubation (n = 25)	Combined spinal-epidural anesthesia (n = 25)	General anesthesia with LMA/nerve block (n = 25)	P
Heart rate	0.47 (0.44–0.54)#*	0.31 (0.30–0.33 *	0.22 (0.21–0.24)	< 0.001
Systolic blood pressure	0.45 (0.39–0.48)#*	0.35 (0.32–0.37)*	0.23 (0.21–0.26)	< 0.001
Diastolic blood pressure	0.46 (0.41–0.49)#*	0.32 (0.30–0.35)*	0.25 (0.23–0.29)	< 0.001

LMA Laryngeal mask airway. #vs combined spinal-epidural anesthesia, P < 0.001; *vs general anesthesia with LMA/nerve block, P < 0.001.

Table 3 Evaluation of perioperative pain.

VAS score	General anesthesia with intubation ($n = 25$)	Combined spinal-epidural anesthesia ($n = 25$)	General anesthesia with LMA/nerve block ($n = 25$)	P
Preoperative	6.72 ± 0.79	6.84 ± 0.75	6.76 ± 0.72	0.849
Postoperative 2 h	6.96 ± 0.73#*	2.52 ± 0.51*	1.48 ± 0.51	< 0.001
Postoperative 4 h	6.48 ± 0.65#*	2.72 ± 0.46*	1.48 ± 0.51	< 0.001
Postoperative 6 h	6.24 ± 0.52#*	3.72 ± 0.94*	2.36 ± 0.64	< 0.001
Postoperative 8 h	6.04 ± 0.54#*	5.44 ± 0.77*	2.76 ± 0.44	< 0.001
Postoperative 24 h at rest	5.72 ± 0.54*	6.16 ± 0.62*	3.40 ± 0.50	< 0.001
Postoperative 24 h during ambulation	7.24 ± 0.44*	7.16 ± 0.37*	5.00 ± 0.58	< 0.001

VAS Visual analog scale, *LMA* Laryngeal mask airway. #vs combined spinal-epidural anesthesia, $P < 0.001$; *vs general anesthesia with LMA/nerve block, $P < 0.001$.

with intubation group and the combined spinal-epidural anesthesia group.

There was no significant difference in preoperative MMSE scores between the three groups. The MMSE scores postoperative 15 min and 45 min differed significantly between the three groups (general anesthesia with intubation < combined spinal-epidural anesthesia < general anesthesia with LMA and nerve block, all $P < 0.001$, Table 4). The MMSE scores postoperative 120 min in the general anesthesia with intubation group were the lowest among the three groups. However, it did not differ significantly between the combined spinal-epidural anesthesia group and the general anesthesia with LMA/nerve block group.

There was no significant difference in the incidence of respiratory infection postoperative 24 h, 48 h, and 72 h between the three groups (Table 5).

Discussion

Our study found that general anesthesia with LMA and nerve block was associated with less significant intraoperative hemodynamic variations compared to general anesthesia with intubation and combined spinal-epidural anesthesia. In addition, patients receiving general anesthesia with LMA and nerve block also had significantly less postoperative pain and significantly better postoperative cognitive function than those receiving the other two anesthesia methods.

Hemodynamic instability during intubation and extubation, such as changes in heart rate and blood pressure, can increase the risk of vascular events, especially in elderly patients [7]. In our study, patients receiving the combined spinal-epidural anesthesia also had significantly greater hemodynamic variations compared to those receiving general anesthesia with LMA and nerve block. Spinal anesthesia can inhibit the sympathetic nerves, leading to peripheral vascular dilation and hypotension [8–10]. In addition, vagus nerve dominance and slow heart rate during spinal anesthesia may also result in significant hemodynamic variations. On the contrary, general anesthesia with LMA and nerve block has been shown to have less effect on hemodynamics [5, 11, 12].

Our study found that patients receiving general anesthesia with LMA and nerve block had generally less postoperative pain compared to those receiving general anesthesia with intubation or combined spinal-epidural anesthesia. Spinal anesthesia and nerve block both can

Table 4 Assessment of perioperative cognitive function

MMSE score	General anesthesia with intubation ($n = 25$)	Combined spinal-epidural anesthesia ($n = 25$)	General anesthesia with LMA/nerve block ($n = 25$)	P
Preoperative	28.56 ± 1.00	28.48 ± 0.77	28.64 ± 0.57	0.780
Postoperative 15 min	16.60 ± 1.35#*	22.68 ± 1.07*	24.72 ± 0.98	< 0.001
Postoperative 45 min	20.92 ± 1.22#*	24.96 ± 1.21*	27.48 ± 0.65	< 0.001
Postoperative 120 min	26.20 ± 1.15#*	28.20 ± 0.71	28.48 ± 0.59	< 0.001

MMSE Mini-Mental State Exam, *LMA* Laryngeal mask airway. #vs combined spinal-epidural anesthesia, $P < 0.001$; *vs general anesthesia with LMA/nerve block, $P < 0.001$.

Table 5 Perioperative respiratory infection.

	General anesthesia with intubation (n = 25)	Combined spinal-epidural anesthesia (n = 25)	General anesthesia with LMA/nerve block (n = 25)	P
Preoperative, n	0	0	0	
Postoperative 24 h, n	0	0	0	
Postoperative 48 h, n	2	1	0	0.769
Postoperative 72 h, n	3	1	0	0.315

LMA laryngeal mask airway.

effectively stop the peripheral afferent pain pathways and provide good analgesic effect. However, spinal anesthesia was not as good as lumbar plexus/sciatic nerve block in terms of analgesic effect and duration in our study. This might be explained by the relatively small doses of anesthetic agents used in spinal anesthesia, which was resulted from controlling the level of anesthesia.

The MMSE is widely used for screening cognitive dysfunction. It is easy to use and has a sensitivity of 87% and a specificity of 82% in diagnosing postoperative cognitive dysfunction [6, 13–15]. Our study found that general anesthesia with LMA and nerve block was associated with generally better postoperative cognitive function compared to general anesthesia with intubation and combined spinal-epidural anesthesia. In addition, combined spinal-epidural anesthesia was also superior to general anesthesia with intubation in terms of postoperative cognitive function. We speculate that the relatively poor postoperative cognitive function of patients receiving general anesthesia with intubation was associated with the residual systemic analgesics, which might inhibit the central nervous system [16–19]. In addition to analgesics, pain may also contribute to the development of postoperative cognitive dysfunction [20–22]. The relatively less postoperative pain in patients receiving general anesthesia LMA and nerve block might be a reason for the higher MMSE scores in this group of patients.

During postoperative 72 h, there were 3 cases of respiratory infection in the group of general anesthesia with intubation. However, none of the patients had respiratory infection in the general anesthesia with LMA/nerve block group, and only 1 patient had this condition in the combined spinal-epidural anesthesia group. Although no airway device was used in the combined spinal-epidural anesthesia group, still 1 case of respiratory infection occurred in this group. This might be related to the high level of anesthesia and respiratory paralysis. Intratracheal intubation is more invasive than LMA and may increase the risk of respiratory infection. Two meta-analysis showed that LMA is superior to, or as good as, intratracheal intubation regarding respiratory infection [23, 24].

Our study is not without limitations. First, the sample size is small. Second, our study is a single-center study and may lack representativeness. Third, data was collected from a short postoperative period.

In conclusion, general anesthesia with LMA and nerve block was associated with less postoperative pain and less disturbances on intraoperative hemodynamics and postoperative cognitive function for elderly patients undergoing intertrochanteric fracture surgeries. LMA might also be associated with reduced risks of respiratory infection.

Abbreviations

ASA: American Society of Anesthesiologists; LMA: Laryngeal mask airway; MMSE: Mini-Mental State Exam; VAS: Visual analog scale

Acknowledgements

Not applicable.

Authors' contributions

YL, MS, WL, and HY collected and analyzed the data. CY analyzed the data and drafted the manuscript. All authors read and approved the final manuscript.

Author details

[1]Department of Orthopedics, Chengdu Aerospace Hospital, Chengdu 610100, China. [2]Department of Anesthesia, Chengdu Aerospace Hospital, Chengdu 610100, China.

References

1. Gragasin FS, Bourque SL, Davidge ST. Vascular aging and hemodynamic stability in the intraoperative period. Front Physiol. 2012;3:74.
2. Li L, Wang Z. Ovarian Aging and Osteoporosis. Adv Exp Med Biol. 2018; 1086:199–215.
3. Major K, et al. Unknown osteoporosis in older patients admitted to post-acute rehabilitation. Aging Clin Exp Res. 2019. https://doi.org/10.1007/s40520-019-01302-7.
4. Neuman MD, et al. Anesthesia technique, mortality, and length of stay after hip fracture surgery. Jama. 2014;311(24):2508–17.
5. Chen WQ, et al. General laryngeal mask airway anesthesia with lumbar plexus and sciatic block provides better outcomes than general anesthesia and endotracheal intubation in elderly patients undergoing hip surgery. Arch Gerontol Geriatr. 2018;78:227–32.
6. Chi YL, et al. Evaluation of the postoperative cognitive dysfunction in elderly patients with general anesthesia. Eur Rev Med Pharmacol Sci. 2017; 21(6):1346–54.
7. Ezhar Y, D'Aragon F, Echave P. Hemodynamic responses to tracheal intubation with Bonfils compared to C-MAC videolaryngoscope: a randomized trial. BMC Anesthesiol. 2018;18(1):124.

8. Kondo Y, et al. Relationship between changes in regional cerebral blood volume and oxygenation and changes in cardiac output and systemic vascular resistance during spinal anesthesia in women undergoing cesarean section. J Anesth. 2019;33:579–86.
9. Hofhuizen C, et al. Spinal anesthesia-induced hypotension is caused by a decrease in stroke volume in elderly patients. Local Reg Anesth. 2019;12:19–26.
10. Saranteas T, et al. The Utility of Echocardiography for the Prediction of Spinal-Induced Hypotension in Elderly Patients: Inferior Vena Cava Assessment Is a Key Player. J Cardiothorac Vasc Anesth. 2019;33(9):2421–7.
11. Song Z, et al. Comparison of laryngeal mask airway and endotracheal intubation in gynecological cancer operation. Oncol Lett. 2019;17(2):2344–50.
12. Mao S, et al. A comparison between laryngeal mask airway and endotracheal intubation for anaesthesia in adult patients undergoing NUSS procedure. J Thorac Dis. 2018;10(6):3216–24.
13. Kilaru P, et al. Postoperative Cognitive Dysfunction in Indian Patients Undergoing Total Knee Replacement Under Spinal Anesthesia. Anesth Essays Res. 2018;12(1):116–8.
14. Konishi Y, et al. Postoperative cognitive dysfunction after sevoflurane or propofol general anaesthesia in combination with spinal anaesthesia for hip arthroplasty. Anaesth Intensive Care. 2018;46(6):596–600.
15. Kulason K, et al. Indication of Cognitive Change and Associated Risk Factor after Thoracic Surgery in the Elderly: A Pilot Study. Front Aging Neurosci. 2017;9:396.
16. Zhang J, et al. Analysis of postoperative cognitive dysfunction and influencing factors of dexmedetomidine anesthesia in elderly patients with colorectal cancer. Oncol Lett. 2019;18(3):3058–64.
17. Li LQ, et al. Effects of dexamethasone on post-operative cognitive dysfunction and delirium in adults following general anaesthesia: a meta-analysis of randomised controlled trials. BMC Anesthesiol. 2019;19(1):113.
18. Yan W, Mao H, Qiu P. Effects of different analgesia regimens on early post-operative cognitive dysfunction in elderly patients undergoing radical resection of cervical carcinoma. Exp Ther Med. 2019;18(2):1465–9.
19. Ezhevskaya AA, et al. Relationship among anesthesia technique, surgical stress, and cognitive dysfunction following spinal surgery: a randomized trial. J Neurosurg Spine. 2019:1–8. https://doi.org/10.3171/2019.4.SPINE184.
20. Wang Y, et al. The effects of postoperative pain and its management on postoperative cognitive dysfunction. Am J Geriatr Psychiatry. 2007;15(1):50–9.
21. Kraychete DC, et al. Postoperative persistent chronic pain: what do we know about prevention, risk factors, and treatment. Braz J Anesthesiol. 2016; 66(5):505–12.
22. Gu H, et al. Preoperational chronic pain impairs the attention ability before surgery and recovery of attention and memory abilities after surgery in non-elderly patients. J Pain Res. 2019;12:151–8.
23. Li L, et al. The impact of laryngeal mask versus other airways on perioperative respiratory adverse events in children: A systematic review and meta-analysis of randomized controlled trials. Int J Surg. 2019;64:40–8.
24. de Carvalho ALR, et al. Laryngeal Mask Airway Versus Other Airway Devices for Anesthesia in Children With an Upper Respiratory Tract Infection: A Systematic Review and Meta-analysis of Respiratory Complications. Anesth Analg. 2018;127(4):941–50.

13

Bilateral thoracic paravertebral block combined with general anesthesia vs. general anesthesia for patients undergoing off-pump coronary artery bypass grafting

Lixin Sun[1†], Qiujie Li[1†], Qiang Wang[1], Fuguo Ma[1], Wei Han[2*] and Mingshan Wang[1]

Abstract

Background: Whether thoracic paravertebral block (PVB) is useful in patients undergoing off-pump coronary artery bypass grafting (OPCABG) remains unknown. This study aimed to investigate the feasibility of bilateral PVB combined with general anesthesia (GA) in patients undergoing OPCABG.

Methods: This feasibility study assessed 60 patients scheduled for OPCABG at the Qingdao Municipal Hospital in 2016–2017. Patients were randomly assigned to receive nerve stimulator-guided bilateral PVB combined with GA (PVB + GA) or GA alone (*n* = 30/group). Patients were asked to rate rest and cough pain hourly after the surgery. The primary endpoint was the visual analogue scale (VAS) pain score within 48 h postoperatively. Secondary endpoints were rescue analgesia and morphine consumption, fentanyl dose within 48 h postoperatively, as well as operative time, time to extubation, intensive care unit (ICU) stay, hospital stay and other postoperative adverse events.

Results: Both rest and cough pains were lower in the PVB + GA group at 12, 24, 36, and 48 h after surgery compared with the GA group. There were fewer patients who needed rescue analgesia in the PVB + GA group at 12 and 24 h than in the GA group. Morphine consumptions at 24 and 48 h were lower in the PVB + GA group compared with the GA group. Time to extubation ($P = 0.035$) and ICU stay ($P = 0.028$) were shorter in the PVB + GA group compared with the GA group. AEs showed no differences between the two groups.

Conclusions: Nerve stimulator-guided bilateral thoracic PVB combined with GA in OPCABG is associated with a reduced rescue analgesia and morphine consumption, compared to GA.

Keywords: Nerve block, Thoracic vertebra, Anesthesia, General

Background

Off-pump coronary artery bypass grafting (OPCABG) is a type of bypass surgery performed on beating heart, without cardiopulmonary bypass (CPB). OPCABG has been developed in Russia mainly to avoid the complications of CPB [1]. The popularity of OPCABG has been declining over the past years in developed countries, but the rate of OPCABG is currently increasing in some countries such as China and India [2]. Nevertheless, the benefits of OPCABG are debatable [3] and it could benefit only some selected patients [4–6].

Thoracic epidural anesthesia (TEA) has been successfully applied in heart surgery and confirmed to have a myocardial protective effect [7–10]. Nevertheless, a cardiac surgery is usually performed in patients receiving anticoagulant therapy and may be associated with an increased risk of an epidural hematoma. The incidence of epidural hematoma has been estimated to be between 1:150,000 and 1:1528 [11]. Furthermore, TEA may also be

* Correspondence: sallyhan1@163.com
†Lixin Sun and Qiujie Li contributed equally to this work.
[2]Department of Respiratory Medicine, Qingdao Municipal Hospital, 1 Jiaozhou Road, Qingdao 266011, Shandong, China

complicated by hypotension, urinary retention and pulmonary complications related to respiratory muscle blockade in some patients [12, 13]. Although a clinical study [14] has revealed important benefits for TEA in cardiac surgery, its use is still debatable because of the potential risks.

Recently, there has been increasing interest in alternative regional techniques, particularly thoracic paravertebral block (PVB), which offers optimal pain control with a better side effects profile [15, 16]. Compared with TEA, PVB can provide comparable pain relief, fewer complications, faster recovery, shorter hospitalization, and lower incidence of postoperative chronic pain [17, 18].

The safety and efficacy of segmental PVB has been reported for postoperative analgesia after modified minimally invasive Heart-Port access cardiac surgery [19], but whether bilateral thoracic paravertebral block can be safely and effectively used in OPCABG remains unknown. We hypothesized that PVB could be useful in patients undergoing OPCABG. Therefore, this study aimed to investigate the feasibility of bilateral PVB combined with general anesthesia (GA) in patients undergoing OPCABG, assessing pain (visual analogue scale [VAS] as primary endpoint and rescue analgesia and morphine consumption within 48 h postoperatively, operative time, dose of fentanyl, time to extubation, intensive care unit (ICU) stay, hospital stay, intraoperative parameters (e.g. bradycardia, tachycardia, hypotension and hypertension) and postoperative adverse events (AEs) as secondary endpoints. This was a pilot study comparing PVB combined with GA vs. GA alone in order to observe the advantages and disadvantages of PVB.

Methods

Patients and study design

This was a feasibility study of patients scheduled to undergo OPCABG at the Qingdao Municipal Hospital between July 2016 and May 2017. All patients received preoperative physical examination and plain X-ray. The inclusion criteria were: 1) planned to undergo OPCABG; 2) 50–75 years old; 3) body mass index (BMI) < 30 kg/m^2; 4) ASA II or III; and 5) elective surgery. The exclusion criteria were: 1) spine malformation; 2) vertebral space-occupying lesion; 3) infection at the site of paravertebral injection; 4) left ventricular ejection fraction (LVEF) < 40%; 5) endocrine disease; 6) metabolic disease; 7) extracorporeal circulation; 8) allergies; 9) severe hepatic (alanine transaminase [ALT] or aspartate transaminase [AST] > 3 times the upper limit of normal) or renal dysfunction (serum creatinine [SCr] > 178 mmol/L and blood urea nitrogen [BUN] > 9 mmol/L); 10) valvular disease; 11) intra-aortic balloon pump; or 12) neurologic or psychotic disorders. The study was approved by the ethics committee of Qingdao Municipal Hospital (No. 20140806–1). Each patient provided a written informed consent.

Randomization and blinding

The patients were randomized using sequential sealed envelopes prepared by an independent statistician using a computer-generated random number table. Patients were randomly divided into two groups: the bilateral thoracic PVB combined with GA group (PVB + GA group), and the GA group (GA group). The postoperative assessors were blinded to grouping.

Anesthesia

All patients received their usual medication on the day of operation, followed by premedication with intramuscular morphine 0.1 mg/kg and midazolam 0.05 mg/kg. Upon arrival in the operating room, 100% oxygen was administered, and peripheral vein Ringer lactate solution was infused at 6–8 ml/kg/h.

The patients were monitored with radial artery pressure, heart rate (HR), electrocardiogram (ECG), oxygen saturation (SpO_2), end-tidal carbon dioxide ($ETCO_2$), and other hemodynamic parameters using a Datex multi-parameter monitor (GE Healthcare, Waukesha, WI, USA). The flow-directed pulmonary artery catheter and central venous catheter (Arrow International Inc., Asheboro, NC, USA) were placed through the right internal jugular vein in both groups.

In the PVB + GA group, bilateral thoracic PVB was performed according to the nerve stimulator-guided technique [20–23] combined with the loss of resistance technique for proper location of the paravertebral space (PVS). Briefly, patients in the right lateral decubitus position received intradermal lidocaine (1%) at T_{3-4} PVS. An insulated needle attached to a nerve stimulator was advanced between the transverse process of the third and fourth vertebrae, and the current intensity of the nerve stimulator was set to 2–5 mA during initial simulation, and subsequently reduced to 0.4–0.8 mA. PVS could also be identified with the "loss-of-resistance" technique to ensure technical success [23, 24], but neuromuscular stimulation was the primary criterion in cases in which loss of resistance could not be felt. After ensuring the absence of blood, air, or cerebrospinal fluid, a 20G catheter was passed through the needle, with 3 cm of the catheter left in the PVS.

After the catheters had been secured, the patient was turned onto the supine position. 0.375% of ropivacaine 20 ml were injected by 2 time with 5 min interval (5 ml in the first time and 15 ml in the second time), followed by 0.375% of ropivacaine infused at 5 ml/h until 30 min before the end of operation [25]. Analgesia block levels were tested by the pinprick method at the middle of the chest. If analgesia block level was less than 2 dermatomes, the patient was withdrawn. Bilateral thoracic PVB was not performed in the GA group.

All patients in both groups received GA. GA was induced by midazolam 0.05 mg/kg, etomidate 0.3 mg/kg, fentanyl 4 µg/kg, and vecuronium 0.1 mg/kg. After endotracheal intubation, patients were mechanically ventilated to maintain $ETCO_2$ between 35 and 40 mmHg. The nasopharyngeal temperature and urine volume were monitored. Warming blankets were used to maintain the nasopharyngeal temperature at 36.5–37.5 °C. Anesthesia was maintained by sevoflurane 1 MAC. Fentanyl 10–20 µg/kg and vecuronium 0.1 mg/kg were given when indicated. At the end of the operation, the catheter was removed in the PVB + GA group in order to observe the effect of PVB on postoperative morphine use. All patients in both groups were transferred to the intensive care unit (ICU) without extubation. Beginning at the end of the operation, all patients in both groups received patient-controlled analgesia (PCA) using morphine (1 mg/ml) for 48 h at a loading dose of 2 mg, continuous infusion dose of 0.5 mg/h, bolus of 1 mg, locking time of 10 min, and maximum dose of 20 mg/4 h.

Assessments

Using the visual analogue scale (VAS; 0 mm = no pain, 100 mm = worst pain imaginable), the patients were asked to rate their pain at rest and during coughing every hour after their arrival and return to consciousness in ICU. If the VAS score was > 5 at rest, rescue analgesia was given with morphine 5 mg IV.

Intraoperative adverse events (AEs), including bradycardia, tachycardia, hypotension, hypertension, and postoperative AEs were recorded. Bradycardia was defined as a heart rate < 50 bpm and treated with intravenous atropine 0.01 mg/kg. Tachycardia was defined as a heart rate > 90 bpm and treated with intravenous esmolol 20 mg. Hypotension was defined as a 20% decrease in systolic blood pressure (SBP) from baseline and treated with intravenous noradrenaline 5 µg. Hypertension was defined as a 20% increase in SBP from baseline and treated with intravenous urapidil hydrochloride 10 mg. All hemodynamic drugs were repeated as required.

Endpoints

The primary endpoint was the pain scores within 48 h postoperatively. The secondary endpoints were the rescue analgesia and morphine consumption, dose of fentanyl within 48 h postoperatively, as well as operative time, time to extubation (defined as the time from the end of surgery to the extubation), ICU stay, hospital stay and postoperative AEs (including bradycardia, tachycardia, hypotension and hypertension).

Statistical analysis

Since this was a pilot study, the sample size was estimated by referring to similar studies [26] rather than an accurate calculation. Continuous data (age, BMI, morphine consumption, operative time, dose of fentanyl, time to extubation, ICU stay, and hospital stay) were expressed as mean ± standard deviation (SD) and analyzed using Student t test for intergroup comparisons. Categorical data (gender, ASA score, diabetes mellitus, chronic obstructive pulmonary disease, renal dysfunction, hypertension, rescue analgesia, and intraoperative and postoperative AEs) were expressed as frequency (percentage) and analyzed using the chi-square test. Ranked data (rest pain score and cough pain score) were expressed as median [IQR] and analyzed using the Wilcoxon rank sum test. All variables, except for pain scores, were baseline characteristics or secondary endpoints. Statistical analysis was performed using PASW Statistics 18.0 (SPSS Inc., Chicago, NY, USA). Two-sided P-values < 0.05 were considered statistically significant.

Results

Patients

Figure 1 presents the patient flowchart. One hundred and fifty-two patients met the inclusion criteria and 92 of them were excluded from the study, including 27 patients due to BMI over 30 kg/m^2, 18 patients due to LVEF < 40%, 12 patients due to severe hepatic or renal dysfunction, 10 patients due to carotid artery stenosis or other vascular diseases, 6 patients due to neurologic disorders and 19 patients due to withdrawal of consent. Sixty patients underwent randomization, with 30 patients in each group. One patient was withdrawn from the study due to the failure of PVB on one side and received GA alone. Table 1 presents the baseline characteristics of the patients.

Postoperative pain

Both rest and cough pain scores were lower in the PVB + GA group at 12, 24, 36, and 48 h after surgery compared with the GA group (rest pain: 12 h: 3 [2, 3] vs. 3 [3, 3], $P = 0.004$; 24 h: 3 [2, 3] vs. 3 [3, 4], $P = 0.007$; 36 h: 3 [2, 3] vs. 3 [2, 4], $P = 0.018$; 48 h: 2 [2, 3] vs. 3 [3, 4], $P = 0.010$; cough pain: 12 h: 4 [3, 4] vs. 4 [4, 5], P = 0.007; 24 h: 3 [3, 5] vs. 4 [4, 5], $P = 0.017$; 36 h: 4 [3, 5] vs. 5 [3, 6], $P = 0.048$; 48 h: 4 [3, 4] vs. 5 [3, 6], $P = 0.023$). There were fewer patients who received rescue analgesia at 12 and 24 h in the PVB + GA group than in the GA group (12 h: 0% vs. 16.7%, $P = 0.034$; 24 h: 3.4% vs. 20.0%, $P = 0.049$). The number of patients who received rescue analgesia at 36 and 48 h in the two groups were similar. Morphine consumption at 24 and 48 h was lower in the PVB + GA group compared with the GA group (24 h:

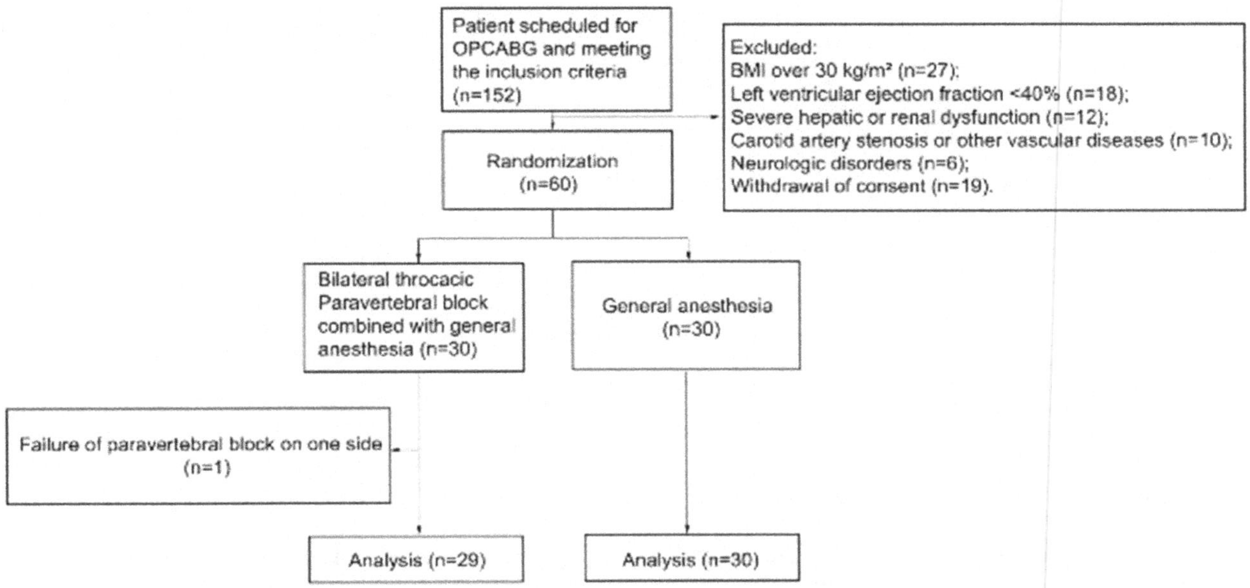

Fig. 1 Study flowchart. BMI, body mass index; OPCABG, off-pump coronary artery bypass grafting

25.6 ± 7.3 vs. 30.7 ± 9.0 mg, $P = 0.033$; 48 h: 47.6 ± 13.5 vs. 54.3 ± 16.1 mg, $P = 0.041$) (Table 2).

Clinical characteristics

Table 3 shows that the time to extubation was shorter in the PVB + GA group compared with the GA group (5.8 ± 1.5 vs. 7.3 ± 1.7 h, $P = 0.035$), as well as the ICU stay (16.3 ± 3.7 vs. 20.2 ± 4.1 h, $P = 0.028$). The dose of fentanyl was lower in the PVB + GA group compared with the GA group (1.2 ± 0.2 vs. 1.5 ± 0.3 mg, $P = 0.022$). There were no differences in operative time and hospital stay between the two groups.

Table 1 Baseline characteristics of the patients

Characteristics	PVB + GA (n = 29)	GA (n = 30)
Male, n (%)	23 (79.3)	21 (70.0)
Age (years)	68.2 ± 10.5	70.6 ± 11.7
BMI (kg/m^2)	23.0 ± 6.6	24.2 ± 5.1
ASA (II/III)	7/10	9/9
LVEF (%)	55.8 ± 8.1	56.6 ± 10.7
DM, n (%)	13 (44.8)	15 (50.0)
COPD, n (%)	3 (10.3)	5 (16.7)
Renal dysfunction, n (%)	3 (10.3)	2 (6.7)
Hypertension, n (%)	20 (69.0)	18 (60.0)

PVB Paravertebral block, *GA* General anesthesia, *BMI* Body mass index, *ASA* American Standards Association, *LVEF* Left ventricular ejection fraction, *DM* Diabetes mellitus, *COPD* Chronic obstructive pulmonary disease. There were no significant differences between the two groups

Adverse events

Table 4 presents the intraoperative and postoperative AEs in the two groups. The occurrences of tachycardia (3.4% vs. 27.8%, P = 0.035) and hypertension (0% vs. 16.7%, $P = 0.008$) were lower in the PVB + GA group compared with the GA group. There were no differences in the occurrences of bradycardia, hypotension, and postoperative AEs between the two groups.

Discussion

It is unknown whether thoracic PVB can be used in patients undergoing OPCABG. Therefore, this pilot study aimed to investigate the feasibility of bilateral PVB combined with GA in patients undergoing OPCABG. The results showed that nerve stimulator-guided bilateral thoracic PVB combined with GA could be efficient in OPCABG to provide high-quality analgesia. However, these findings should be interpreted with caution as non-anticoagulated patients were not assessed in this study. In addition, the risk of AEs is rather difficult to estimate, especially in case of small sample size.

Thoracic spinal nerve block has been clinically used since as early as 1905 and has become more popular in recent years due to a number of advantages: simple application, low failure rate, satisfactory analgesia, and less influence on respiration and circulation [26–28]. Previous studies reported unilateral thoracic nerve block combined with GA applied as analgesia in minimally invasive direct coronary artery bypass (MIDCAB) [29–31]. Satisfyingly, unilateral thoracic nerve block combined with GA exhibited remarkable efficacy in postoperative pain relief, while maintaining stable hemodynamics and

Table 2 Comparison of VAS scores, rescue analgesia and morphine consumption between groups

Variable	Group	n	PCA 12 h	PCA 24 h	PCA 36 h	PCA 48 h
Rest pain	PVB + GA	29	3 [2, 3]	3 [2, 3]	3 [2, 3]	2 [2, 3]
	GA	30	3 [3, 3]	3 [3, 4]	3 [2, 4]	3 [3, 4]
	P		0.015	0.023	0.026	0.042
Cough pain	PVB + GA	29	3 [2, 3]	3 [2, 3]	3 [2, 3]	2 [2, 3]
	GA	30	3 [3, 3]	3 [3, 4]	3 [2, 4]	3 [3, 4]
	P		0.023	0.030	0.027	0.034
Rescue analgesia	PVB + GA	29	0 (0)	1 (3.4)	3 (10.3)	2 (6.9)
	GA	30	5 (16.7)	6 (20.0)	6 (20.0)	7 (23.3)
	P		0.034	0.049	0.302	0.079
Morphine consumption	PVB + GA	29	–	25.6 ± 7.3	–	47.6 ± 13.5
	GA	30	–	30.7 ± 9.0	–	54.3 ± 16.1
	P			0.033		0.041

VAS Visual analogue scale, *PCA* Patient-controlled analgesia, *PVB* Paravertebral block, *GA* General anesthesia

less postoperative complications [29–31]. In this study, both rest and cough pain scores were lower in patients undergoing OPCABG and fewer patients received rescue analgesia within 24 h postoperatively in the PVB + GA group compared with the GA group. However, it should be noted that similar numbers of patients received rescue analgesia at 36 h and 48 h in both groups. These findings indicate some improvement in analgesia with PVB + GA compared with GA alone. Therefore, PVB may exert beneficial effects in patients undergoing OPCABG, which deserves further investigation.

Our study is the first comparative study to evaluate bilateral preoperative thoracic paravertebral block applied to patients undergoing OPCABG. We found that the thoracic nerve block segment was about 5 dermatomes in the PVB + GA group, which is in accordance with the imaging results from Christopher et al. [25] Our results also showed that a lower dosage of fentanyl was used during the operation and less PCA morphine was consumed at 24 and 48 h postoperatively. The extubation time and length of stay in the ICU were shorter in the PVB + GA group, but these factors have little clinical impact, if any.

As is well known, pneumothorax, puncturing of blood vessels, local hematoma, hypotension, and epidural block are common complications of thoracic PVB [32, 33]. Fortunately, no local anesthetic toxicity event occurred in the present study. The rate of AEs was not different in both groups. It is worth noting that the biggest PVS is close to the T_{1-2} or T_{2-3} intervertebral space, so it is safest to puncture at this site, as the risk for pneumothorax will be lower due to the greater distance between the parietal pleura and pyramis. That is also the reason why we chose T_{3-4} as the puncture point, which is close to T_{1-2} or T_{2-3} PVS, as it increased puncture reliability and reduced AE occurrence. In addition, anesthesia was terminated at 30 min before the end of the operation in this study, for the following reasons: 1) to achieve better postoperative analgesia; 2) to assess safety issues due to a high level of monitoring after cardiac surgery; and 3) since 15 ml of drug was injected on each side, PVB was

Table 3 Clinical characteristics of the patients

Variable	PVB + GA (n = 29)	GA (n = 30)	P*
Operative time (min)	168 ± 23	176 ± 28	0.279
Dose of fentanyl (mg)	1.2 ± 0.2	1.5 ± 0.3	0.022
Time to extubation (h)	5.8 ± 1.5	7.3 ± 1.7	0.035
ICU stay (h)	16.3 ± 3.7	20.2 ± 4.1	0.028
Hospital stay (d)	9.6 ± 2.1	10.1 ± 2.3	0.459

PVB Paravertebral block, *GA* General anesthesia, *ICU* Intensive care unit. *All variables were analyzed using Student t test

Table 4 Intraoperative and postoperative AEs

Variable, n (%)	PVB + GA (n = 29)	GA (n = 30)	P*
Intraoperative AE			
Bradycardia	5 (17.2)	3 (10.0)	0.334
Tachycardia	1 (3.4)	5 (27.8)	0.035
Hypotension	13 (44.8)	10 (33.3)	0.262
Hypertension	0 (0)	5 (16.7)	0.008
Postoperative AE			
Nausea	1 (3.4)	3 (10.0)	0.612
Vomiting	0 (0)	1 (3.3)	1.000
Pulmonary infection	0 (0)	1 (3.3)	1.000
Atelectasis	1 (3.4)	1 (3.3)	1.000
Reoperation	0 (0)	1 (3.3)	1.000
Paresthesia	1 (3.4)	0 (0)	0.492

AE Adverse event, *PVB* Paravertebral block, *GA* General anesthesia. *All variables were analyzed using chi-square test prone to exert minimal impact on hemodynamics, ensuring stable circulation.

Hypotension is an AE that occurs in about 4% of pediatric patients [32]. In breast cancer surgery, PVB did not induce hypotension in any of the patients [34, 35]. Similar results were observed in healthy volunteers [36]. Nevertheless, PVB has a lower risk of hypotension than thoracic epidural analgesia [26, 37, 38]. In the present study, no hypotension occurred in the PVB + GA group, suggesting that hypotension is not a major risk in these patients. Nevertheless, this could vary among different populations of patients with different conditions. This warrants additional study.

In the present study, neuromuscular stimulation was used for PVB instead of the ultrasound-guided approach, which is now considered the best approach for PVB [39]. Nevertheless, neuromuscular stimulation is still a valid approach for PVB [22, 23, 40]. China is a developing country that is still adapting to modern approaches. Our hospital has just purchased the ultrasonography (USG) equipment, and the Anesthesiologist have not yet grasped the USG-guided technique. In addition, the learning curve of USG is steep [41]. Hence, even the nerve stimulator has been used in our hospital for many years, the nerve stimulator-guided technique was adopted in the present study until recently.

The present study is not without limitations. Despite the randomization, blinding, and control group, this was a pilot study with a small sample size from a single center. Since this was a pilot study, the sample size was estimated by referring to similar studies [26] rather than accurate calculation. In addition, our reduced sample does not allow any conclusions to be drawn about the safety of the procedure, whether for the morbidity of the technique or for the toxicity of local anesthetics. Our future multicenter randomized controlled trial will have a rigorous sample size calculation based on the results of the present study. Additional studies are necessary to confirm the effect of PVB for OPCABG.

Conclusions

In conclusion, nerve stimulator-guided bilateral thoracic PVB combined with GA could be used efficiently in OPCABG with reduced rescue analgesia and morphine consumption. Additional studies are necessary to examine the potential AEs.

Abbreviations

AE: Adverse event; ALT: Alanine transaminase; ANOVA: Analysis of variance; AST: Aspartate transaminase; BMI: Body mass index; BUN: Blood urea nitrogen; CI: Cardiac index; CPB: Cardiopulmonary bypass; CVP: Central venous pressure; ECG: Electrocardiogram; $ETCO_2$: End-tidal carbon dioxide; GA: General anesthesia; HR: Heart rate; ICU: Intensive care unit; LVEF: Left ventricular ejection fraction; MAP: Mean arterial pressure; MIDCAB: Minimally invasive direct coronary artery bypass; MPAP: Mean pulmonary arterial pressure; OPCABG: Off-pump coronary artery bypass grafting; PCA: Patient-controlled analgesia; PCWP: Pulmonary capillary wedge pressure; PVB: Paravertebral block; PVRI: Pulmonary vascular resistance index; PVS: Paravertebral space; SBP: Systolic blood pressure; SCr: Serum creatinine; SD: Standard deviation; SpO_2: Oxygen saturation; SVRI: Systemic vascular resistance index; TEA: Thoracic epidural anesthesia; USG: ultrasonography; VAS: Visual analogue scale

Acknowledgements
Not applicable.

Authors' contributions

LXS carried out the studies, and drafted the manuscript. QJL, QW and FGM performed the statistical analysis and helped to collect the data. WH and MSW helped to revise the manuscript. All authors read and approved the final manuscript.

Author details
[1]Department of Anesthesiology, Qingdao Municipal Hospital, Qingdao 266011, Shandong, China. [2]Department of Respiratory Medicine, Qingdao Municipal Hospital, 1 Jiaozhou Road, Qingdao 266011, Shandong, China.

References

1. Jensen BO, Hughes P, Rasmussen LS, Pedersen PU, Steinbruchel DA. Cognitive outcomes in elderly high-risk patients after off-pump versus conventional coronary artery bypass grafting: a randomized trial. Circulation. 2006;113:2790–5.
2. Taggart DP. Off-pump coronary artery bypass grafting (OPCABG)-a 'personal' European perspective. J Thorac Dis. 2016;8:S829–S31.
3. Moller CH, Penninga L, Wetterslev J, Steinbruchel DA, Gluud C. Off-pump versus on-pump coronary artery bypass grafting for ischaemic heart disease. Cochrane Database Syst Rev. 2012;14:CD007224.
4. Shroyer AL, Grover FL, Hattler B, Collins JF, McDonald GO, Kozora E, et al. On-pump versus off-pump coronary-artery bypass surgery. N Engl J Med. 2009;361:1827–37.
5. Lamy A, Devereaux PJ, Prabhakaran D, Taggart DP, Hu S, Paolasso E, et al. Effects of off-pump and on-pump coronary-artery bypass grafting at 1 year. N Engl J Med. 2013;368:1179–88.
6. Diegeler A, Borgermann J, Kappert U, Breuer M, Boning A, Ursulescu A, et al. Off-pump versus on-pump coronary-artery bypass grafting in elderly patients. N Engl J Med. 2013;368:1189–98.
7. Neskovic V, Milojevic P. High thoracic epidural anesthesia in coronary surgery. Med Pregl. 2003;56:152–6.
8. Palomero Rodriguez MA, Suarez Gonzalo L, Villar Alvarez F, Varela Crespo C, Moreno Gomez Limon I, Criado Jimenez A. Thoracic epidural anesthesia decreases C-reactive protein levels in patients undergoing elective coronary artery bypass graft surgery with cardiopulmonary bypass. Minerva Anestesiol. 2008;74:619–26.
9. Kessler P, Neidhart G, Bremerich DH, Aybek T, Dogan S, Lischke V, et al. High thoracic epidural anesthesia for coronary artery bypass grafting using two different surgical approaches in conscious patients. Anesth Analg. 2002;95: 791–7 table of contents.
10. Salvi L, Sisillo E, Brambillasca C, Juliano G, Salis S, Marino MR. High thoracic epidural anesthesia for off-pump coronary artery bypass surgery. J Cardiothorac Vasc Anesth. 2004;18:256–62.
11. Ho AM, Chung DC, Joynt GM. Neuraxial blockade and hematoma in cardiac surgery: estimating the risk of a rare adverse event that has not (yet) occurred. Chest. 2000;117:551–5.
12. Conlon NP, Shaw AD, Grichnik KP. Postthoracotomy paravertebral analgesia: will it replace epidural analgesia? Anesthesiol Clin. 2008;26:369–80 viii.
13. Olivier JF, Bracco D, Nguyen P, Le N, Noiseux N, Hemmerling T, et al. A novel approach for pain management in cardiac surgery via median sternotomy: bilateral single-shot paravertebral blocks. Heart Surg Forum. 2007;10:E357–62.
14. Hemmerling TM, Le N, Olivier JF, Choiniere JL, Basile F, Prieto I. Immediate extubation after aortic valve surgery using high thoracic epidural analgesia or opioid-based analgesia. J Cardiothorac Vasc Anesth. 2005;19:176–81.
15. Richardson J, Lonnqvist PA. Thoracic paravertebral block. Br J Anaesth. 1998; 81:230–8.
16. Tighe SQ. Paravertebral block. Anaesthesia. 2002;57:511–2 author reply 2.
17. Joshi GP, Bonnet F, Shah R, Wilkinson RC, Camu F, Fischer B, et al. A systematic review of randomized trials evaluating regional techniques for postthoracotomy analgesia. Anesth Analg. 2008;107:1026–40.

18. Davies RG, Myles PS, Graham JM. A comparison of the analgesic efficacy and side-effects of paravertebral vs epidural blockade for thoracotomy--a systematic review and meta-analysis of randomized trials. Br J Anaesth. 2006;96:418–26.
19. Carmona P, Llagunes J, Casanova I, Mateo E, Canovas S, Martin E, et al. Continuous paravertebral analgesia versus intravenous analgesia in minimally invasive cardiac surgery by mini-thoracotomy. Rev Esp Anestesiol Reanim. 2012;59:476–82.
20. Wheeler LJ. Peripheral nerve stimulation end-point for thoracic paravertebral block. Br J Anaesth. 2001;86:598–9.
21. Boezaart AP, Raw RM. Continuous thoracic paravertebral block for major breast surgery. Reg Anesth Pain Med. 2006;31:470–6.
22. Naja MZ, Ziade MF, Lonnqvist PA. General anaesthesia combined with bilateral paravertebral blockade (T5-6) vs. general anaesthesia for laparoscopic cholecystectomy: a prospective, randomized clinical trial. Eur J Anaesthesiol. 2004;21:489–95.
23. Naja ZM, Raf M, El Rajab M, Ziade FM, Al Tannir MA, Lonnqvist PA. Nerve stimulator-guided paravertebral blockade combined with sevoflurane sedation versus general anesthesia with systemic analgesia for postherniorrhaphy pain relief in children: a prospective randomized trial. Anesthesiology. 2005;103:600–5.
24. Canto M, Sanchez MJ, Casas MA, Bataller ML. Bilateral paravertebral blockade for conventional cardiac surgery. Anaesthesia. 2003;58:365–70.
25. Harle CC, Su G. Paravertebral analgesia for cardiac surgery. Tech Reg Anesth Pain Manag. 2008;12:57–63.
26. Baidya DK, Khanna P, Maitra S. Analgesic efficacy and safety of thoracic paravertebral and epidural analgesia for thoracic surgery: a systematic review and meta-analysis. Interact Cardiovasc Thorac Surg. 2014;18:626–35.
27. Thavaneswaran P, Rudkin GE, Cooter RD, Moyes DG, Perera CL, reports MGJB. Paravertebral block for anesthesia: a systematic review. Anesth Analg. 2010;110:1740–4.
28. Junior Ade P, Erdmann TR, Santos TV, Brunharo GM, Filho CT, Losso MJ, et al. Comparison between continuous thoracic epidural and paravertebral blocks for postoperative analgesia in patients undergoing thoracotomy: systematic review. Braz J Anesthesiol. 2013;63:433–42.
29. Dhole S, Mehta Y, Saxena H, Juneja R, Trehan N. Comparison of continuous thoracic epidural and paravertebral blocks for postoperative analgesia after minimally invasive direct coronary artery bypass surgery. J Cardiothorac Vasc Anesth. 2001;15:288–92.
30. Mehta Y, Arora D, Sharma KK, Mishra Y, Wasir H, Trehan N. Comparison of continuous thoracic epidural and paravertebral block for postoperative analgesia after robotic-assisted coronary artery bypass surgery. Ann Card Anaesth. 2008;11:91–6.
31. Mehta Y, Swaminathan M, Mishra Y, Trehan N. A comparative evaluation of intrapleural and thoracic epidural analgesia for postoperative pain relief after minimally invasive direct coronary artery bypass surgery. J Cardiothorac Vasc Anesth. 1998;12:162–5.
32. Naja Z, Lonnqvist PA. Somatic paravertebral nerve blockade. Incidence of failed block and complications. Anaesthesia. 2001;56:1184–8.
33. Richardson J, Lonnqvist PA, Naja Z. Bilateral thoracic paravertebral block: potential and practice. Br J Anaesth. 2011;106:164–71.
34. Weltz CR, Greengrass RA, Lyerly HK. Ambulatory surgical management of breast carcinoma using paravertebral block. Ann Surg. 1995;222:19–26.
35. Pusch F, Freitag H, Weinstabl C, Obwegeser R, Huber E, Wildling E. Single-injection paravertebral block compared to general anaesthesia in breast surgery. Acta Anaesthesiol Scand. 1999;43:770–4.
36. Saito T, Den S, Cheema SP, Tanuma K, Carney E, Carlsson C, et al. A single-injection, multi-segmental paravertebral block-extension of somatosensory and sympathetic block in volunteers. Acta Anaesthesiol Scand. 2001;45:30–3.
37. Koyyalamudi VB, Arulkumar S, Yost BR, Fox CJ, Urman RD, Kaye AD. Supraclavicular and paravertebral blocks: are we underutilizing these regional techniques in perioperative analgesia? Best Pract Res Clin Anaesthesiol. 2014;28:127–38.
38. Bigeleisen PE, Goehner N. Novel approaches in pain management in cardiac surgery. Curr Opin Anaesthesiol. 2015;28:89–94.
39. Okajima H, Tanaka O, Ushio M, Higuchi Y, Nagai Y, Iijima K, et al. Ultrasound-guided continuous thoracic paravertebral block provides comparable analgesia and fewer episodes of hypotension than continuous epidural block after lung surgery. J Anesth. 2015;29:373–8.
40. Naja MZ, Ziade MF, Lonnqvist PA. Nerve-stimulator guided paravertebral blockade vs. general anaesthesia for breast surgery: a prospective randomized trial. Eur J Anaesthesiol. 2003;20:897–903.
41. Stolz LA, Cappa AR, Minckler MR, Stolz U, Wyatt RG, Binger CW, Amini R, Adhikari S. Prospective evaluation of the learning curve for ultrasound-guided peripheral intravenous catheter placement. J Vasc Access. 2016;17:366–70.

14

Anesthesiology and cognitive impairment: A narrative review of current clinical literature

Jillian C. Belrose* and Ruediger R. Noppens*

Abstract

Background: The impact of general anesthesia on cognitive impairment is controversial and complex. A large body of evidence supports the association between exposure to surgery under general anesthesia and development of delayed neurocognitive recovery in a subset of patients. Existing literature continues to debate whether these short-term effects on cognition can be attributed to anesthetic agents themselves, or whether other variables are causative of the observed changes in cognition. Furthermore, there is conflicting data on the relationship between anesthesia exposure and the development of long-term neurocognitive disorders, or development of incident dementia in the patient population with normal preoperative cognitive function. Patients with pre-existing cognitive impairment present a unique set of anesthetic considerations, including potential medication interactions, challenges with cooperation during assessment and non-general anesthesia techniques, and the possibility that pre-existing cognitive impairment may impart a susceptibility to further cognitive dysfunction.

Main body: This review highlights landmark and recent studies in the field, and explores potential mechanisms involved in perioperative cognitive disorders (also known as postoperative cognitive dysfunction, POCD). Specifically, we will review clinical and preclinical evidence which implicates alterations to tau protein, inflammation, calcium dysregulation, and mitochondrial dysfunction. As our population ages and the prevalence of Alzheimer's disease and other forms of dementia continues to increase, we require a greater understanding of potential modifiable factors that impact perioperative cognitive impairment.

Conclusions: Future research should aim to further characterize the associated risk factors and determine whether certain anesthetic approaches or other interventions may lower the potential risk which may be conferred by anesthesia and/or surgery in susceptible individuals.

Keywords: Alzheimer's disease, Dementia, Anesthesia, Postoperative cognitive dysfunction, Neurocognitive disorder, Elderly, Sevoflurane, Desflurane, Isoflurane, Propofol

Background

A growing body of evidence has explored the whether exposure to anesthesia might cause temporary or long-term cognitive dysfunction. The specific impact of anesthesia on individuals with pre-existing cognitive impairment is also gaining attention. Dementia presents with impaired learning, memory, and reasoning. The worldwide prevalence of dementia in 2015 was 46.8 million, with a projected increase to 131.5 million by 2050 [1]. The estimated worldwide cost of dementia in 2015 was US$818 billion [2]. Dementia impacts length of hospital stay, morbidity, and mortality [3, 4]. Alzheimer's disease (AD) accounts for 60–80% of dementia cases [3]. The projected increased prevalence suggests that anesthesiologists will be confronted with managing more patients diagnosed with AD and other forms of dementia. A greater understanding of the relationship between cognitive impairment with surgery and anesthesia is critical to guiding our clinical practice. This review will summarize key existing evidence in individuals with and without pre-existing cognitive impairment and will

* Correspondence: rnoppens@uwo.ca
Department of Anesthesia & Perioperative Medicine, Western University, London Health Sciences Center, 339 Windermere Rd, London, ON N6A 5A5, Canada

review potential pathways which may play a role in postoperative cognitive impairment.

Main body

Postoperative cognitive dysfunction

Postoperative cognitive impairment and the potential association with surgery under general anesthesia exposure was first described in 1955 [5]. Since this time, a substantial amount of research has been published which focuses on cognitive effects including delirium, postoperative cognitive dysfunction (POCD), development of dementia, and a decline in cognitive function in pre-existing dementia. POCD is often defined as a measurable impairment in cognition measured with neuropsychological testing in an individual over time, which may affect memory, attention, and psychomotor function [6]. In 2018, recommendations for nomenclature used to further define POCD were developed [7]. These definitions are summarized in Table 1. The implementation of more consistent terminology will allow for easier identification of trials assessing cognitive changes diagnosed up to 30 days after an operation (delayed neurocognitive recovery) vs. cognitive decline persisting beyond the 30-day recovery period (postoperative neurocognitive disorder). Due to variability in previous studies, the term POCD will be used interchangeably with the updated nomenclature throughout this review. In addition to updated nomenclature, the recent recommendations propose that screening cognitive tests are not sufficient for a diagnosis of a perioperative neurocognitive disorder, and instead diagnosis should involve assessment of performance on one or more cognitive domains. Prior literature has also exhibited wide variation in methodology employed to assess cognition, and differences in statistical analyses [6, 8–11]. The consequence of this is study heterogeneity which makes it challenging to draw definitive conclusions about various interventions or risk factors for perioperative neurocognitive disorders. Interestingly, individuals who self-report alterations in cognition postoperatively do not consistently demonstrate impairment on neuropsychological testing. Instead, some of these individuals may have higher levels of depression or anxiety [12]. This again highlights the need for the appropriate application of cognitive tests, and in the importance of considering a broad differential when patients report postoperative cognitive impairment.

Initial research on POCD revealed that patients undergoing coronary artery bypass graft (CABG) procedures with cardiopulmonary bypass were more likely to develop intellectual dysfunction when compared with a similar subset of patients undergoing peripheral vascular surgery [13]. One week following cardiac surgery, cognitive decline is observed in 50–70% of patients [14]. Long lasting cognitive decline has also been observed, with 13–40% of individuals affected ≥1 year postoperatively [15–17]. One potential contributing factor to the high incidence of POCD in this population is the presence of microemboli from cardiopulmonary bypass [18]. In addition to microemboli, several other factors have been proposed, many of which are highlighted throughout this review. Interestingly, the progression of cerebrovascular disease itself in this patient population has also

Table 1 Nomenclature used for cognitive impairment at different perio-operative time periods

Time Period	Nomenclature	Definition
Preoperative	Mild Neurocognitive Disorder (NCD)	DSM-5 definition: (1) cognitive concern from the individual/informant/clinician + (2) objective evidence of decline of 1–2 SD compared to normative group + (3) maintained iADLs &/or ADLs
	Major NCD	DSM-5 definition: (1) cognitive concern from the individual/informant/clinician + (2) objective evidence of decline of ≥2 SD + (3) impaired iADLs &/or ADLs
Emergence	Emergence excitation or delirium	
After operation to postoperative day 30	Postoperative delirium	Fluctuating changes in attention, mental status, or level of consciousness which occur in hospital up to 1 week following surgery
	Delayed neurocognitive recovery	Cognitive decline meeting DSM-5 criteria for mild or major NCD, diagnosed within the 30 day recovery period
From expected recovery (30 days) to 12 months	Postoperative mild neurocognitive disorder (POCD) Postoperative major NCD (POCD)	Criteria as per DSM-5 for mild and major NCD Assumes decline cannot be accounted for by any other condition. Postoperative specifier implies temporal relationship. It does not imply causation. POCD is included as a specifier in parentheses while transitioning to the new nomenclature
Greater than 12 months postoperatively	Routine DSM-5 nomenclature	Postoperative specifier is NO LONGER attached if neurocognitive disorder is first diagnosed after this time.

The above nomenclature has been recently proposed to further define neurocognitive disorders associated with the perioperative period. Abbreviations: *DSM-5* diagnostic and statistical manual of mental disorders, *NCD* neurocognitive disorder, *SD* standard deviation, *iADL* instrumental activities of daily living, *ADL* activities of daily living; Objective evidence: tests of complex attention, executive function, learning and memory, language, perceptual-motor, or social cognition. Objective evidence cannot be limited to screening tools. This table is adapted from Evered et al. (2018) [7]

been proposed as a major contributor to the high incidence of neurocognitive disorder identified postoperatively. In support of this hypothesis, a prospective study comparing a group of patients undergoing CABG to patients undergoing medical management for CAD over a 6 year study demonstrated that patients in both groups showed a similar degree of cognitive decline over the study period [19].

The International Study of Post-Operative Cognitive Dysfunction (ISPOCD1) from 1998 increased interest in the association between surgery and perioperative neurocognitive disorders in non-cardiac surgery. The study enrolled 1218 patients aged 60 and older. Delayed neurocognitive recovery was present in 25% of patients 1 week after surgery, and postoperative neurocognitive disorder was present in 10% of patients 3 months after surgery [20]. Several risk factors for POCD were identified at the 1 week time point including age, level of education, duration of surgery/anesthesia exposure, a second operation, and postoperative infection or respiratory complications. At the 3 month time point, age was the only significant risk factor for POCD. Hypoxemia and hypotension were not identified as risk factors at either time point. Multiple trials have since been published to identify risk factors or interventions which can help to mitigate the potential impact on cognitive function.

The effects of anesthetic agents on POCD

Several studies have aimed to determine whether general anesthesia itself is a risk factor for POCD. Many of these studies have chosen to compare general anesthesia (GA) to non-GA techniques such as neuraxial, regional, local anesthesia, and sedation. A meta-analysis published in 2010 looked at the existing literature on the topic. In their analysis, non-GA techniques included spinal, epidural, regional, and combination GA plus neuraxial or regional. POCD was defined by any objectively measured cognitive impairment. There was a non-significant trend toward increased POCD with GA vs. non-GA, with a 95% confidence interval (CI) of 0.93–1.95 [21]. Since the publication of this meta-analysis, a randomized controlled trial was published which compared GA to spinal without co-administration of confounding sedative medications. The trial population was patients ≥55 years of age undergoing extracorporeal shock wave lithotripsy. The authors concluded that the type of anesthesia did not impact rates of POCD at 7 days or 3 months postoperatively [22]. Of note, the trial did conduct an interim analysis and the trial was stopped early for futility at 50% of the a priori calculated required sample size. Furthermore, the mean age of the study population was 63.9 and 66.9 in the GA and spinal groups, respectively, and patients with pre-existing cognitive dysfunction were excluded from the study, which limits generalizability of the findings to individuals of advanced age and individuals with dementia. Indeed, the practice guidelines for perioperative brain health published in 2018 concluded that, based on current available data, there is insufficient evidence to recommend the use of regional anesthesia instead of general anesthesia [23].

Several studies have also been designed to assess whether the risk of POCD differs with general anesthesia using inhalational agents, vs. GA with TIVA (total intravenous anesthesia). A recent meta-analysis combined data from seven studies, and concluded that TIVA may reduce the risk of POCD, with an odds ratio (OR) of 0.52; however, this certainty of this conclusion is low due to heterogeneity of diagnostic tools utilized, variability in time of assessment, and inconsistent data reporting [24]. Furthermore, the authors reported that there were 11 ongoing studies on the topic at the time of the meta-analysis in 2018. At this time, it would be premature to conclude superiority of one mode of anesthetic.

The effect of depth of anesthesia on cognitive impairment has also been proposed as a potential risk factor for POCD. A meta-analysis recently compared cognitive outcomes in patients receiving low vs. high depth anesthesia as measured by bispectral index (BIS) monitoring. Included studies used either Propofol or Isoflurane. The authors concluded that depth of anesthesia did not significantly impact risk of POCD [25]. This conclusion was based on only 3 RCTs, and in one study the age of the participants was 45 ± 7.93 in the low BIS group, and 48.8 ± 10.2 in the high BIS group, which is unlikely to represent a patient population at risk for perioperative cognitive disorders. Furthermore, Hou and colleagues identified that there may have been variations in analgesic requirements between groups in the studies included in the meta-analysis which could confound results. Hou et al. (2018) proceeded to investigate patients aged 60 and older without pre-existing dementia scheduled to undergo elective total knee replacement. They randomized these patients to different depths of anesthesia as measured by BIS monitoring, with analgesic requirements controlled for using femoral and sciatic nerve blocks in both groups. Hemodynamic targets and induction doses were standardized. All patients received sevoflurane at 0.3MAC and a Propofol infusion titrated to target the appropriate BIS. On postoperative day 1, cognitive performance as measured by the Montreal cognitive assessment (MoCA) was significantly lower in the group with a target BIS of 40–50, when compared with the group with a target BIS of 55–65, indicating that a greater depth of anesthesia may increase POCD in the immediate postoperative period when other factors are carefully controlled [26]. There was no difference in cognition measured on postoperative days 3 or 7 which brings into questions whether a lower BIS has any meaningful clinical or economic significance. It should also be noted that the validity of BIS and other EEG-based depth of anesthesia monitoring does not correct for age or the presence of underlying cognitive dysfunction, and therefore may not serve as a reliable surrogate of depth of anesthesia in this patient population [27, 28]. Additional studies are required to validate depth of anesthesia monitoring in the elderly patient population, and also to investigate whether depth of anesthesia impacts the risk for cognitive impairment in the elderly population.

The effect of perioperative dexmedetomidine has been explored as a potential intervention to reduce the risk of POCD. The precise mechanism is still under investigation, but may relate to decreased requirements of other sedative and anesthetic medications, decreased opioids, modulation of the systemic stress response, promotion of natural sleep patterns, and potentially direct neuroprotective effects [29–31]. A landmark study published in 2016 demonstrated reduced delirium when low dose dexmedetomidine was administered postoperatively to elderly patients admitted to the intensive care unit following elective non-cardiac surgery [31]. The role of dexmedetomidine in prevention of POCD is less well studied, but has been the focus of a 2016 meta-analysis which concluded that dexmedetomidine may reduce the incidence of delayed neurocognitive recovery, and improve scores on the mini-mental state exam (MMSE) on postoperative day one [32]. This meta-analysis was limited by a small number of included studies with a small overall sample size, and study heterogeneity relating to patient inclusion and exclusion criteria and variations in dexmedetomidine administration. Since this time, many more studies have been designed to assess the impact of intraoperative and postoperative dexmedetomidine infusions in a variety of patient populations. Many of these studies are still underway. In the published literature, Deiner and colleagues (2017) randomized 404 elderly patients undergoing major elective non-cardiac surgery to dexmedetomidine infusion intraoperatively and 2 h postoperatively vs. placebo, with a primary outcome of delirium. A secondary outcome of cognitive impairment at 3 and 6 months postoperatively was also investigated. There were no differences in either delirium or cognitive performance; however, the study was designed and powered for the primary outcome of delirium, and the study was stopped for futility prior to reaching the calculated sample size of 706 [33]. Further high quality studies designed to assess cognitive function as the primary outcome are required to determine whether dexmedetomidine administration reduces the risk for perioperative neurocognitive disorders.

Cerebral perfusion and cerebral oxygen saturation have been implicated in the development of POCD. Chernov and colleagues (2006) utilized seven neuropsychological tests prior to and following CABG, and defined POCD as a 20% or greater reduction in score on 2 or more tests. Regional cerebral blood flow (rCBF) was measured with single photon emission computed tomography (SPECT) imaging. The study identified a relationship between reduced rCBF and cognitive performance [34]. Similarly, in patients who underwent CABG under hypothermic nonpulsatile cardiopulmonary bypass(CPB), a relationship was identified between reduced cognitive performance on the incidental memory assessment with cerebral blood flow measured by ^{131}Xe clearance [35]. In another study, regional cerebral oxygen saturation was monitored with the INVOS cerebral oximeter in patients undergoing CABG. Patients were randomized to either a blinded control group or to an unblinded intervention group in which providers could intervene to improve cerebral oxygenation. Although there was no difference in cognitive decline between the groups, the study demonstrated that prolonged cerebral desaturation was associated with a higher risk of POCD [36]. Notably, there has also been research which has not replicated the relationship between cerebral blood flow and POCD. Specifically, Abildstrom and colleagues (2002) identified a global reduction in CBF following CABG using SPECT imaging, without any associated regional differences in CBF. In this study, there was no correlation between performance on neuropsychological testing and either global or regional CBF [37]. In the non-cardiac surgery population, a cohort study of elderly patients measured intraoperative cerebral autoregulation using bilateral transcranial doppler probes, and cerebral oxygenation using near-infrared spectroscopy (NIRS). Due to a large number of patients lost to follow-up, only the pre-operative and 1-week postoperative data was analyzed. The primary endpoint was assessed with a multivariable regression analysis, and did not identify an association between impaired intraoperative cerebral oxygenation or perfusion with POCD; however, a secondary analysis using a univariable logistic regression model did reveal a potential relationship between cerebral autoregulation and POCD [38]. Whether the potential association between cerebral perfusion or oxygenation with POCD is causative, or whether other confounds may explain the association observed is still unclear.

Limited available data also demonstrates mixed results regarding the impact of other modifiable factors on POCD risk including hypothermia [39, 40] and preoperative and intraoperative glycemic control [41, 42]. Further prospective RCT evidence is required to evaluate the contribution of these factors to delayed neurocognitive recovery.

Although there is a need for further research and additional data to guide perioperative management of elderly individuals, recommendations have been developed based on current evidence [23]. The fifth international perioperative neurotoxicity working groups included over 30 experts who developed recommendations specific to postoperative brain health in individuals > 65 years of age. This article focused on pre-procedural consent, preoperative cognitive assessment, intraoperative management, and postoperative follow-up. We direct readers to the article by the working group for a more detailed description of their recommendations. Their recommendations are briefly summarized below:

(1) Consent: Individuals over the age of 65 should be informed of the risk of postoperative delirium and perioperative neurocognitive disorder prior to their procedure;

(2) Baseline cognitive assessment: Cognitive function should be assessed preoperatively using a brief screening tool. Examples of screening tools provided included the Minicog, MoCA, MMSE, clock-drawing test, verbal fluency test, or the cognitive disorder examination;

(3) Intraoperative management: Current literature is insufficient to define a specific anesthetic regimen to decrease risk of perioperative neurocognitive disorder; however, cautious use or avoidance of medications such as first-generation antihistamines, centrally acting anticholinergics, benzodiazepines, and meperidine was recommended. The authors also suggest avoiding relative hypotension, maintenance of normothermia, use age-adjusted minimal alveolar concentration (MAC) of volatile anesthetic agents, and use EEG-based depth of anesthesia monitoring to titrate anesthetic delivery.

(4) Postoperative follow-up: additional research is required to determine feasibility, efficacy, and cost-effectiveness of postoperative follow-up to assess cognitive outcomes [23].

In our opinion, the above recommendations reflect the evidence, as well as the continued uncertainty in the field. We do recognize that baseline cognitive assessment is often challenging to implement with limited time for preoperative assessment. Furthermore, without established postoperative follow-up, the utility of baseline cognitive assessment could be questioned. This highlights the need to establish assessments with strong reliability and validity which are relatively easy to administer, and which can be applied postoperatively to identify patients with impaired cognition in the perioperative period.

As summarized above, there is a large body of evidence which supports the existence of delayed neurocognitive recovery and postoperative neurocognitive disorder. Perioperative neurocognitive disorder is a distinct clinical presentation which is separate from Alzheimer's disease and other forms of dementia. Based on our current knowledge, it is unclear whether the presence of delayed neurocognitive recovery or postoperative neurocognitive disorder confers an increased susceptibility to Alzheimer's disease or other dementia. Indeed, the pathological mechanisms may be distinct from those involved in Alzheimer's disease and other forms of dementia. Furthermore, it is currently unclear whether surgery and/or anesthesia increases the risk of subsequent diagnosis of dementia. A meta-analysis published in 2017 showed no significant association between GA and incident dementia (95% CI 0.90–1.19). Importantly, reporting bias may impact study results as patients may be unsure of the type of anesthesia they received. Indeed, a subgroup analysis did show a small but significant association between GA and risk of dementia when only studies using anesthesia records to collect exposure data were included (OR1.22; 95% CI 1.01–1.47) [43]. Since the publication of this metanalysis, a large prospective cohort study using data from the Korean National Health Insurance Service – National Sample Database was published which adds to the debate in the field [44]. The study followed patients 50 years of age and older without pre-existing dementia over a 12 year period and assessed for incident dementia as defined by an ICD-10 code of dementia and documented history of dementia medication. There were 44,956 individuals in the GA group, and 174,469 in the control group. The authors used a time-varying Cox hazard model to minimize time-dependent bias, and utilized propensity score matching to reduce potential confounding biases between groups. Exposure to GA was determined by a general anesthesia operation code in NHIS-NSC database. Individuals who did not have a general anesthesia operation code were assigned to the control group. Similar to prior studies, this study design would not be able to separate the effects of anesthesia exposure from the effects of surgical stress and other potential confounders (for example, perioperative hypothermia or administration of narcotics and other medications). After adjusting for important covariates, a multivariable survival analysis determined there was a 1.285-fold increased risk for developing dementia in the GA group when compared with controls [44]. The authors also conducted a multivariable analysis which demonstrated that the risk of incident dementia was increased with desflurane with a hazards ratio (HR) of 1.27, and isoflurane (HR 1.33), but was decreased with sevoflurane (HR 0.71) [44]. Although the difference hazards ratio of the inhalational agents is intriguing, the observational study design may include unaccounted for confounding variables which influenced choice of anesthetic agent, and independently increase the risk of dementia. A randomized controlled trial would be required to compare the risk profile of various anesthetic agents on cognition and risk for incident dementia. If a difference between volatile agents can be reproduced with a well designed RCT, further research would be required to explore the biological mechanisms differentially altered by various volatile agents.

In summary, it still unclear whether anesthesia itself causes POCD, or whether other surgical or patient factors might explain the observed cognitive impairment. Conflicting data also exists regarding the potential link between anesthesia exposure and risk of developing AD or other forms of dementia. Research assessing the risk profile of various anesthetic techniques is heterogeneous, and there is no strong evidence in favour of one technique over another. The debate in the field highlights the need for further high-quality research. Furthermore, whether there are additional considerations that should be applied to the individual with pre-existing cognitive impairment is unclear.

Anesthesia in individuals with cognitive impairment

Alzheimer's disease accounts for the majority of cases of dementia [3]. AD is a fatal progressive neurodegenerative disorder, characterized by neuronal degeneration in the basal forebrain, entorhinal cortex, hippocampus, and cortex [45–47]. Pathological hallmarks include the presence of senile plaques which contain Amyloid-β (Aβ), and neurofibrillary tangles which form in the presence of pathological modifications to the microtubule-associated protein, tau. The pathways underlying neurodegeneration are complex and involve many players including soluble and insoluble Aβ, hyperphosphorylated tau, neuroinflammation and microglia dysfunction, cholinergic deficits, and oxidative stress [48–53].

AD and other forms of dementia can impact the ability of anesthesiologists to collect a detailed history and elicit appropriate cooperation for physical examination. The potential for confusion and limited cooperation may make approaches such as neuraxial anesthesia, peripheral nerve blocks, or sedation more challenging. In terms of pharmacologic management, it is commonly accepted that short-acting medications should be used, and medications which may increase risk of postoperative confusion should be avoided [23, 54, 55]. Available evidence does not support the hypothesis that these patients are more sensitive to anesthetic agents; however, the sample size employed in these studies and use of the BIS monitor as a surrogate of anesthetic depth make it challenging to draw any definitive conclusion [27, 56].

Anesthesiologists must also be aware of drug-drug interactions, such as the interaction between neuromuscular blocking agents and acetylcholinesterase inhibitors [57, 58]. Donepezil (Aricept), a commonly prescribed medication in AD, is a reversible non-competitive cholinesterase inhibitor. It has a half-life of approximately 72 h, and requires 2–3 weeks for complete wash out [59]. Published case reports demonstrate that patients on donepezil may exhibit high intraoperative requirements for non-depolarizing neuromuscular blockers including atracurium, rocuronium, and vecuronium [57, 60]. In contrast, prolonged paralysis has been described with administration of succinylcholine to a patient on donepezil, potentially due to reduced pseudocholinesterase inhibitor activity [58]. In addition to these anesthetic considerations, it is also important to consider the potential long-term impact of anesthesia on cognition, morbidity, and mortality in patients with dementia.

The prevalence of preoperative dementia varies in different patient groups requiring surgery. For example, in the vascular surgery population, 3.8% of individuals have a pre-operative diagnosis of dementia [61]. In patients undergoing hip fracture surgery, an estimated 20% of individuals have a diagnosis of dementia [62]. In the vascular surgery population, dementia was identified as the strongest predictor for postoperative complications, increased hospital expenditures and was an independent predictor of increased mortality (HR 1.37) [61]. In a retrospective study, a multivariate analysis identified pre-existing dementia as an independent predictor of 30-day mortality following hip fracture surgery ($p = 0.01$) [63]. In a population-based retrospective cohort study, individuals with dementia who received GA were matched to similar patients receiving regional anesthesia. The type of anesthetic did not affect postoperative 30 day mortality, length of stay, or measured postoperative complications [64].

A meta-analysis published in 2014 concluded that there is an association between carrier status of the APOEε4 allele, a gene implicated in AD susceptibility, and risk of POCD one-week postoperatively [65]. This correlation was no longer present at 1–3 months or 1 year postoperatively [65]. A recent longitudinal cohort study assessed the interaction between gender and APOEε4 carrier status, and proposed that men carrying the APOEε4 allele have a more rapid decline in performance on tests of global cognitive function and memory when compared with women carrying the APOEε4 allele [66]. In individuals with pre-existing cognitive impairment, there is limited evidence to demonstrate whether exposure to anesthesia increases the risk of further cognitive decline. In one RCT, 180 patients with amnestic mild cognitive impairment (MCI) undergoing lumbar spinal surgery were randomized to sevoflurane, Propofol, or epidural analgesia. There was no difference in the risk of developing AD between groups after a 2 year follow-up; however, there was accelerated progression of amnestic MCI to progressive MCI in the group exposed to sevoflurane [67]. One study utilized data from 394 patients in the Oxford Project to Investigate Memory and Ageing (OPTIMA) cohort. Patients had at least two documented Cambridge Cognition Examination

(CAMCOG) scores, had joined the study as controls or with MCI, and had been followed for at least 3 years. A total of 109 patients underwent surgery. Mixed-effects modeling was used to assess the association between CAMCOG scores and multiple variables, including exposure to surgery and anesthesia. The study identified a correlation between more rapid cognitive decline after surgery if cognitive impairment was diagnosed postoperatively ($p = 0.0001$) [68].

The preceding studies suggest that pre-existing cognitive impairment may impact postoperative morbidity, mortality, and/or health care costs. Furthermore, exposure to surgery and anesthesia may increase cognitive decline in these patients. Further research is required to better characterize this association, the resulting functional impact, and assess whether certain anesthetic approaches or other interventions can reduce the potential risk of morbidity in patients with pre-existing cognitive impairment.

Potential mechanisms

In the clinical literature, it is challenging to isolate the contributions of surgical stress, various anesthetic options, and other confounding variables which may occur during the perioperative period. Therefore, elucidating mechanisms involved requires integration of knowledge gained from both the preclinical as well as the clinical literature. In this section, we will focus on key experiments which help us better understanding the multitude of factors which may be involved in development of POCD.

In animal studies, research has shown that surgery increases the risk of cognitive impairment when compared with exposure to anesthesia alone [69, 70]. One study established a model of abdominal surgery under local anesthesia alone to assess the effects of surgery without the confounding risk of sedative or anesthesia exposure. This group demonstrated that surgery alone, in the absence of a general anesthetic, produced cognitive impairment in 18 month old WT mice [71].

Exposure to anesthesia in the absence of a surgical stress does not reliably impair cognition when younger animals are utilized [72]. When aged animals are employed, there has been conflicting evidence assessing whether anesthesia exposure can lead to cognitive impairment [73–76]. The variability in results is likely impacted by heterogeneity in study design, including choice of animal models, age of animals, choice of anesthesia agent, dose, duration of exposure, and the choice of cognitive test and timing of assessment relative to anesthesia exposure. Despite the conflicting data on a single exposure, it does appear that repeat exposure to anesthesia may increase the risk for cognitive impairment in animal studies [77–79]. The use of transgenic animal models of Alzheimer's disease also appears to increase the likelihood of cognitive impairment following surgery and anesthesia. This has been reviewed elsewhere [80]. Of interest, the timing of the exposure relative to the disease process may be important. For example, one study demonstrated that isoflurane exposure produced cognitive impairment in wild type (WT) mice at 12 months of age, but not in the Tg2576 AD mouse model at the same age [81]. It has been postulated that this may because the disease process was advanced in the AD animal model, and further impairment could not be induced with exposure to anesthesia. Furthermore, cognitive impairments were also not observed in 3xTgAD mice exposed to isoflurane at a 2, 4, or 6 months of age, prior to onset of pathology [82].

One hypothesis underlying the mechanism for postoperative cognitive impairment is that exposure to surgery and/or anesthesia will produce changes in Aβ and tau levels which mirror the changes observed in patients with MCI and AD. To examine this hypothesis, we will first review some evidence on antemortem biomarkers observed in AD and MCI. In patients with AD, several studies have demonstrated an increase in Total Tau (T-Tau), phosphorylated Tau (pTau), and neurofilament light levels in cerebral spinal fluid (CSF), and a decrease in CSF $A\beta_{1-42}$ [83]. In plasma, concentrations of Aβ to not appear to be associated with the diagnosis of AD or the severity of cognitive impairment measured by MMSE [84, 85]. The ratio of $A\beta_{1-40}$ / $A\beta_{1-42}$ may be more reliable than the absolute concentration of these markers independently at predicting progression from MCI to AD, or differentiating early onset sporadic AD from age-matched controls [86, 87]. In a recent meta-analysis, only an increase in plasma T-tau could be used to differentiate between control and AD plasma samples (AD: control ratio of 1.95) [83].

There is a small amount of evidence exploring the effects of anesthesia on these biomarkers in individuals without pre-existing cognitive impairment. In one study, 11 patients without cognitive impairment were recruited who were scheduled to undergo endoscopic nasal surgery to correct idiopathic CSF leaks. The procedure requires placement of a lumbar drain which is left in situ for 24–48 h, or until accidental extradural placement. Over a 24-h period following surgery, there was no change in CSF $A\beta_{1-42}$ concentration; however, there was an increase in the CSF concentration of total tau by more than 200%, and an increase in levels of $pTau^{181}$ [88]. In a subsequent study, patients undergoing procedures that required the placement of a lumbar drain were randomized to either inhalational anesthesia with isoflurane or to TIVA using Propofol for maintenance [89]. The authors found no changes in CSF $A\beta_{1-42}$ levels but did identify an increase in total tau levels 24 h postoperatively when compared with the time of drain insertion. In contrast to prior research, this study identified a decrease in pTau over time [89]. There was no interaction between the type of anesthesia employed and the biomarker levels in CSF; however, the authors appropriately point out that all patients underwent surgical manipulation of a dura and blood brain barrier, and this confound may outweigh any potential effects from the choice of anesthesia technique. Of note, this study did not examine the effects of isoflurane or propofol on cognition postoperatively Furthermore, neither this study nor the 2011 study mentioned whether a phosphatase inhibitor was included in the CSF at the time of collection, which may make any alterations in level of phosphorylated proteins less reliable, and/or more difficult to interpret. Pikwer and colleagues (2017) did not identify a changes in CSF Aβ or tau levels with a Propofol and remifentanil based TIVA; however, the mean age in this study was 50 years, and the follow-up time for CSF analysis was at 0, 2, and 5 h following spinal catheter placement, which raises the question of whether an older study population or later timepoint may have demonstrated changes in biomarker levels [90]. Separate studies have also examined whether preoperative biomarkers predict development of delirium or POCD. Indeed, plasma levels of $A\beta_{1-42}$ were significantly lower in patients scheduled for CABG who developed POCD [15]. In another study, CSF was collected during spinal anesthesia for total hip or knee replacement. Lower CSF Aβ/Tau ratios were associated with a higher incidence of delirium as measured by the confusion assessment method and memorial delirium assessment scale [91].

These same pathways have also been explored in preclinical studies using animal models. In one landmark paper, Planel and colleagues (2007) demonstrated that tau hyperphosphorylation occurred when anesthesia was induced with either chloral hydrate or isoflurane. Interestingly, both of these agents also cause hypothermia, and maintenance of normothermic conditions was able to attenuate the hyperphosphorylation of tau [92]. In a separate study, maintenance of normothermia was shown to abolish tau hyperphosphorylation following exposure to anesthesia in aged mice, and also attenuated cognitive impairment in the animals [93]. Although these papers show that maintenance of normothermia is an important consideration, there are likely several other factors involved. Indeed, when animal models of AD are employed, exposure to anesthetic agents promotes tau hyperphosphorylation even when normothermia is maintained [82, 94–97]. This suggests that the susceptible brain may be more prone to pathological changes following exposure to anesthesia and/or surgery. In support of the link between pathologic modifications to tau and development of POCD, animal studies have shown that modulation of tau pathology using transgenic approaches or pharmacological approaches may decrease the risk of cognitive impairment following anesthesia and surgery [98, 99].

Inflammation has also been associated with POCD. An increase in various cytokines including IL-6, TNF-α, IL-8, and IL-10 have been correlated with postoperative cognitive impairment [88, 100, 101]. Recently, a meta-analysis was conducted which assessed for the association between various inflammatory biomarkers and POCD. The meta-analysis found that higher postoperative c-reactive protein ($n = 11$ studies) and interleukin-6 (IL-6) ($n = 17$ studies) are associated with POCD [102]. In the endoscopic nasal surgery study mentioned previously, the authors compared CSF from patients receiving anesthesia with sevoflurane to those who received TIVA and noted a significant increase in postoperative concentration of IL-6 in the patients receiving sevoflurane. Importantly, the study is limited by a small sample size and the fact that anesthetic approach was not randomized [88]. The increase in inflammatory markers has also been correlated with an increase in high rates of insulin resistance as calculated by the homeostasis model assessment 2, raising the possibility of a potential combined impact of inflammation and insulin resistance with development of POCD [100].

In animal studies, there is mixed evidence regarding whether volatile agents increase pro-inflammatory cytokines and/or microglial activation in the absence of surgery. Although an increase in inflammation has been observed by some groups [75, 103–105], other groups have reported no effect of isoflurane or sevoflurane anesthesia alone on microglial activation and/or proinflammatory cytokine expression [70, 82, 106, 107]. The mechanism for induction of neuroinflammation following exposure to anesthesia with or without surgery continues to be actively investigated. Potential factors involved include P2X7 receptors, NFκB, and increased blood brain barrier permeability [107–109].

Significant preclinical data has also explored the effects of anesthetic agents on synapse structure and function and calcium homeostasis. For example, volatile anesthetic agents, with or without surgery, have been shown to alter expression of post-synaptic density 95 (PSD-95) [73, 110–112]. Exposure to volatile agents has also been shown to impact expression of the extrasynaptic N-methyl-D-aspartate (NMDA) receptor GluN2B subunit, trafficking of the GluA1 subunit of the α-amino-3-hydroxy-5-methyl-4-isoxazoleproprionic acid (AMPA) receptor, and expression of the α5-γ-Aminobutyric acid A ($\alpha 5GABA_A$) receptor [113–115]. Electrophysiological assessment of synaptic plasticity following exposure to volatile agents has also demonstrated impaired long-term potentiation and facilitated long-term depression [114, 116]. A summary of the potential role of calcium dysregulation downstream of anesthetic exposure has also previously been published [117]. In vivo preclinical evidence suggesting that calcium dysregulation participates in anesthesia-mediated neurotoxicity includes the finding that nimodipine, an L-type calcium channel antagonist, protects against sevoflurane or isoflurane-induced cognitive deficits, neuroinflammation, and apoptosis [103, 118, 119]. Inhibition of the NMDA receptor with memantine has also been shown to protect against the isoflurane-mediated increase in cytosolic calcium, caspase-3 activation and cytotoxicity in vitro [120].

Preclinical research has also focused on mitochondrial dysfunction and oxidative stress as a potential contributor to POCD. To examine this hypothesis, one study used animals with a knockout of Cyclophilin D (CypD), a protein which contributes to opening of the mitochondrial permeability transition pores. Knockout of CypD improves mitochondrial function and stability. These animals were crossed with an Alzheimer's disease mouse model. Knockout of CypD resulted in improved cognitive performance following exposure to sevoflurane and laparotomy when compared with AD transgenic mice exposed to the same conditions [112]. Pharmacological targeting of the pathway with SS-31 pre-treatment, a mitochondrial targeted peptide anti-oxidant, similarly attenuates cognitive deficits and biochemical changes induced by a 2 hour exposure to isoflurane in aged mice [73].

In summary, several molecular pathways likely participate in the development of POCD. Clinical and preclinical evidence points toward a possible role for pathological modifications to tau, as well as neuroinflammation. Preclinical data also suggests that altered synapse structure or function, calcium dysregulation, and mitochondrial dysfunction may participate in the development of cognitive impairment following exposure to anesthesia and/or surgery. Elucidation of pathways upstream and downstream of these observed changes are under active investigation.

Conclusions

This review summarizes previous findings relevant to the potential relationship between surgery, anesthesia exposure and POCD. AD or similar underlying pathology may make individuals more susceptible to the potential neurotoxic effects of the surgical stress and/or anesthesia exposure and increase the risk of progression of cognitive impairment. Several mechanisms have been implicated including altered Aβ processing or accumulation, pathological modifications to tau, neuroinflammation, calcium dysregulation, and mitochondrial dysfunction.

Review of the literature identifies several areas which require further investigation. First, additional high-quality clinical studies are required which focus on individuals with a pre-operative diagnosis of MCI, AD or other forms of dementia. Consistency in the evaluation of anesthesia exposure and measurement of cognitive function will be an asset to determine the true effect of anesthesia exposure. Second, well controlled RCTs are required to determine whether particular agents or anesthetic approaches have a more favorable risk profile. Third, additional clinical work and basic science research investigating molecular mechanisms at play will help to identify susceptible individuals, and possible interventions which could eventually be incorporated into clinical practice to minimize the risk of POCD. With the expected increase in AD prevalence and associated cost, and in the absence of effective disease modifying therapeutic agents to treat AD, clinicians and scientists must aim to identify and modify factors which may contribute to cognitive impairment in this subset of patients.

Abbreviations

AD: Alzheimer's disease; AMPA: α-amino-3-hydroxy-5-methyl-4-isoxazoleproprionic acid; Aβ: Amyloid-β; BIS: Bispectral index; CABG: Coronary artery bypass graft; CAMCOG: Cambridge Cognition Examination; CI: Confidence interval; CPB: Cardiopulmonary bypass; CSF: Cerebral spinal fluid; CypD: Cyclophilin D; GA: General anesthesia; HR: Hazards ratio; IL: Interleukin; MAC: Minimal alveolar concentration; MCI: Mild cognitive impairment; MMSE: Mini-mental state exam; MoCA: Montreal cognitive assessment; NIRS: Near-infrared spectroscopy; NMDA: N-methyl-D-aspartate; OR: Odds ratio; POCD: Postoperative cognitive dysfunction; PSD-95: Post-synaptic density 95; pTau: Phosphorylated tau; rCBF: Regional cerebral blood flow; SPECT: Single photon emission computed tomography; TIVA: Total intravenous anesthesia; T-Tau: Total tau; WT: Wild type; α5GABA$_A$: α5-γ-Aminobutyric acid A

Acknowledgements

We thank Rachel Sandison, MME; Education, Research & Innovation Coordinator for proof -reading this manuscript.

Authors' contributions

J.C.B. and R.R.N. contributed to the literature review, writing, and editing of the manuscript. Both authors read and approved the final manuscript.

References

1. Prince M, Wimo A, Guerchet M, Ali GC, Wu Y-T, Prina M. World Alzheimer Report 2015, The Global Impact of Dementia: An analysis of prevalence, incidence, cost and trends. Alzheimer's Dis Int ADI Lond. 2015;87. https://www.alz.co.uk/research/world-report-2015. (last accessed 10/2018).
2. Wimo A, Guerchet M, Ali G-C, Wu Y-T, Prina AM, Winblad B, et al. The worldwide costs of dementia 2015 and comparisons with 2010. Alzheimers Dement J Alzheimers Assoc. 2017;13:1–7.
3. Alzheimer's Association. 2018 Alzheimer's disease facts and figures. Alzheimers Dement J Alzheimers Assoc. 2018;14:367–429.
4. Möllers T, Stocker H, Wei W, Perna L, Brenner H. Length of hospital stay and dementia: a systematic review of observational studies. Int J Geriatr Psychiatry. 2018;34:8–21.
5. Bedford PD. Adverse cerebral effects of anaesthesia on old people. Lancet Lond Engl. 1955;269:259–63.
6. Symes E, Maruff P, Ajani A, Currie J. Issues associated with the identification of cognitive change following coronary artery bypass grafting. Aust N Z J Psychiatry. 2000;34:770–84.
7. Evered L, Silbert B, Knopman DS, Scott DA, DeKosky ST, Rasmussen LS, et al. Recommendations for the nomenclature of cognitive change associated with Anaesthesia and Surgery-20181. J Alzheimers Dis JAD. 2018;66:1–10.
8. Lewis M, Maruff P, Silbert B. Statistical and conceptual issues in defining postoperative cognitive dysfunction. Neurosci Biobehav Rev. 2004;28:433–40.

9. Murkin JM, Newman SP, Stump DA, Blumenthal JA. Statement of consensus on assessment of neurobehavioral outcomes after cardiac surgery. Ann Thorac Surg. 1995;59:1289–95.
10. Murkin JM, Stump DA, Blumenthal JA, McKhann G. Defining dysfunction: group means versus incidence analysis--a statement of consensus. Ann Thorac Surg. 1997;64:904–5.
11. Ghoneim MM, Block RI. Clinical, methodological and theoretical issues in the assessment of cognition after anaesthesia and surgery: a review. Eur J Anaesthesiol. 2012;29:409–22.
12. Newman S, Klinger L, Venn G, Smith P, Harrison M, Treasure T. Subjective reports of cognition in relation to assessed cognitive performance following coronary artery bypass surgery. J Psychosom Res. 1989;33:227–33.
13. Shaw PJ, Bates D, Cartlidge NE, French JM, Heaviside D, Julian DG, et al. Neurologic and neuropsychological morbidity following major surgery: comparison of coronary artery bypass and peripheral vascular surgery. Stroke. 1987;18:700–7.
14. Newman MF, Mathew JP, Grocott HP, Mackensen GB, Monk T, Welsh-Bohmer KA, et al. Central nervous system injury associated with cardiac surgery. Lancet Lond Engl. 2006;368:694–703.
15. Evered LA, Silbert BS, Scott DA, Maruff P, Laughton KM, Volitakis I, et al. Plasma amyloid beta42 and amyloid beta40 levels are associated with early cognitive dysfunction after cardiac surgery. Ann Thorac Surg. 2009;88:1426–32.
16. Gao L, Taha R, Gauvin D, Othmen LB, Wang Y, Blaise G. Postoperative cognitive dysfunction after cardiac surgery. Chest. 2005;128:3664–70.
17. Newman MF, Kirchner JL, Phillips-Bute B, Gaver V, Grocott H, Jones RH, et al. Longitudinal assessment of neurocognitive function after coronary-artery bypass surgery. N Engl J Med. 2001;344:395–402.
18. Pugsley W, Klinger L, Paschalis C, Treasure T, Harrison M, Newman S. The impact of microemboli during cardiopulmonary bypass on neuropsychological functioning. Stroke. 1994;25:1393–9.
19. Selnes OA, Grega MA, Bailey MM, Pham LD, Zeger SL, Baumgartner WA, et al. Cognition 6 years after surgical or medical therapy for coronary artery disease. Ann Neurol. 2008;63:581–90.
20. Moller JT, Cluitmans P, Rasmussen LS, Houx P, Rasmussen H, Canet J, et al. Long-term postoperative cognitive dysfunction in the elderly ISPOCD1 study. ISPOCD investigators. International study of postoperative cognitive dysfunction. Lancet Lond Engl. 1998;351:857–61.
21. Mason SE, Noel-Storr A, Ritchie CW. The impact of general and regional anesthesia on the incidence of postoperative cognitive dysfunction and postoperative delirium: a systematic review with meta-analysis. J Alzheimers Dis JAD. 2010;22(Suppl 3):67–79.
22. Silbert BS, Evered LA, Scott DA. Incidence of postoperative cognitive dysfunction after general or spinal anaesthesia for extracorporeal shock wave lithotripsy. Br J Anaesth. 2014;113:784–91.
23. Berger M, Schenning KJ, Brown CH, Deiner SG, Whittington RA, Eckenhoff RG, et al. Best practices for postoperative brain health: recommendations from the fifth international perioperative neurotoxicity working group. Anesth Analg. 2018;127:1406–13.
24. Miller D, Lewis SR, Pritchard MW, Schofield-Robinson OJ, Shelton CL, Alderson P, et al. Intravenous versus inhalational maintenance of anaesthesia for postoperative cognitive outcomes in elderly people undergoing non-cardiac surgery. Cochrane Database Syst Rev. 2018;8:CD012317.
25. Lu X, Jin X, Yang S, Xia Y. The correlation of the depth of anesthesia and postoperative cognitive impairment: a meta-analysis based on randomized controlled trials. J Clin Anesth. 2018;45:55–9.
26. Hou R, Wang H, Chen L, Qiu Y, Li S. POCD in patients receiving total knee replacement under deep vs light anesthesia: a randomized controlled trial. Brain Behav. 2018;8:e00910.
27. Erdogan MA, Demirbilek S, Erdil F, Aydogan MS, Ozturk E, Togal T, et al. The effects of cognitive impairment on anaesthetic requirement in the elderly. Eur J Anaesthesiol. 2012;29:326–31.
28. Purdon PL, Pavone KJ, Akeju O, Smith AC, Sampson AL, Lee J, et al. The ageing brain: age-dependent changes in the electroencephalogram during propofol and sevoflurane general anaesthesia. Br J Anaesth. 2015;115(Suppl 1):i46–57.
29. Ma D, Rajakumaraswamy N, Maze M. alpha2-Adrenoceptor agonists: shedding light on neuroprotection? Br Med Bull. 2004;71:77–92.
30. Mo Y, Zimmermann AE. Role of dexmedetomidine for the prevention and treatment of delirium in intensive care unit patients. Ann Pharmacother. 2013;47:869–76.
31. Su X, Meng Z-T, Wu X-H, Cui F, Li H-L, Wang D-X, et al. Dexmedetomidine for prevention of delirium in elderly patients after non-cardiac surgery: a randomised, double-blind, placebo-controlled trial. Lancet Lond Engl. 2016; 388:1893–902.
32. Zhou C, Zhu Y, Liu Z, Ruan L. Effect of dexmedetomidine on postoperative cognitive dysfunction in elderly patients after general anaesthesia: a meta-analysis. J Int Med Res. 2016;44:1182–90.
33. Deiner S, Luo X, Lin H-M, Sessler DI, Saager L, Sieber FE, et al. Intraoperative infusion of Dexmedetomidine for prevention of postoperative delirium and cognitive dysfunction in elderly patients undergoing major elective noncardiac surgery: a randomized clinical trial. JAMA Surg. 2017;152: e171505.
34. Chernov VI, Efimova NY, Efimova IY, Akhmedov SD, Lishmanov YB. Short-term and long-term cognitive function and cerebral perfusion in off-pump and on-pump coronary artery bypass patients. Eur J Cardio-Thorac Surg Off J Eur Assoc Cardio-Thorac Surg. 2006;29:74–81.
35. Paolin A, Michielon P, Betetto M, Sartori G, Valfré C, Rodriguez G, et al. Lower perfusion pressure during hypothermic cardiopulmonary bypass is associated with decreased cerebral blood flow and impaired memory performance 6 months postoperatively. Heart Surg Forum. 2010;13:E7–12.
36. Slater JP, Guarino T, Stack J, Vinod K, Bustami RT, Brown JM, et al. Cerebral oxygen desaturation predicts cognitive decline and longer hospital stay after cardiac surgery. Ann Thorac Surg. 2009;87:36–44 discussion 44-45.
37. Abildstrom H, Høgh P, Sperling B, Moller JT, Yndgaard S, Rasmussen LS. Cerebral blood flow and cognitive dysfunction after coronary surgery. Ann Thorac Surg. 2002;73:1174–8 discussion 1178-1179.
38. Goettel N, Burkhart CS, Rossi A, Cabella BCT, Berres M, Monsch AU, et al. Associations between impaired cerebral blood flow autoregulation, cerebral oxygenation, and biomarkers of brain injury and postoperative cognitive dysfunction in elderly patients after major noncardiac surgery. Anesth Analg. 2017;124:934–42.
39. Gong G-L, Liu B, Wu J-X, Li J-Y, Shu B-Q, You Z-J. Postoperative cognitive dysfunction induced by different surgical methods and its risk factors. Am Surg. 2018;84:1531–7.
40. Shoair OA, Grasso Ii MP, Lahaye LA, Daniel R, Biddle CJ, Slattum PW. Incidence and risk factors for postoperative cognitive dysfunction in older adults undergoing major noncardiac surgery: a prospective study. J Anaesthesiol Clin Pharmacol. 2015;31:30–6.
41. Kadoi Y, Kawauchi C, Kuroda M, Takahashi K, Saito S, Fujita N, et al. Association between cerebrovascular carbon dioxide reactivity and postoperative short-term and long-term cognitive dysfunction in patients with diabetes mellitus. J Anesth. 2011;25:641–7.
42. Puskas F, Grocott HP, White WD, Mathew JP, Newman MF, Bar-Yosef S. Intraoperative hyperglycemia and cognitive decline after CABG. Ann Thorac Surg. 2007;84:1467–73.
43. Jiang J, Dong Y, Huang W, Bao M. General anesthesia exposure and risk of dementia: a meta-analysis of epidemiological studies. Oncotarget. 2017;8: 59628–37.
44. Kim CT, Myung W, Lewis M, Lee H, Kim SE, Lee K, et al. Exposure to general anesthesia and risk of dementia: a Nationwide population-based cohort study. J Alzheimers Dis JAD. 2018;63:395–405.
45. Coyle JT, Price DL, DeLong MR. Alzheimer's disease: a disorder of cortical cholinergic innervation. Science. 1983;219:1184–90.
46. Gómez-Isla T, Price JL, McKeel DW, Morris JC, Growdon JH, Hyman BT. Profound loss of layer II entorhinal cortex neurons occurs in very mild Alzheimer's disease. J Neurosci. 1996;16:4491–500.
47. Whitehouse PJ, Price DL, Struble RG, Clark AW, Coyle JT, Delon MR. Alzheimer's disease and senile dementia: loss of neurons in the basal forebrain. Science. 1982;215:1237–9.
48. Douchamps V, Mathis C. A second wind for the cholinergic system in Alzheimer's therapy. Behav Pharmacol. 2017;28:112–23.
49. Francis PT, Palmer AM, Snape M, Wilcock GK. The cholinergic hypothesis of Alzheimer's disease: a review of progress. J Neurol Neurosurg Psychiatry. 1999;66:137–47.
50. Guerrero-Muñoz MJ, Gerson J, Castillo-Carranza DL. Tau oligomers: the toxic player at synapses in Alzheimer's disease. Front Cell Neurosci. 2015;9:464.
51. Krstic D, Knuesel I. The airbag problem-a potential culprit for bench-to-bedside translational efforts: relevance for Alzheimer's disease. Acta Neuropathol Commun. 2013;1:62.
52. Markesbery WR. Oxidative stress hypothesis in Alzheimer's disease. Free Radic Biol Med. 1997;23:134–47.

53. Selles MC, Oliveira MM, Ferreira ST. Brain inflammation connects cognitive and non-cognitive symptoms in Alzheimer's disease. J Alzheimers Dis JAD. 2018;64: S313–27.
54. Di Nino G, Adversi M, Samolsky Dekel BG, Fodale V, Rosa G, Melotti RM. Peri-operative risk management in patients with Alzheimer's disease. J Alzheimers Dis JAD. 2010;22(Suppl 3):121–7.
55. Fernandez CR, Fields A, Richards T, Kaye AD. Anesthetic considerations in patients with Alzheimer's disease. J Clin Anesth. 2003;15:52–8.
56. Perez-Protto S, Geube M, Ontaneda D, Dalton JE, Kurz A, Sessler DI. Sensitivity to volatile anesthetics in patients with dementia: a case-control analysis. Can J Anaesth J Can Anesth. 2014;61:611–8.
57. Baruah J, Easby J, Kessell G. Effects of acetylcholinesterase inhibitor therapy for Alzheimer's disease on neuromuscular block. Br J Anaesth. 2008;100:420.
58. Crowe S, Collins L. Suxamethonium and donepezil: a cause of prolonged paralysis. Anesthesiology. 2003;98:574–5.
59. Dooley M, Lamb HM. Donepezil: a review of its use in Alzheimer's disease. Drugs Aging. 2000;16:199–226.
60. Bhardwaj A, Dharmavaram S, Wadhawan S, Sethi A, Bhadoria P. Donepezil: a cause of inadequate muscle relaxation and delayed neuromuscular recovery. J Anaesthesiol Clin Pharmacol. 2011;27:247–8.
61. Mehaffey JH, Hawkins RB, Tracci MC, Robinson WP, Cherry KJ, Kern JA, et al. Preoperative dementia is associated with increased cost and complications after vascular surgery. J Vasc Surg. 2018;68(4):1203–208
62. Evered LA, Silbert BS, Scott DA, Maruff P, Ames D, Choong PF. Preexisting cognitive impairment and mild cognitive impairment in subjects presenting for total hip joint replacement. Anesthesiology. 2011;114:1297–304.
63. Khan MA, Hossain FS, Ahmed I, Muthukumar N, Mohsen A. Predictors of early mortality after hip fracture surgery. Int Orthop. 2013;37:2119–24.
64. Seitz DP, Gill SS, Bell CM, Austin PC, Gruneir A, Anderson GM, et al. Postoperative medical complications associated with anesthesia in older adults with dementia. J Am Geriatr Soc. 2014;62:2102–9.
65. Cao L, Wang K, Gu T, Du B, Song J. Association between APOE epsilon 4 allele and postoperative cognitive dysfunction: a meta-analysis. Int J Neurosci. 2014;124:478–85.
66. Schenning KJ, Murchison CF, Mattek NC, Kaye JA, Quinn JF. Sex and genetic differences in postoperative cognitive dysfunction: a longitudinal cohort analysis. Biol Sex Differ. 2019;10:14.
67. Liu Y, Pan N, Ma Y, Zhang S, Guo W, Li H, et al. Inhaled sevoflurane may promote progression of amnestic mild cognitive impairment: a prospective, randomized parallel-group study. Am J Med Sci. 2013;345:355–60.
68. Patel D, Lunn AD, Smith AD, Lehmann DJ, Dorrington KL. Cognitive decline in the elderly after surgery and anaesthesia: results from the Oxford project to investigate memory and ageing (OPTIMA) cohort. Anaesthesia. 2016;71:1144–52.
69. Wan Y, Xu J, Ma D, Zeng Y, Cibelli M, Maze M. Postoperative impairment of cognitive function in rats: a possible role for cytokine-mediated inflammation in the hippocampus. Anesthesiology. 2007;106:436–43.
70. Kawano T, Yamanaka D, Aoyama B, Tateiwa H, Shigematsu-Locatelli M, Nishigaki A, et al. Involvement of acute neuroinflammation in postoperative delirium-like cognitive deficits in rats. J Anesth. 2018;32(4):506–17.
71. Xu Z, Dong Y, Wang H, Culley DJ, Marcantonio ER, Crosby G, et al. Age-dependent postoperative cognitive impairment and Alzheimer-related neuropathology in mice. Sci Rep. 2014;4. https://doi.org/10.1038/srep03766.
72. Crosby C, Culley DJ, Baxter MG, Yukhananov R, Crosby G. Spatial memory performance 2 weeks after general anesthesia in adult rats. Anesth Analg. 2005;101:1389–92.
73. Wu J, Zhang M, Li H, Sun X, Hao S, Ji M, et al. BDNF pathway is involved in the protective effects of SS-31 on isoflurane-induced cognitive deficits in aging mice. Behav Brain Res. 2016;305:115–21.
74. Liu W, Xu J, Wang H, Xu C, Ji C, Wang Y, et al. Isoflurane-induced spatial memory impairment by a mechanism independent of amyloid-beta levels and tau protein phosphorylation changes in aged rats. Neurol Res. 2012;34:3–10.
75. Callaway JK, Wood C, Jenkins TA, Royse AG, Royse CF. Isoflurane in the presence or absence of surgery increases hippocampal cytokines associated with memory deficits and responses to brain injury in rats. Behav Brain Res. 2016;303:44–52.
76. Xu X, Zhang Q, Tian X, Wang G. Sevoflurane anesthesia induces neither contextual fear memory impairment nor alterations in local population connectivity of medial prefrontal cortex local field potentials networks in aged rats. Fundam Clin Pharmacol. 2016;30:338–46.
77. Le Freche H, Brouillette J, Fernandez-Gomez F-J, Patin P, Caillierez R, Zommer N, et al. Tau phosphorylation and sevoflurane anesthesia: an association to postoperative cognitive impairment. Anesthesiology. 2012; 116:779–87.
78. Ji M, Dong L, Jia M, Liu W, Zhang M, Ju L, et al. Epigenetic enhancement of brain-derived neurotrophic factor signaling pathway improves cognitive impairments induced by isoflurane exposure in aged rats. Mol Neurobiol. 2014;50:937–44.
79. Guo S, Liu L, Wang C, Jiang Q, Dong Y, Tian Y. Repeated exposure to sevoflurane impairs the learning and memory of older male rats. Life Sci. 2018;192:75–83.
80. Tang JX, Eckenhoff MF. Anesthetic effects in Alzheimer transgenic mouse models. Prog Neuro-Psychopharmacol Biol Psychiatry. 2013;47:167–71.
81. Bianchi SL, Tran T, Liu C, Lin S, Li Y, Keller JM, et al. Brain and behavior changes in 12-month-old Tg2576 and nontransgenic mice exposed to anesthetics. Neurobiol Aging. 2008;29:1002–10.
82. Tang JX, Mardini F, Caltagarone BM, Garrity ST, Li RQ, Bianchi SL, et al. Anesthesia in presymptomatic Alzheimer's disease: a study using the triple-transgenic mouse model. Alzheimers Dement J Alzheimers Assoc. 2011;7:521–31 e1.
83. Olsson B, Lautner R, Andreasson U, Öhrfelt A, Portelius E, Bjerke M, et al. CSF and blood biomarkers for the diagnosis of Alzheimer's disease: a systematic review and meta-analysis. Lancet Neurol. 2016;15:673–84.
84. Mehta PD, Pirttilä T, Mehta SP, Sersen EA, Aisen PS, Wisniewski HM. Plasma and cerebrospinal fluid levels of amyloid beta proteins 1-40 and 1-42 in Alzheimer disease. Arch Neurol. 2000;57:100–5.
85. Fukumoto H, Tennis M, Locascio JJ, Hyman BT, Growdon JH, Irizarry MC. Age but not diagnosis is the main predictor of plasma amyloid beta-protein levels. Arch Neurol. 2003;60:958–64.
86. Fei M, Jianghua W, Rujuan M, Wei Z, Qian W. The relationship of plasma Aβ levels to dementia in aging individuals with mild cognitive impairment. J Neurol Sci. 2011;305:92–6.
87. Kim HJ, Park KW, Kim TE, Im JY, Shin HS, Kim S, et al. Elevation of the plasma Aβ40/Aβ42 ratio as a diagnostic marker of sporadic early-onset Alzheimer's disease. J Alzheimers Dis JAD. 2015;48:1043–50.
88. Tang JX, Baranov D, Hammond M, Shaw LM, Eckenhoff MF, Eckenhoff RG. Human Alzheimer and inflammation biomarkers after anesthesia and surgery. Anesthesiology. 2011;115:727–32.
89. Berger M, Nadler JW, Friedman A, McDonagh DL, Bennett ER, Cooter M, et al. The effect of Propofol versus Isoflurane anesthesia on human cerebrospinal fluid markers of Alzheimer's disease: results of a randomized trial. J Alzheimers Dis JAD. 2016;52:1299–310.
90. Pikwer A, Castegren M, Namdar S, Blennow K, Zetterberg H, Mattsson N. Effects of surgery and propofol-remifentanil total intravenous anesthesia on cerebrospinal fluid biomarkers of inflammation, Alzheimer's disease, and neuronal injury in humans: a cohort study. J Neuroinflammation. 2017;14:193.
91. Xie Z, Swain CA, Ward SAP, Zheng H, Dong Y, Sunder N, et al. Preoperative cerebrospinal fluid β-amyloid/tau ratio and postoperative delirium. Ann Clin Transl Neurol. 2014;1:319–28.
92. Planel E, Richter KEG, Nolan CE, Finley JE, Liu L, Wen Y, et al. Anesthesia leads to tau hyperphosphorylation through inhibition of phosphatase activity by hypothermia. J Neurosci. 2007;27:3090–7.
93. Xiao H, Run X, Cao X, Su Y, Sun Z, Tian C, et al. Temperature control can abolish anesthesia-induced tau hyperphosphorylation and partly reverse anesthesia-induced cognitive impairment in old mice. Psychiatry Clin Neurosci. 2013;67:493–500.
94. Dong Y, Wu X, Xu Z, Zhang Y, Xie Z. Anesthetic isoflurane increases phosphorylated tau levels mediated by caspase activation and Aβ generation. PLoS One. 2012;7:e39386.
95. Feng C, Liu Y, Yuan Y, Cui W, Zheng F, Ma Y, et al. Isoflurane anesthesia exacerbates learning and memory impairment in zinc-deficient APP/PS1 transgenic mice. Neuropharmacology. 2016;111:119–29.
96. Li C, Liu S, Xing Y, Tao F. The role of hippocampal tau protein phosphorylation in isoflurane-induced cognitive dysfunction in transgenic APP695 mice. Anesth Analg. 2014;119:413–9.
97. Tang JX, Mardini F, Janik LS, Garrity ST, Li RQ, Bachlani G, et al. Modulation of murine Alzheimer pathogenesis and behavior by surgery. Ann Surg. 2013;257:439–48.
98. Tao G, Zhang J, Zhang L, Dong Y, Yu B, Crosby G, et al. Sevoflurane induces tau phosphorylation and glycogen synthase kinase 3β activation in young mice. Anesthesiology. 2014;121:510–27.
99. Tan W-F, Cao X-Z, Wang J-K, Lv H-W, Wu B-Y, Ma H. Protective effects of lithium treatment for spatial memory deficits induced by tau

hyperphosphorylation in splenectomized rats. Clin Exp Pharmacol Physiol. 2010;37:1010–5.
100. Tang N, Jiang R, Wang X, Wen J, Liu L, Wu J, et al. Insulin resistance plays a potential role in postoperative cognitive dysfunction in patients following cardiac valve surgery. Brain Res. 1657;2017:377–82.
101. Kline R, Wong E, Haile M, Didehvar S, Farber S, Sacks A, et al. Peri-operative inflammatory cytokines in plasma of the elderly correlate in prospective study with postoperative changes in cognitive test scores. Int J Anesthesiol Res. 2016;4:313–21.
102. Liu X, Yu Y, Zhu S. Inflammatory markers in postoperative delirium (POD) and cognitive dysfunction (POCD): a meta-analysis of observational studies. PLoS One. 2018;13:e0195659.
103. Cui R-S, Wang K, Wang Z-L. Sevoflurane anesthesia alters cognitive function by activating inflammation and cell death in rats. Exp Ther Med. 2018;15: 4127–30.
104. Perucho J, Rubio I, Casarejos MJ, Gomez A, Rodriguez-Navarro JA, Solano RM, et al. Anesthesia with isoflurane increases amyloid pathology in mice models of Alzheimer's disease. J Alzheimers Dis JAD. 2010;19:1245–57.
105. Wu X, Lu Y, Dong Y, Zhang G, Zhang Y, Xu Z, et al. The inhalation anesthetic isoflurane increases levels of proinflammatory cytokine TNF-α, IL-6 and IL-1β. Neurobiol Aging. 2012;33:1364–78.
106. Cibelli M, Fidalgo AR, Terrando N, Ma D, Monaco C, Feldmann M, et al. Role of interleukin-1beta in postoperative cognitive dysfunction. Ann Neurol. 2010;68:360–8.
107. Zheng J-W, Meng B, Li X-Y, Lu B, Wu G-R, Chen J-P. NF-κB/P65 signaling pathway: a potential therapeutic target in postoperative cognitive dysfunction after sevoflurane anesthesia. Eur Rev Med Pharmacol Sci. 2017; 21:394–407.
108. Acharya NK, Goldwaser EL, Forsberg MM, Godsey GA, Johnson CA, Sarkar A, et al. Sevoflurane and Isoflurane induce structural changes in brain vascular endothelial cells and increase blood-brain barrier permeability: possible link to postoperative delirium and cognitive decline. Brain Res. 1620;2015:29–41.
109. Zheng B, Lai R, Li J, Zuo Z. Critical role of P2X7 receptors in the neuroinflammation and cognitive dysfunction after surgery. Brain Behav Immun. 2017;61:365–74.
110. Ling Y, Ma W, Yu L, Zhang Y, Liang Q. Decreased PSD95 expression in medial prefrontal cortex (mPFC) was associated with cognitive impairment induced by sevoflurane anesthesia. J Zhejiang Univ Sci B. 2015;16:763–71.
111. Miao H, Dong Y, Zhang Y, Zheng H, Shen Y, Crosby G, et al. Anesthetic Isoflurane or Desflurane Plus Surgery Differently Affects Cognitive Function in Alzheimer's Disease Transgenic Mice. Mol Neurobiol. 2018;55(7):5623–638.
112. Zhang C, Zhang Y, Shen Y, Zhao G, Xie Z, Dong Y. Anesthesia/surgery induces cognitive impairment in female Alzheimer's disease transgenic mice. J Alzheimers Dis JAD. 2017;57:505–18.
113. Li L, Li Z, Cao Y, Fan D, Chui D, Guo X. Increased extrasynaptic GluN2B expression is involved in cognitive impairment after isoflurane anesthesia. Exp Ther Med. 2016;12:161–8.
114. Uchimoto K, Miyazaki T, Kamiya Y, Mihara T, Koyama Y, Taguri M, et al. Isoflurane impairs learning and hippocampal long-term potentiation via the saturation of synaptic plasticity. Anesthesiology. 2014;121:302–10.
115. Zurek AA, Yu J, Wang D-S, Haffey SC, Bridgwater EM, Penna A, et al. Sustained increase in α5GABAA receptor function impairs memory after anesthesia. J Clin Invest. 2014;124:5437–41.
116. Zhang D-X, Jiang S, Yu L-N, Zhang F-J, Zhuang Q, Yan M. The effect of sevoflurane on the cognitive function of rats and its association with the inhibition of synaptic transmission. Int J Clin Exp Med. 2015;8:20853–60.
117. Wei H, Xie Z. Anesthesia, calcium homeostasis and Alzheimer's disease. Curr Alzheimer Res. 2009;6:30–5.
118. Qi Z, Tianbao Y, Yanan L, Xi X, Jinhua H, Qiujun W. Pre-treatment with nimodipine and 7.5% hypertonic saline protects aged rats against postoperative cognitive dysfunction via inhibiting hippocampal neuronal apoptosis. Behav Brain Res. 2017;321:1–7.
119. Zhang Q, Li Y, Bao Y, Yin C, Xin X, Guo Y, et al. Pretreatment with nimodipine reduces incidence of POCD by decreasing calcineurin mediated hippocampal neuroapoptosis in aged rats. BMC Anesthesiol. 2018;18:42.
120. Zhang G, Dong Y, Zhang B, Ichinose F, Wu X, Culley DJ, et al. Isoflurane-induced caspase-3 activation is dependent on cytosolic calcium and can be attenuated by memantine. J Neurosci. 2008;28:4551–60.

15

Association of Mallampati scoring on airway outcomes in women undergoing general anesthesia with supreme™ laryngeal mask airway in cesarean section

Hon Sen Tan[1], Shi Yang Li[2], Wei Yu Yao[2], Yong Jing Yuan[3], Rehena Sultana[4], Nian-Lin R. Han[5], Alex Tiong Heng Sia[1,6] and Ban Leong Sng[1,6*]

Abstract

Background: Obstetric dfficult airway is a leading cause of maternal morbidity and mortality. The laryngeal mask airway (LMA) is often used as a rescue airway device after failed intubation, however, little is known about predictors of cifficult LMA insertion, particularly in obstetrics. Since Mallampati scores of III/IV has been associated with difficult tracheal intubation, our present study aims to investigate if Mallampati score (MP) could predict airway outcomes for LMA use in obstetrics.

Methods: This prospective cohort study was performed at a single-center: Quanzhou Women's and Children's Hospital, Fujian Province, China. Five hundred and eighty-four parturients undergoing elective cesarean section under general anesthesia were recruited. The primary outcome was time to effective ventilation, and secondary outcomes included first attempt insertion success, seal pressure, ventilation and hemodynamic parameters, occurrence of clinical aspiration, and maternal and fetal outcomes.

Results: The parturients were classified into two groups based on MP of III/IV (High MP: 61) versus I/II (Low MP: 523). BMI was higher in the High MP group than in the Low MP group (mean (SD) 29.3 (7.0) vs 26.8 (3.1), $p < 0.0001$). There was no difference in maternal age, ASA status and gestational age. There was similar time to effective ventilation (mean (SD) High MP: 14.9 (4.5) vs Low MP: 15.7 (4.4) seconds, $p = 0.2172$), and first attempt success rate, seal pressure, and peak airway pressure. No clinical aspiration was noted. The incidence of blood on SLMA was higher in the High MP group than in Low MP (4 (6.6%) vs 4 (0.8%), $p = 0.001$). There was no difference in sore throat, voice hoarseness, maternal satisfaction and fetal outcomes.

Conclusion: High MP was not associated with reduced SLMA airway outcomes in cesarean section under general anesthesia, but may increase the risk of blood found on SLMA upon removal.

Keywords: Laryngeal mask, Obstetrics, Cesarean section, Airway

* Correspondence: sng.ban.leong@singhealth.com.sg
Presentation: The results has been presented at the Difficult Airway Society Meeting, London, 2017.
[1]Department of Women's Anaesthesia, KK Women's and Children's Hospital, 100 Bukit Timah Road, Singapore, Singapore
[6]Anaesthesiology and Perioperative Sciences Academic Clinical Program, Duke-NUS Medical School, 8 College Road, Singapore, Singapore

Background

Airway complication is one of the main causes of anesthesia-related obstetric adverse events. There are several complex clinical challenges faced in managing the parturient including the risk of pulmonary aspiration, physiological changes of pregnancy, urgent nature of cesarean section, and balancing the potentially conflicting needs of the mother and fetus. Endotracheal intubation has long been considered standard of care for obstetric airway management [1, 2], but comes with the concomitant risk of difficult intubation; a potentially life-threatening situation. The Mallampati score and other bedside airway assessments have been used to predict difficult intubation in adult patients. A recent Cochrane systematic review reported the specificity and sensitivity of the modified Mallampati score in diagnosing difficult tracheal intubation as 0.87 and 0.51, respectively [3].

With the additional risk of failed intubation posed by the obstetric airway (estimated at 0.4%), the laryngeal mask airway (LMA) has emerged as a second-line airway device [4–8]. Additionally, the viability of second-generation LMAs with a double-lumen specifically designed to physically isolate the alimentary tract and reduce the risk of aspiration [9–12] was highlighted by its inclusion in the obstetric-specific guideline jointly released by Obstetric Anaesthetists' Association (OAA) and Difficult Airway Society (DAS) [13]. Our group has also demonstrated the efficacy of LMA use for obstetric airway management in several prospective cohort studies [12, 14].

Notwithstanding its utility as a rescue airway device, we should be cognizant that the incidence of first-attempt LMA failure in obstetrics is approximately 2% [12, 14]. Additionally, the efficacy of bedside tests to predict LMA failure is poorly elucidated in the general population, with a paucity of obstetric-specific data. Despite its widespread use in predicting difficult intubations, the modified Mallampati score in non-obstetric cases has been shown to predict LMA failure by some authors [15], whereas others reported otherwise [16, 17]. This gap in knowledge, especially relating to parturients, is concerning, as the ability to accurately and rapidly predict LMA failure a priori is essential in obstetrics, due to the reliance on the LMA as a rescue airway device, as well as the limited time available before the risk of maternal or fetal morbidity increases.

Therefore, it is vital to predict when LMA failure is likely to occur, and formulate an alternate airway plan. Additionally, to be an effective rescue airway the factors associated with LMA failure could be different from those predicting failure to intubate. This prospective cohort study aims to investigate the association between the modified Mallampati score and airway outcomes of Supreme™ LMA insertion for cesarean section under general anesthesia.

Methods

This is a secondary analysis of a previously-published prospective cohort study [14], which was approved by the Quanzhou Women's and Children's Hospital Institutional Review Board (dated 11 November 2013) and registered at Clinicaltrials.gov registry (NCT02026882). The study was conducted at Quanzhou Women's and Children's Hospital, Fujian Province, China, and patient recruitment occurred between December 2013 and November 2014. Largely due to patient preference, approximately 35% of parturients undergo cesarean section at the study center, with the majority performed under general anesthesia using the Supreme™ LMA (SLMA). Hence, the SLMA has been established as part of the routine airway management at the study center.

Parturients who were healthy or with well-controlled medical conditions (American Society of Anesthesiologists (ASA) physical status classification II) undergoing elective cesarean section under general anesthesia were recruited. We excluded patients with BMI > 35 kg/m^2, upper respiratory tract or neck pathology, or self-reported reflux disease. After fasting for a minimum of 4 h, the modified Mallampati score was determined by an independent assessor and the patients divided into two groups: Mallampati III/IV (High MP) and Mallampati I/II (Low MP).

The induction of anesthesia and SLMA insertion reflects the clinical practice at the study center, as well as the cohort study that forms the basis for this secondary analysis [14]. As per institutional standard, all parturients were premedicated with intravenous ranitidine, and monitored with electrocardiogram, pulse oximetry, capnography and non-invasive blood pressure monitor. The chosen SLMA size was based on the manufacturer's guidelines and the discretion of the attending anesthesiologist. All SLMA were inserted by three investigators (Yao, Li, and Yuan), each with at least five years of experience in its use for cesarean delivery. Anesthesia was commenced via rapid sequence induction with the application of cricoid pressure by a trained anesthetic assistant, and administration of propofol and succinylcholine, followed by SLMA insertion using the recommended rotational technique. After cuff inflation to 60 cmH_2O via a manometer, assessment of successful SLMA placement was made by auscultation of breath sounds and the capnographic evidence of end-tidal carbon dioxide, and cricoid pressure was released. The use of additional maneuvers such as chin lift, jaw thrust, or head tilt were permitted. Rocuronium was used to maintain intraoperative muscle relaxation, and fentanyl was administered for analgesia after delivery of the fetus.

We recorded (1) the number of insertion attempts required, with each attempt defined as insertion and complete removal of the SLMA; and (2) the time to effective airway placement, from when the SLMA was picked up until the first end-tidal carbon dioxide capnogram appeared. Subsequently, a pre-mounted #14 orogastric tube was inserted through the gastric drainage port, and placement confirmed by aspiration of gastric contents and auscultation of a "swoosh" over the epigastrium with air injection, followed by suctioning of the orogastric tube before surgery commenced. Finally, oropharyngeal leak pressure was measured by shutting the adjustable pressure-limiting valve and maintaining 3 L/min fresh gas flow into the closed circuit. Cesarean section was allowed to commence if the following were met: presence of square-wave capnogram, cuff pressure of 60 cmH_2O, positioning of the SLMA bite block between the incisors, successful orogastric tube insertion, and leak pressure > $20cmH_2O$. If successful SLMA insertion was not accomplished (1) after two attempts, (2) within one minute, or (3) before desaturation ensued, endotracheal intubation would be performed.

Perioperative anesthesia management during the original cohort study [14] reflects the clinical practice at the study center. With all parturients positioned left lateral tilt using a wedge, anesthesia was maintained with 1.5 to 2% sevoflurane and 50:50 mix of nitrous oxide in oxygen. We recorded the incidence of airway complications including airway obstruction, inadequate oxygenation or ventilation, and the presence of signs of clinical aspiration such as hypoxemia, auscultation of wheezing or crepitations, and postoperative dyspnea. Parturients were ventilated with tidal volume of 6 to 10 ml/kg, and respiratory rate of 10 to 16 breaths/min. The obstetricians were advised to avoid excessive fundal pressure during fetal delivery. Upon completion of surgery, suctioning and removal of the orogastric tube was performed, and the SLMA was withdrawn and inspected for blood. An independent assessor determined the incidence of sore throat and voice hoarseness prior to discharge from the post anesthesia care unit.

Our primary outcome was time to effective ventilation, as defined above. Secondary outcomes included the rate of successful first-attempt SLMA insertion, oropharyngeal leak pressure, ventilation parameters such as tidal volume and respiratory rate, hemodynamic parameters including heart rate and blood pressure at 2 and 5 min after induction, amount and pH of gastric aspirate, the pH of the SLMA laryngeal surface, and the presence of clinical aspiration. Obstetric and fetal outcomes included neonatal weight, Apgar scores, and umbilical venous pH.

Statistical analysis

All demographic, anesthetic, and clinical categorical data were summarized as frequency with corresponding proportion, and continuous variables were expressed as mean (standard deviation (SD)) or median [interquartile range (IQR)], whichever appropriate. The difference between categorical data was tested using the Chi-Square test, while Student's t-test and Mann-Whitney U test were used for parametric and non-parametric continuous data, respectively. Simple linear and multivariable linear regression methods were utilized to determine associated risk factors for our primary outcome of time to effective ventilation. Associations identified from linear regression were expressed as estimate (β) with 95% confidence interval (95%CI). Significance level was set at $p < 0.05$ and all tests were two-sided. Data analysis was generated using SAS 9.3 software (SAS Institute Inc., Cary, NC, USA).

We performed a sample size calculation based on the following assumptions: a meaningful clinical difference of at least 10 s in time to effective ventilation between "High MP" and "Low MP" groups, pooled SD of 4.5, allocation ratio of 1:8, use of two-sample independent t-test, level of significance of 5% and > 95% power. The study was adequately powered (> 95%) with 584 parturients.

Results

We recruited 584 parturients. Of these, 61 were found to have Mallampati III/IV (High MP) and 523 with Mallampati I/II (Low MP) (Table 1). There was no withdrawal or dropout. Demographic and clinical characteristics are summarized in Table 2. The BMI in the High MP group was higher than in the Low MP group (mean (SD) 29.3 (7.1) vs 26.8 (3.1), $p = 0.0001$), but there was no significant difference in maternal age, fetal weight, or gestational age. The duration of surgery was similar, with mean (SD) 31.0 (11.1) minutes in the High MP group vs 29.3 (9.2) minutes in the Low MP group ($p = 0.4159$).

Anesthetic outcomes are presented in Table 3. There was no significant difference in our primary outcome of time to effective ventilation, with 14.9 (4.5) seconds for the High MP group versus 15.7 (4.4) for the Low MP group ($p = 0.2172$). Similarly, there was no difference in first attempt insertion success rate of 98.4% for the High MP group versus 98.3% for the Low MP group. The lowest SpO_2, seal pressure and peak airway pressures were similar between the groups. No episodes of hypoxemia,

Table 1 Distribution of modified Mallampati score among participants undergoing cesarean section under general anesthesia

	Frequency, $n = 584$	Proportion (%)
Mallampati I	226	38.70
Mallampati II	297	50.86
Mallampati III	56	9.59
Mallampati IV	5	0.86

Table 2 Baseline patient demographics and clinical characteristics of participants with either modified Mallampati scores of III/IV versus I/II undergoing cesarean section under general anesthesia

	Mallampati Score		*p*-value
	III to IV	I to II	
Age (years), mean (SD)	28.8 (5.4)	28.9 (4.0)	0.5315
BMI (kg/m^2), mean (SD)	29.3 (7.1)	26.8 (3.1)	**0.0001**
Duration of surgery (min), mean (SD)	31.0 (11.1)	29.3 (9.2)	0.4159
Gestation (weeks), median [IQR]	38.0 [37.1 to 39.0]	38.3 [37.1 to 39.0]	0.1024
Fetal weight (g), mean (SD)	2995 (580)	3017 (532)	0.3608

Values are presented as mean (SD) or median [IQR]
Significance level was set at $P < 0.05$

laryngospasm, or bronchospasm were observed intraoperatively.

Maternal and fetal outcomes are summarized in Table 4. There was no clinical aspiration noted, and the volume of gastric aspirate was similar between the groups. However, the pH of the SLMA laryngeal surface was statistically lower in the Low MP group: 7.2 (0.4) for High MP versus 7.0 (0.5) for Low MP ($p = 0.0191$). The presence of blood on the SLMA was more frequently noted in the High MP group with 4 (6.6%) versus 4 (0.8%) in the Low MP group ($p = 0.0010$), but there were no significant differences in sore throat ($p = 0.6071$), voice hoarseness ($p = 0.1585$), or maternal satisfaction ($p = 0.5131$). Fetal outcomes, including Apgar scores at 1 and 5 min, and venous cord pH were similar between the groups.

Univariate linear regression method showed that age and baseline systolic blood pressure were significantly associated with time to effective ventilation (Table 5); while multivariable linear regression showed that age (β (95%CI): 0.012 (0.007, 0.017)) and baseline systolic blood pressure (β (95%CI): – 0.004 (– 0.006, – 0.002)) were significantly associated with time to effective ventilation (Table 5).

Discussion

This prospective cohort study of 584 parturients undergoing cesarean section under general anesthesia compared the airway outcomes of the SLMA in patients with lower Mallampati scores (I or II) versus higher scores (III or IV). Out of 584 patients, 61 (10.4%) had Mallampati scores of III or IV. We found no association between Mallampati scores and time to effective ventilation, first attempt success rate, or SLMA seal pressure. There was no clinical aspiration detected, and the pH of the SLMA laryngeal surface was not indicative of gastric regurgitation. However, higher Mallampati scores was associated with increased risk of blood found on the SLMA, which may indicate increased risk of oropharyngeal trauma on insertion, but without

Table 3 Anesthetic outcomes of participants with either modified Mallampati scores of III/IV versus I/II while undergoing cesarean section under general anesthesia

	Mallampati Score		*p*-value
	III to IV	I to II	
Time to effective ventilation (s), mean (SD)	14.9 (4.5)	15.7 (4.4)	0.2172
No. of insertion attempts of LMA > 1, n (%)	1 (1.6%)	9 (1.7%)	0.6373
No. of insertion attempts of gastric tube, median [IQR]	1 [1–1]	1 [1–1]	1.0000
Seal pressure (cmH2O), median [IQR]	27 [26–31]	27 [25–30]	0.5811
Peak airway pressure (cmH2O), median [IQR]	18 [16–23]	18 [15–21]	0.1134
Lowest SpO_2 (%), median [IQR]	99 [98–99]	99 [98–99]	0.5812
Baseline systolic blood pressure (mmHg), mean (SD)	128.8 (15.7)	121.8 (12.4)	**0.0001**
Systolic blood pressure 2 min after induction (mmHg), mean (SD)	126.9 (21.2)	115.9 (17.3)	**< 0.0001**
Systolic blood pressure 5 min after induction (mmHg), mean (SD)	111.9 (13.4)	108.5 (14.6)	0.0802
Baseline heart rate (beats/min), mean (SD)	89.0 (12.0)	87.4 (11.3)	0.2866
Heart rate 2 min after induction (beats/min), mean (SD)	94.0 (15.4)	94.4 (17.2)	0.8725
Heart rate 5 min after induction (beats/min), mean (SD)	86.1 (13.1)	88.4 (18.2)	0.3481

Values are presented as mean (SD), n(%) or median [IQR]
Significance level was set at $P < 0.05$

Table 4 Maternal and fetal outcomes of participants with either modified Mallampati scores of III/IV versus I/II undergoing cesarean section under general anesthesia

	Mallampati Score		*p*-value
	III to IV	I to II	
Gastric aspirate volume (mL), mean (SD)	18.3 (27.9)	13.7 (11.7)	0.4256
pH of gastric aspirate, mean (SD)	2.6 (1.0)	2.3 (0.8)	**0.0314**
pH of SLMA laryngeal surface, mean (SD)	7.2 (0.4)	7.0 (0.5)	**0.0191**
Blood on SLMA, n (%)	4 (6.6%)	4 (0.8%)	**0.0010**
Sore throat, n (%)	4 (6.6%)	34 (6.5%)	0.6071
Voice hoarseness, n (%)	0	4 (0.8%)	0.1585
Maternal satisfaction (%), mean (SD)	86.8 (9.2)	86.0 (8.5)	0.5131
Fetal Apgar at 1 min, mean (SD)	9.2 (1.2)	9.2 (1.1)	0.8250
Fetal Apgar at 5 min, mean (SD)	9.6 (0.9)	9.7 (0.7)	0.5198
Venous cord pH, mean (SD)	7.3 (0.1)	7.3 (0.1)	0.4969

Values are presented as mean (SD) or n (%)
Significance level was set at $P < 0.05$

corresponding change in sore throat, voice hoarseness, or maternal satisfaction.

Our results suggest that LMA outcomes in obstetric general anesthesia was not significantly affected by higher Mallampati scores. The Mallampati score is postulated to be related to the size of the tongue base during difficult laryngoscopy due to occlusion of the view of pharyngeal structures [15]. This is supported by Cormack and Lehane, who cited large or poorly mobile tongue and anterior larynx as potential causes of difficult laryngoscopy [18].

Although previous studies associated higher Mallampati scores with increased LMA failure rates [15], our findings concur with studies demonstrating poor relation between Mallampati score and LMA outcomes [16, 17]. Furthermore, the time to effective ventilation and first attempt SLMA insertion success rate reported here is comparable to other LMA studies in obstetric general anesthesia [12], despite application of cricoid pressure which may impede LMA insertion into the post-cricoid hypopharyngeal space. This excellent success rate despite high Mallampati scores may be stem from the postulation by Brain that intubation difficulties were associated with anteriorly sited larynx and therefore predicted by higher Mallampati scores, whereas a posteriorly sited larynx may increase LMA failure by blocking downward progress of the LMA tip [19]. Other attenuating factors include (1) routine use of SLMA for cesarean delivery at the study center, (2) insertion by experienced anesthetists, and (3) the relative rigidity of the SLMA.

A common concern of LMA use in obstetrics relates to the inherently higher risk of gastric regurgitation and pulmonary aspiration, exacerbated by concomitant obesity, labor pain, or opioid analgesia. In this study, we did not detect any clinical aspiration or regurgitation, likely due to (1) the ability of second-generation LMAs to isolate the alimentary tract and facilitate gastric decompression, (2) better pharyngeal seal that prevents stomach insufflation and regurgitated gastric contents from entering the airway, (3) use of rapid-sequence induction and cricoid pressure, and (4) careful patient selection with exclusion of patients at high risk for regurgitation. However, this study was not powered to investigate the risk of pulmonary aspiration.

There are several limitations in this study. First, we are cognizant that bedside tests, including the Mallampati

Table 5 Univariate and multivariable linear regression to find associated risk factors for time to effective ventilation

Variables	Univariate linear regression		Multivariable linear regression	
	Estimate (95%CI)	*P* - value	Estimate (95%CI)	*P* - value
Age (years)	0.17 (0.08, 0.25)	**0.0001**	0.012 (0.007, 0.017)	**< 0.0001**
BMI (kg/m^2)	0.02 (−0.07, 0.12)	0.6074		
Gestation (weeks)	0.19 (0, 0.38)	0.0537		
Fetal weight (g)	0.0004 (−0.0003, 0.0011)	0.2252		
Baseline systolic blood pressure (mmHg)	−0.05 (− 0.08, − 0.03)	**0.0002**	−0.004 (− 0.006, − 0.002)	**< 0.0001**
Heart rate (bpm)	0.003 (− 0.029, 0.035)	0.8514		

Significance level was set at $P < 0.05$

score, are considered by some to be poor predictors of difficult intubation especially if used in isolation [20, 21]. However, a recent meta-analysis by Lee et al. reported a five-fold increase in accuracy of the modified Mallampati score for predicting difficult laryngoscopy in obstetric patients [20], thus lending weight to its use in parturients. Additionally, we investigated the Mallampati score independently instead of in combination with other bedside tests for difficult intubation due to scarce data of the utility of such tests in obstetrics, and concerns that a possible correlation with SLMA failure may be hidden if several predictive factors were summated.

Second, we utilized clinical markers of SLMA airway outcomes, such as time to ventilation, first attempt insertion success rate, and seal pressure, in contrast to other studies that assessed LMA position via a fiberoptic grading scale [17]. Several studies utilizing fibreoptic grading have reported a 50% incidence of suboptimal anatomical positioning, allegedly resulting in gastric air insufflation [17, 22]. While we agree that fiberoptic grading would provide additional information on SLMA placement, our routine practice does not include fiberoptic assessment, and this study was a pragmatic evaluation of the use SLMA in obstetrics, hence our focus was on its ability to achieve adequate ventilation. Furthermore, gastric insufflation may be attenuated by our reported average seal pressure being 9cmH_2O greater than the average peak airway pressure regardless of Mallampati score, as well as gastric decompression via an orogastric tube.

Third, we deliberately excluded patients at high risk of gastric regurgitation, including parturients with BMI of 35 kg/m^2 or higher. The retrospective study by Ramachandran et al. reported that elevated BMI of 29.3 versus 26.9 was associated with LMA Unique failure, but Mallampati scores of III to IV were not [23]. Despite the "High MP" group having significantly higher mean BMI of 29.3 versus 26.8 kg/m^2 in the "Low MP" group, we did not find any corresponding increased SLMA failure, although we were not specifically assessing the effects of increasing BMI on SLMA outcomes. Finally, we did not directly correlate failed intubation with LMA failure, and therefore cannot comment on the use of SLMA as a rescue airway.

Conclusion

Our prospective cohort study suggests that higher Mallampati score is not associated with longer time to effective ventilation when using the Supreme LMA in parturients undergoing elective cesarean delivery under general anesthesia, with similar time to effective ventilation, first attempt SLMA success rate, and seal pressure. More work is required to evaluate the accuracy of other bedside tests on predicting LMA airway outcomes in obstetrics.

Abbreviations

ASA: American Society of Anesthesiologists; BMI: Body mass index; DAS: Difficult Airway Society; LMA: Laryngeal mask airway; MP: Mallampati Score; OAA: Obstetric Anaesthetists' Association; SD: Standard deviation; SLMA: Supreme™ LMA

Acknowledgements

The authors would like to acknowledge the staff of Quanzhou Women's and Children's Hospital for their help in patient care for this study.

Authors' contributions

BLS: study design, data collection, data analysis, revising the article critically for important intellectual content and final approval of the version to be submitted. HST: data analysis, revising the article and final approval of the version to be submitted. SYL: study design, data collection, patient recruitment and final approval of the version to be submitted. WYY: data collection, patient recruitment and final approval of the version to be submitted. YJY: data collection, patient recruitment and final approval of the version to be submitted. RS: data analysis, revising the article and final approval of the version to be submitted. NLH: data analysis, revising the article and final approval of the version to be submitted. ATS: study design, data analysis, revising the article critically for important intellectual content and final approval of the version to be submitted. All authors read and approved the final manuscript.

Author details

[1]Department of Women's Anaesthesia, KK Women's and Children's Hospital, 100 Bukit Timah Road, Singapore, Singapore. [2]Department of Anesthesiology and Perioperative Medicine, Quanzhou Macare Women's Hospital, Quanzhou, Fujian Province, China. [3]Department of Anesthesiology, Qinghai University Affiliated Hospital, Xining, Qinghar Province, China. [4]Center for Quantitative Medicine, Duke-NUS Medical School, 8 College Road, Singapore, Singapore. [5]Division of Clinical Support Services, KK Women's and Children's Hospital, 100 Bukit Timah Road, Singapore, Singapore. [6]Anaesthesiology and Perioperative Sciences Academic Clinical Program, Duke-NUS Medical School, 8 College Road, Singapore, Singapore.

References

1. Harmer M. Difficult and failed intubation in obstetrics. Int J Obstet Anesth. 1997;6:25–31.
2. Mushambi MC, Kinsella SM. Obstetric Anaesthetists' Association/difficult airway society difficult and failed tracheal intubation guidelines--the way forward for the obstetric airway. Br J Anaesth. 2015;115:815–8.
3. Roth D, Pace NL, Lee A, Hovhannisyan K, Warenits AM, Arrich J, Herkner H. Airway physical examination tests for detection of difficult airway management in apparently normal adult patients. Cochrane Database Syst Rev. 2018;5:CD008874.
4. Barnardo PD, Jenkins JG. Failed tracheal intubation in obstetrics: a 6-year review in a UK region. Anaesthesia. 2000;55:690–4.
5. Hawthorne L, Wilson R, Lyons G, Dresner M. Failed intubation revisited: 17-yr experience in a teaching maternity unit. Br J Anaesth. 1996;76:680–4.
6. McDonnell NJ, Paech MJ, Clavisi OM, Scott KL. Group AT. Difficult and failed intubation in obstetric anaesthesia: an observational study of airway management and complications associated with general anaesthesia for caesarean section. Int J Obstet Anesth. 2008;17:292–7.
7. Quinn AC, Milne D, Columb M, Gorton H, Knight M. Failed tracheal intubation in obstetric anaesthesia: 2 yr national case-control study in the UK. Br J Anaesth. 2013;110:74–80.
8. Rahman K, Jenkins JG. Failed tracheal intubation in obstetrics: no more frequent but still managed badly. Anaesthesia. 2005;60:168–71.
9. Bercker S, Schmidbauer W, Volk T, Bogusch G, Bubser HP, Hensel M, et al. A comparison of seal in seven supraglottic airway devices using a cadaver model of elevated esophageal pressure. Anesth Analg. 2008;106:445–8.
10. Keller C, Brimacombe J, Kleinsasser A, Loeckinger A. Does the ProSeal laryngeal mask airway prevent aspiration of regurgitated fluid? Anesth Analg. 2000;91:1017–20.

11. Lim Y, Goel S, Brimacombe JR. The ProSeal laryngeal mask airway is an effective alternative to laryngoscope-guided tracheal intubation for gynaecological laparoscopy. Anaesth Intensive Care. 2007;35:52–6.
12. Yao WY, Li SY, Sng BL, Lim Y, Sia AT. The LMA supreme in 700 parturients undergoing cesarean delivery: an observational study. Can J Anaesth. 2012; 59:648–54.
13. Mushambi MC, Kinsella SM, Popat M, Swales H, Ramaswamy KK, Winton AL, et al. Obstetric Anaesthetists' Association and difficult airway society guidelines for the management of difficult and failed tracheal intubation in obstetrics. Anaesthesia. 2015;70:1286–306.
14. Li SY, Yao WY, Yuan YJ, Tay WS, Han NLR, Sultana R, et al. Supreme™ laryngeal mask airway use in general anesthesia for category 2 and 3 cesarean delivery: a prospective cohort study. BMC Anesthesiol. 2017;17:169.
15. McCrory CR, Moriarty DC. Laryngeal mask airway positioning is related to Mallampati grading in adults. Anesth Analg. 1995;81:1001–4.
16. Brimacombe J. Analysis of 1500 laryngeal mask uses by one anaesthetist in adults undergoing routine anaesthesia. Anaesthesia. 1996;51:76–80.
17. Joo HJ, Jong HK, Hee JB, Youn JK, Doo GY. Analysis of predictive factors for difficult ProSeal laryngeal mask airway insertion and suboptimal positioning. Anesth Pain Med. 2013;8:271–8.
18. Cormack RS, Lehane J. Difficult tracheal intubation in obstetrics. Anaesthesia. 1984;39:1105–11.
19. Brain AI. Three cases of difficult intubation overcome by the laryngeal mask airway. Anaesthesia. 1985;40:353–5.
20. Lee A, Fan LT, Gin T, Karmakar MK, Ngan Kee WD. A systematic review (meta-analysis) of the accuracy of the Mallampati tests to predict the difficult airway. Anesth Analg. 2006;102:1867–78.
21. Shiga T, Wajima Z, Inoue T, Sakamoto A. Predicting difficult intubation in apparently normal patients: a meta-analysis of bedside screening test performance. Anesthesiology. 2005;103:429–37.
22. Brimacombe J, Keller C, Fullekrug B, Agrò F, Rosenblatt W, Dierdorf SF, et al. A multicenter study comparing the ProSeal and classic laryngeal mask airway in anesthetized, nonparalyzed patients. Anesthesiology. 2002;96:289–95.
23. Ramachandran SK, Mathis MR, Tremper KK, Shanks AM, Kheterpal S. Predictors and clinical outcomes from failed laryngeal mask airway unique: a study of 15,795 patients. Anesthesiology. 2012;116:1217–26.

16

Effect of caudal ketamine on minimum local anesthetic concentration of ropivacaine in children

Huai-Zhen Wang[†], Ling-Yu Wang[†], Hui-Hong Liang, Yan-Ting Fan, Xing-Rong Song and Ying-Jun She[*]

Abstract

Background: Caudal ketamine has been shown to provide an effective and prolonged post-operative analgesia with few adverse effects. However, the effect of caudal ketamine on the minimum local anesthetic concentration (MLAC) of ropivacaine for intra-operative analgesia is unclear.

Methods: One hundred and sixty-nine children were randomized to five groups: Group C (caudal ropivacaine only), Group $K_{0.25}$ (caudal ropivacaine plus 0.25 mg/kg ketamine), Group $K_{0.5}$ (caudal ropivacaine plus 0.5 mg/kg ketamine), Group $K_{0.75}$ (caudal ropivacaine plus 0.75 mg/kg ketamine), and Group $K_{1.0}$ (caudal ropivacaine plus 1.0 mg/kg ketamine). The primary outcome was the MLAC values of ropivacaine with/without ketamine for caudal block.

Results: The MLAC values of ropivacaine were 0.128% (0.028%) in the control group, 0.112% (0.021%) in Group $K_{0.25}$, 0.112% (0.018%) in Group $K_{0.5}$, 0.110% (0.019%) in Group $K_{0.75}$, and 0.110% (0.020%) in Group $K_{1.0}$. There were no significant differences among the five groups for the MLAC values ($p = 0.11$). During the post-operative period the mean durations of analgesia were 270, 381, 430, 494, and 591 min in the control, $K_{0.25}$, $K_{0.\ 5}$, $K_{0.75}$, and $K_{1.0}$ groups respectively, which shown that control group is significantly different from all ketamine groups. Also there were significant differences between $K_{0.25}$ and $K_{0.75}$ groups, and between $K_{1.0}$ groups and the other ketamine groups.

Conclusions: Adding caudal ketamine to ropivacaine prolong the duration of post-operative analgesia; however, it does not decrease the MLAC of caudal ropivacaine for intra-operative analgesia in children.

Keywords: Anesthesia, caudal, Ketamine, Ropivacaine, Analgesia, Anesthetic techniques

* Correspondence: yjsheh@yeah.net
[†]Huai-Zhen Wang and Ling-Yu Wang are contributed equally to this work and should be considered co-first authors.
Department of Anesthesiology and Perioperative Medicine, Guangzhou Women and Children's Medical Center, Guangzhou Medical University, 9# Jinsui Road, Guangzhou 510623, China

Background

A caudal block is commonly used in children during lower abdominal and limb surgeries because it provides safe and effective perioperative analgesia. Single dose caudal levobupivacaine or ropivacaine provides analgesia for 4–8 h and has gained popularity with a high success rate and a low incidence of adverse effects [1, 2]. Also, it has been proved that several additives with local anesthetics can prolong the duration of caudal analgesia [3]. Research discovered that the most commonly used additives were clonidine (42.3%), ketamine (37.5%), opioids (18.1%), adrenaline (1.8%), and midazolam (0.3%) [4].

Caudal block is usually injected by a single high-dose local anesthetic, while decreasing local anesthetic dose reduces local tissue and systemic toxicity. Adjuvants were usually used to decrease the dose of local anesthetic and prolong the duration of analgesia. The minimum local anesthetic concentration (MLAC) has been conventionally used for evaluating the relative efficacy of generally used local anesthetics [5–7]. Many additives have been administrated in order to decrease the concentration of local anesthetics for caudal analgesia, while the effect of some additives on the MLAC values of local anesthetics have been explored in some previous studies [8, 9]. Caudal clonidine and dexmedetomidine produced a local anesthetic sparing effect with a dose-dependent decrease in MLAC of levobupivacaine for caudal anesthesia [8, 9]. As a commonly used additive, caudal ketamine has been shown to provide an effective and prolonged post-operative analgesia with few adverse events. However, the effect of caudal ketamine on the MLAC of ropivacaine is unclear. The aim of this prospective, randomized, and double-blind trial was to observe whether ketamine reduces the MLAC of ropivacaine for caudal block in children.

Methods

This study was approved by the Institutional Review Board of Guangzhou Women and Children's Medical Center (IRB2013053103), and written informed patient consent was attained from the parents or legal guardians of each paediatric patient in this trial. The trial was registered prior to patient enrolment at chictr.org.cn (ChiCTR-TRC-13003492). This study adhered to CONSORT guidelines for randomized trials. One hundred and sixty nine ASA physical status I or II children aged from 1 to 3 years old scheduled to undergo elective hydrocele or inguinal hernia repair were recruited. Exclusion criteria included patients with neurological, psychiatric, cardiovascular, respiratory, hepatic, renal diseases or bleeding disorders; or a known allergy history of anesthetics. Using a computer-generated table and a sealed envelope with sequence of numbers, children were randomly allocated into five groups into one of the five groups: Group C (caudal ropivacaine only), Group $K_{0.25}$ (caudal ropivacaine plus 0.25 mg/ml preservative free ketamine), Group $K_{0.5}$ (caudal ropivacaine plus 0.5 mg/ml preservative free ketamine), Group $K_{0.75}$ (caudal ropivacaine plus 0.75 mg/ml preservative free ketamine), and Group $K_{1.0}$ (caudal ropivacaine plus 1.0 mg/ml preservative free ketamine). The total volume of ropivacaine with/without preservative free ketamine solution for caudal injection in all groups are 1 ml/kg.

All children underwent preoperative fasting for 6 h and received no premedication. Sevoflurane via a face mask was used for anesthesia induction in the children. After securing intravenous access, 3 mg/kg propofol was intravenously administered to maintain sedation in a single dose or repeated doses. A caudal puncture was performed with a 22-gauge catheter by introducing in the caudal space with the patient in the left lateral decubitus position by a consultant anesthesiologist. The mixed solution of caudal injection is prepared by 0.9% saline, ropivacaine and ketamine. After felling the loss of resistance and checking for the negative presence of cerebrospinal fluid or blood, the ropivacaine with/without preservative free ketamine solution (total volume, 1 ml/kg) was administered via the catheter over 60 s. All inhalational agents were discontinued after the finish of the caudal injection. Then the patient was repositioned to supine for surgery. Continuously intravenous infused propofol (8–10 mg/kg/h) was administered to maintain sedation, and the depth of anesthesia was adjusted accordingly with the objective of achieving 80–120% baseline non-invasive mean arterial pressure. Dermatomal heights or upper limits of the caudal block were not formally assessed by pinprick before skin incision which was performed at exactly 20 min after the caudal injection. Baseline vital signs were collected to ensure a stable state and to discriminate slow onset of analgesia which was regarded as a confounding variable. An anesthesiologist who was unaware of the group assignments and the test concentrations of ropivacaine or ketamine maintain intraoperative depth of anesthesia, evaluated analgesic efficacy and collected the data. After skin incision, the patient was observed for at least 60 s for hemodynamic stability and signs of purposeful movement.

The primary outcome was the MLAC of ropivacaine with/without ketamine for caudal block in children. The success of a caudal block was defined as the change in hemodynamic parameters $< 20\%$ of baseline values and the absence of gross purposeful movement after skin incision. The modified Dixon's up-and-down method was used to determine the target concentration of caudal ropivacaine for each pediatric patient, starting from 0.16% in each group, with 0.02% as a step size. According to the response of the previous patient in the same group, the target concentration of caudal ropivacaine was increased or decreased. If it failed, a 0.02% concentration of caudal ropivacaine would be increased for the next patient. If it was successful, the next child could be given caudal ropivacaine where the concentration would be decreased by 0.02%. When a response was determined to be a failure, the surgeon would stop all operations, and a rescue dose of 0.5 mg/kg ketamine would be intravenously administrated immediately to reduce the pain and could be repeated if needed during the surgery. A pair of crossover was defined as the midpoint between failed and successful caudal block in two consecutive children. And the study would be ended after collecting nine pairs of crossover in each group.

The secondary outcomes of the study were durations of analgesia. Postoperative analgesia was assessed by using the "Face, Legs, Activity, Cry, Consoling" tool (FLACC). A FLACC score of more than 4 points was considered as inadequate analgesia and was additional orally administrated 10 mg/kg ibuprofen every 6 h as needed. The duration time of analgesia was defined from caudal block to the first postoperative rescue analgesia. The independent nurses evaluated the pain scale every hour in 8 h after the surgery and then every 6 h as required. Beside these time points, the independent nurses will be on call to assess the pain scale of patients. Side effects like postoperative nausea and vomiting (PONV), urine retention, agitation, hypotension, bradycardia, and respiratory depression were recorded. Emergence agitation evaluation was scored by using a five-point scale. A score of ≥3 was defined as emergence agitation according to five-point scale (0 = falling asleep peacefully; 1 = quiet; 2 = easy to console; 3 = difficult to console with moderate agitation; 4 = combative, excited, and disorientated). On the second day after surgery all children were discharged.

Statistical analysis

Statistical analyses were performed in SPSS 19.0 for Windows (SPSS Inc., USA). Data were expressed as mean (SD) or count, when appropriate. The MLAC was estimated from the up-and-down sequences with the Dixon and Massey method. The MLAC of caudal ropivacaine was analysed by calculating the midpoint concentration of all independent pairs of crossover points in each group. According to the study conducted by Paul and Fisher [10], nine pairs of crossover patients were needed. The variance of age, weight, duration of surgery, propofol doses, recovery time and duration of analgesia was analysed by using analysis of variance followed by a Dunnett t test or Kruskal-Wallis test. A Dunnett *t* test was used to test for normal distribution of the data. The duration of caudal analgesia was also analysed with Kaplan-Meier survival analysis and log-rank test. The type of surgery and adverse effects were analysed with the Chi-square test. $P < 0.05$ was considered statistically significant.

Results

One hundred and eighty-one children were enrolled in this study, 169 were analysed and 12 were excluded. Among the excluded patients, four were excluded because of serious airway symptoms, two were excluded because of data loss, three declined to participate in the study, and three were excluded due to the violation of anesthesia. All caudal block were considered as successful. The CONSORT flow diagram shows the details of patient recruitment (Fig. 1). Patient characteristics, the duration of operation, and the type of surgery were shown in Table 1. There were no significantly difference in incidences of agitation, urine retention, respiratory depression, bradycardia, hypotension, and PONV among groups (Table 1).

The patient responses to the skin incision according to the up-and-down sequence were illustrated in Fig. 2. The MLAC values of ropivacaine were 0.128% (0.028%) in control group, 0.112% (0.021%) in Group $K_{0.25}$, 0.112% (0.018%) in Group $K_{0.5}$, 0.110% (0.019%) in Group $K_{0.75}$, and 0.110% (0.020%) in Group $K_{1.0}$. There were no significant differences of the MLAC values among the five groups ($p = 0.11$).

The durations of analgesia in the five groups were illustrated with Kaplan-Meier survival curves in Fig. 3. The mean durations of analgesia in the postoperative period were 270, 381, 430, 494, and 591 min in the control, $K_{0.25}$, $K_{0.5}$, $K_{0.75}$, and $K_{1.0}$ groups, respectively. There were significant differences between the control group and all ketamine groups (control VS $K_{0.25}$, $p = 0.01$; control VS $K_{0.5}$, control VS $K_{0.75}$, control VS $K_{1.0}$, $p < 0.001$), and also between $K_{1.0}$ groups and the other ketamine groups ($K_{0.25}$ VS $K_{1.0}$, and $K_{0.5}$ VS $K_{1.0}$, $p < 0.001$; $K_{0.75}$ VS $K_{1.0}$, $p = 0.022$). Significant differences were observed between $K_{0.25}$ and $K_{0.75}$ groups ($p = 0.001$), but not between $K_{0.25}$ and $K_{0.5}$ groups ($p = 0.961$), or between $K_{0.5}$ and $K_{0.75}$ groups ($p = 0.222$).

Discussion

The aim of this study was to demonstrate whether caudal ketamine reduces the MLAC of caudal ropivacaine and prolongs the duration of post-operative analgesia in children. Our results showed that combined ketamine with ropivacaine for caudal block would prolong the duration of post-operative analgesia. However, caudal ketamine did not reduce the MLAC of caudal ropivacaine for intra-operative analgesia in children.

Some studies have determined the MLAC value of ropivacaine for caudal blocks in young children. Ingelmo et al. [7] investigated the MLAC of a single dose of

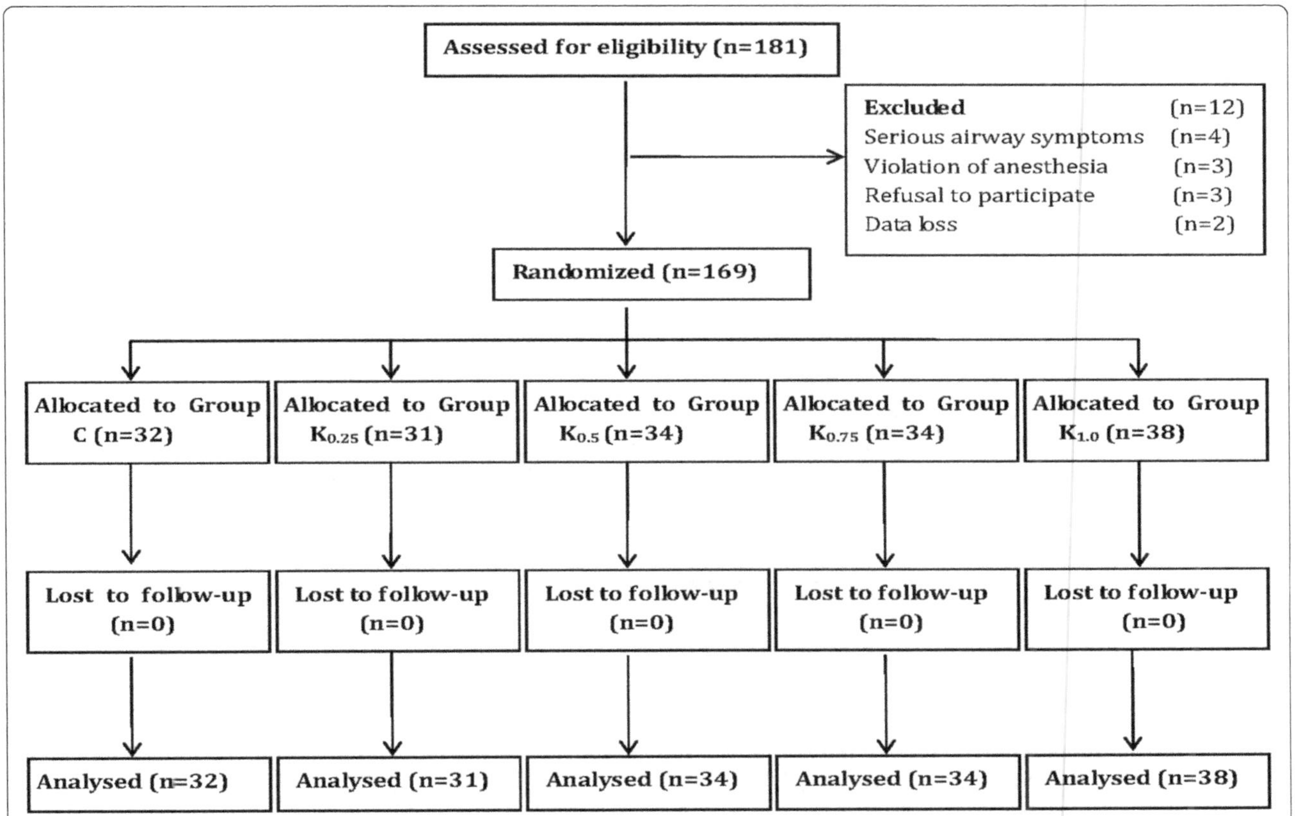

Fig. 1 Consort flow diagram

Table 1 Children's demographic and experimental data and postoperative side effects data

Group	Group C	Group $K_{0.25}$	Group $K_{0.5}$	Group $K_{0.75}$	Group $K_{1.0}$	P
Number of Patients (n)	32	31	34	34	38	/
Age (months)	22 (7)	20 (7)	21 (7)	19 (6)	20 (7)	0.653
Weight (kg)	11.6 (1.6)	11.3 (1.6)	11.8 (1.7)	11.4 (1.7)	11.3 (1.8)	0.737
Duration of surgery (min)	32 (9)	30 (7)	29 (5)	29 (6)	30 (8)	0.378
Recovery time (min)	31 (4)	31 (8)	31 (3)	30 (6)	30 (7)	0.850
Propofol dose (mg)	105 (27)	104 (26)	107 (30)	103 (28)	102 (28)	0.957
Type of surgery						
Inguinal hernia (n)	22	23	24	26	27	0.96
Hydrocele (n)	10	8	10	8	11	
PONV (n)	4	4	5	6	10	0.513
Agitation (n)	0	0	0	0	0	/
Urine retention (n)	1	0	0	0	0	0.366
Bradycardia (n)	1	1	2	1	3	0.822
Hypotension (n)	0	1	0	1	0	0.517
Respiratory depression (n)	0	0	0	0	0	/

Values are mean (SD) or numbers, Data are mean ± SD or numbers of cases (n)

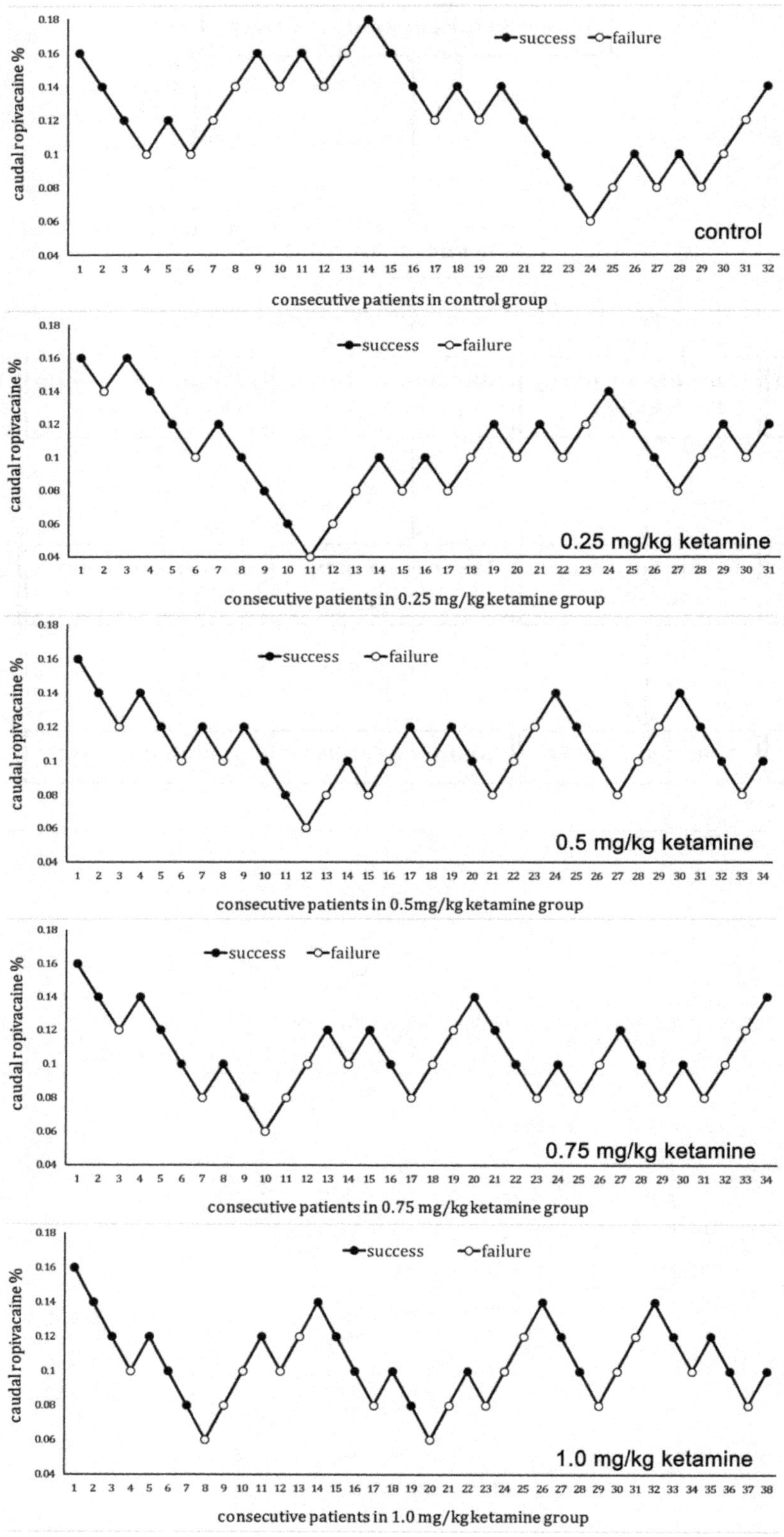

Fig. 2 (See legend on next page.)

(See figure on previous page.)
Fig. 2 The response curve of consecutive children in each of the five groups. Skin incisions were attempted at different concentrations of caudal ropivacaine. The MLAC values of ropivacaine were 0.128% (0.03%) in the control group, 0.112% (0.02%) in Group $K_{0.25}$, 0.112% (0.02%) in Group $K_{0.5}$, 0.110% (0.02%) in Group $K_{0.75}$, and 0.110% (0.02%) in Group $K_{1.0}$. There were no significant differences among the five groups for the MLAC values ($p = 0.11$)

caudal ropivacaine with 1 MAC of sevoflurane in children aged 1–6 years old, and the MLAC of caudal ropivacaine was 0.066%. Deng et al. [5, 11] reported that the MLAC of caudal ropivacaine with 0.5 MAC enflurane was 0.11% in children aged 1–5 years old, and it was 0.107% in preschool age children with 0.7 MAC sevoflurane. The MLAC values of ropivacaine were 0.128% in the present study, and the value reported in our study was consistent with the value reported elsewhere, but it was different from certain other studies. This discrepancy could be mainly attributed to individual factors, the concentration and volume of caudal injection, the use and concentration of inhaled or intravenous anesthetics, methods of measuring MLAC value [9, 10]. Sevoflurane have a much stronger inhibitory effect compared with propofol within concentrations close to their reported 50% effective concentrations [12, 13]. And sevoflurane strongly decrease the required concentrations of local anesthetics compared with midazolam or propofol. Also, MLAC estimates could be influenced by starting concentration, number of crossovers, increment size of concentration when using up-down method for analysis of quantal data [10].

Lots of previous studies had performed to evaluate the effect of different doses of ketamine on the postoperative analgesia. However, to the best of our knowledge, no Chinese or English studies have been designed to evaluate the effect of different dose of caudal ketamine on MLAC of ropivacaine. Our results showed that caudal ketamine did not influence the MLAC of ropivacaine for intra-operative caudal analgesia in young children. However, it prolonged the duration of postoperative analgesia in this study. Our results were consistent with previous studies of caudal ketamine in association with local anesthetics for post-operative analgesia [14–17]. Our results showed that caudal ketamine prolonged the duration of post-operative analgesia in a dose-dependent manner. Caudal ketamine with 0.25% bupivacaine was used in doses of 0.25, 0.5, and 1 mg/kg, obtaining mean postoperative analgesia durations of 7.9, 11, and 16.5 h, respectively [18]. In another study, the mean durations of caudal analgesia in caudal 0.25%

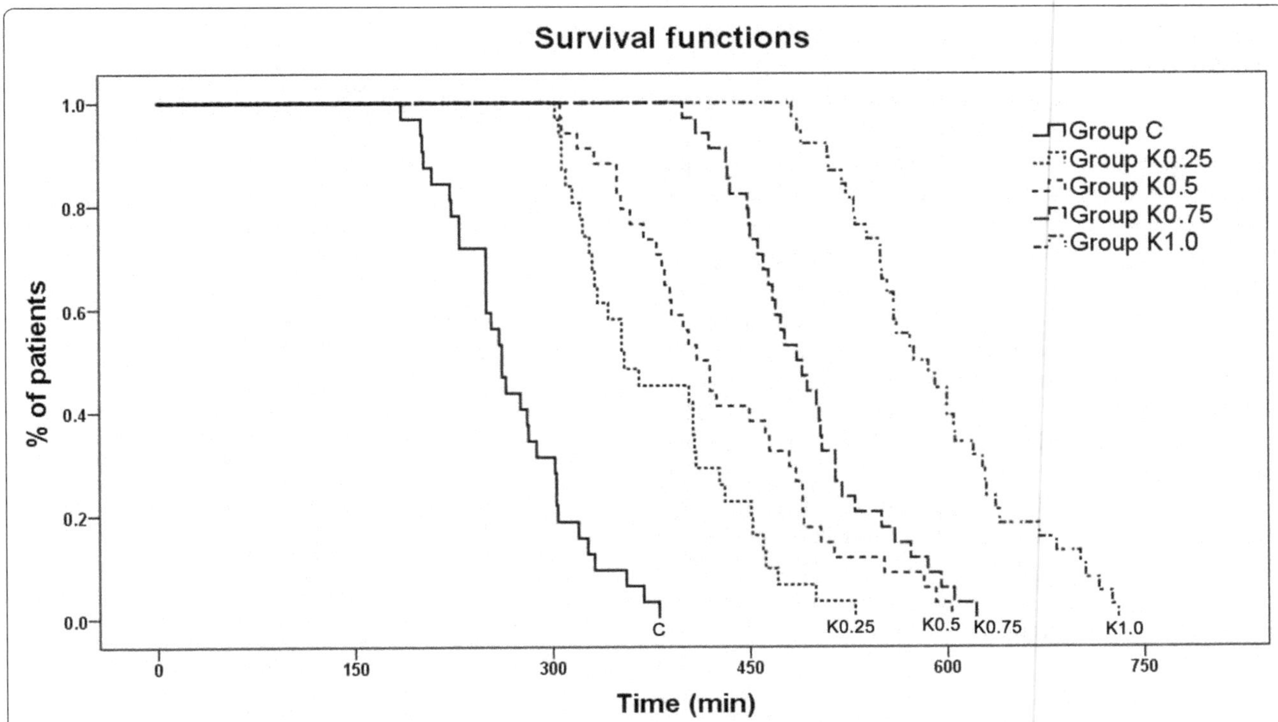

Fig. 3 Results of Kaplan-Meier survival analysis were displayed as survival curves for the five caudal solution. The log-rank test was used to compare the rate of requirement for additional analgesia in the study

bupivacaine with 0.25, 0.5, 1 mg/kg ketamine were 8.8, 22.1, and 25.2 h, respectively [19]. Adequate postoperative analgesia has also been achieved by combining caudal ropivacaine with ketamine. Adding 0.25 mg/kg ketamine to 0.2% ropivacaine provided analgesia up to 9 h in Lee et al. study [14]. Adding 0.5 mg/kg ketamine to 0.2% ropivacaine produced analgesia that extended about 11–17 h [15–17].

Caudal ketamine provide analgesia of central nervous system effects by both a direct effect on the spinal cord and a systemic absorption effect. Ketamine exerts its analgesic and anesthetic effects by binding to a subset of glutamate receptors influenced by the agonist N-methyl-D-asparate (NMDA). Caudal ketamine produced analgesic effects by acting on NMDA receptors in the lumbar spinal cord, or from μ-opioid receptors agonist activity and interaction with voltage-sensitive sodium channels [20, 21]. Koinig et al. [22] showed that the mean time to maximum ketamine plasma concentration after caudal ketamine administration was about 20 min and the maximum ketamine plasma concentrations after caudal injection were significantly lower than that after intramuscular administration of ketamine. Caudal ketamine alone was typically used to provide post-operative analgesia in children in several studies [23, 24]. These suggested that caudal ketamine analgesic effect was provided primarily by a direct effect on the spinal cord. In our study, skin incision was performed at 20 min after caudal injection. And at this time, it was the peak of ketamine plasma concentration, may not be the peak of ketamine concentration in the spinal cord nervous after caudal ketamine injection. It's the limitation in our study and future studies need to confirm this.

Ketamine is a low molecular weight and relatively high lipid soluble drug, and this characteristic of ketamine leads to release slowly from the lipid composition of the spinal cord [25]. Elimination half-life after epidurally administered ketamine was two times longer than that after intravenous ketamine [26]. Hence, the synergistic effect between ketamine and ropivacaine primarily resulted in the prolongation of post-operative caudal analgesia, but not for intra-operative caudal analgesia. The doses of caudal ketamine were from 0 to 1 mg/kg in the present study. This study's limitation is that we're not sure whether ketamine in larger doses than 1 mg/kg could decrease the MLAC of ropivacaine for intra-operative caudal analgesia in children. However, the range of doses in our study is representative of commonly used doses in clinical medicine.

Conclusions

In summary, this study indicated that the addition of caudal ketamine ranged from 0 to 1 mg/kg to ropivacaine prolonged the duration of post-operative analgesia; however, it did not decrease the MLAC of caudal ropivacaine for intra-operative analgesia in children.

Abbreviations

FLACC: Face, Legs, Activity, Cry, Consoling" tool; PONV: Postoperative Nausea and Vomiting; MLAC: Minimum Local Anesthetic Concentration; ASA: American Society of Anesthesiology; NMDA: N-methyl-D-asparate; MAC: Minimal Alveolar Concentration

Acknowledgements

The authors would like to thank the staff of anesthesia nurses at the Department of Anesthesiology and Perioperative Medicine, Guangzhou Women and Children Medical Centre.

Authors' contributions

All authors have read and approved the manuscript. WHZ: Study design, data analysis, writing paper and approval of final manuscript. WLY: data analysis, writing paper and approval of final manuscript. LHH: Study design, data collection and approval of final manuscript. FYT: Study design, data collection, data analysis, manuscript revision and approval of final manuscript. SXR: Study design, manuscript revision and approval of final manuscript. SYJ: Study design, data analysis, writing paper, manuscript revision and approval of final manuscript.

References

1. Locatelli B, Ingelmo P, Sonzogni V, Zanella A, Gatti V, Spotti A, Di Marco S, Fumagalli R. Randomized, double-blind, phase III, controlled trial comparing levobupivacaine 0.25%, ropivacaine 0.25% and bupivacaine 0.25% by the caudal route in children. Br J Anaesth. 2005;94(3):366–71.
2. Kim EM, Lee JR, Koo BN, Im YJ, Oh HJ, Lee JH. Analgesic efficacy of caudal dexamethasone combined with ropivacaine in children undergoing orchiopexy. Br J Anaesth. 2014;112(5):885–91.
3. Ansermino M, Basu R, Vandebeek C, Montgomery C. Nonopioid additives to local anaesthetics for caudal blockade in children: a systematic review. Paediatr Anaesth. 2003;13(7):561–73.
4. Menzies R, Congreve K, Herodes V, Berg S, Mason DG. A survey of pediatric caudal extradural anesthesia practice. Paediatr Anaesth. 2009;19(9):829–36.
5. Deng XM, Xiao WJ, Tang GZ, Luo MP, Xu KL. Minimum local analgesic concentration of ropivacaine for intra-operative caudal analgesia in pre-school and school age children. Anaesthesia. 2010;65(10):991–5.
6. McLeod GA, Dale J, Robinson D, Checketts M, Columb MO, Luck J, Wigderowitz C, Rowley D. Determination of the EC50 of levobupivacaine for femoral and sciatic perineural infusion after total knee arthroplasty. Br J Anaesth. 2009;102(4):528–33.
7. Ingelmo P, Frawley G, Astuto M, Duffy C, Donath S, Disma N, Rosano G, Fumagalli R, Gullo A. Relative analgesic potencies of levobupivacaine and ropivacaine for caudal anesthesia in children. Anesth Analg. 2009;108(3): 805–13.
8. Disma N, Frawley G, Mameli L, Pistorio A, Alberighi OD, Montobbio G, Tuo P. Effect of epidural clonidine on minimum local anesthetic concentration (ED50) of levobupivacaine for caudal block in children. Paediatr Anaesth. 2011;21(2):128–35.
9. She YJ, Zhang ZY, Song XR. Caudal dexmedetomidine decreases the required concentration of levobupivacaine for caudal block in pediatric patients: a randomized trial. Paediatr Anaesth. 2013;23(12):1205–12.
10. Paul M, Fisher DM. Are estimates of MAC reliable? Anesthesiology. 2001; 95(6):1362–70.
11. Deng XM, Xiao WJ, Tang GZ, Luo MP, Xu KL. The minimum local anesthetic concentration of ropivacaine for caudal analgesia in children. Anesthesia Analgesia. 2002;94(6):1465–8 table of contents.
12. Matute E, Rivera-Arconada I, Lopez-Garcia JA. Effects of propofol and sevoflurane on the excitability of rat spinal motoneurones and nociceptive reflexes in vitro. Br J Anaesth. 2004;93(3):422–7.
13. Kammer T, Rehberg B, Menne D, Wartenberg HC, Wenningmann I, Urban BW. Propofol and sevoflurane in subanesthetic concentrations act preferentially on the spinal cord: evidence from multimodal electrophysiological assessment. Anesthesiology. 2002;97(6):1416–25.
14. Lee HM, Sanders GM. Caudal ropivacaine and ketamine for postoperative analgesia in children. Anaesthesia. 2000;55(8):806–10.
15. De Negri P, Ivani G, Visconti C, De Vivo P. How to prolong postoperative analgesia after caudal anaesthesia with ropivacaine in children: S-ketamine

versus clonidine. Paediatr Anaesth. 2001;11(6):679–83.
16. Akbas M, Titiz TA, Ertugrul F, Akbas H, Melikoglu M. Comparison of the effect of ketamine added to bupivacaine and ropivacaine, on stress hormone levels and the duration of caudal analgesia. Acta Anaesthesiol Scand. 2005;49(10):1520–6.
17. Odes R, Erhan OL, Demirci M, Goksu H. Effects of ketamine added to ropivacaine in pediatric caudal block. Agri. 2010;22(2):53–60.
18. Semple D, Findlow D, Aldridge LM, Doyle E. The optimal dose of ketamine for caudal epidural blockade in children. Anaesthesia. 1996;51(12):1170–2.
19. Panjabi N, Prakash S, Gupta P, Gogia AR. Efficacy of three doses of ketamine with bupivacaine for caudal analgesia in pediatric inguinal herniotomy. Reg Anesth Pain Med. 2004;29(1):28–31.
20. Coggeshall RE, Carlton SM. Receptor localization in the mammalian dorsal horn and primary afferent neurons. Brain Res Brain Res Rev. 1997;24(1):28–66.
21. Hirota K, Lambert DG. Ketamine: its mechanism(s) of action and unusual clinical uses. Br J Anaesth. 1996;77(4):441–4.
22. Koinig H, Marhofer P, Krenn CG, Klimscha W, Wildling E, Erlacher W, Nikolic A, Turnheim K, Semsroth M. Analgesic effects of caudal and intramuscular S(+)-ketamine in children. Anesthesiology. 2000;93(4):976–80.
23. Almenrader N, Passariello M, D'Amico G, Haiberger R, Pietropaoli P. Caudal additives for postoperative pain management in children: S(+)-ketamine and neostigmine. Paediatr Anaesth. 2005;15(2):143–7.
24. Passariello M, Almenrader N, Canneti A, Rubeo L, Haiberger R, Pietropaoli P. Caudal analgesia in children: S(+)-ketamine vs S(+)-ketamine plus clonidine. Paediatr Anaesth. 2004;14(10):851–5.
25. Xie H, Wang X, Liu G, Wang G. Analgesic effects and pharmacokinetics of a low dose of ketamine preoperatively administered epidurally or intravenously. Clin J Pain. 2003;19(5):317–22.
26. Pedraz JL, Lanao JM, Calvo MB, Muriel C, Hernandez-Arbeiza J, Dominguez-Gil A. Pharmacokinetic and clinical evaluation of ketamine administered by i.v. and epidural routes. Int J Clin Pharmacol Ther Toxicol. 1987;25(2):77–80.

17

Better haemodynamic stability under xenon anaesthesia than under isoflurane anaesthesia during partial nephrectomy

Patrick Schäfer[1], Astrid Fahlenkamp[2], Rolf Rossaint[1], Mark Coburn[1] and Ana Kowark[1*]

Abstract

Background: Renal dysfunction following intraoperative arterial hypotension is mainly caused by an insufficient renal blood flow. It is associated with higher mortality and morbidity rates. We hypothesised that the intraoperative haemodynamics are more stable during xenon anaesthesia than during isoflurane anaesthesia in patients undergoing partial nephrectomy.

Methods: We performed a secondary analysis of the haemodynamic variables collected during the randomised, single-blinded, single-centre PaNeX study, which analysed the postoperative renal function in 46 patients who underwent partial nephrectomy. The patients received either xenon or isoflurane anaesthesia with 1:1 allocation ratio. We analysed the duration of the intraoperative systolic blood pressure decrease by > 40% from baseline values and the cumulative duration of a mean arterial blood pressure (MAP) of < 65 mmHg as primary outcomes. The secondary outcomes were related to other blood pressure thresholds, the amount of administered norepinephrine, and the analysis of confounding factors on the haemodynamic stability.

Results: The periods of an MAP of < 65 mmHg were significantly shorter in the xenon group than in the isoflurane group. The medians [interquartile range] were 0 [0–10.0] and 25.0 [10.0–47.5] minutes, for the xenon and isoflurane group, respectively ($P = 0.002$). However, the cumulative duration of a systolic blood pressure decrease by > 40% did not significantly differ between the groups ($P = 0.51$). The periods with a systolic blood pressure decrease by 20% from baseline, MAP decrease to values < 60 mmHg, and the need for norepinephrine, as well as the cumulative dose of norepinephrine were significantly shorter and lower, respectively, in the xenon group. The confounding factors, such as demographic data, surgical technique, or anaesthesia data, were similar in the two groups.

Conclusion: The patients undergoing xenon anaesthesia showed a better haemodynamic stability, which might be attributed to the xenon properties. The indirect effect of xenon anaesthesia might be of importance for the preservation of renal function during renal surgery and needs further elaboration.

Keywords: Xenon, Isoflurane, Haemodynamic stability, Renal function, Nephroprotection

* Correspondence: akowark@ukaachen.de
[1]Department of Anaesthesiology, Medical Faculty RWTH Aachen University, Pauwelsstr. 30, 52074 Aachen, Germany

Introduction

The current "gold-standard" for curative surgery of renal cell carcinomas is partial nephrectomy [1]. Although efforts have been made to further reduce the iatrogenic tissue trauma during surgery in the last years, it remains unclear how the anaesthesia could have a lasting effect on the patients' outcome. The intraoperative renal dysfunction frequently induces a postoperative renal insufficiency [2]. Thus, the preservation of the renal perfusion and function has a great value in anaesthesiological management [3]. The risk factors for renal dysfunction are intraoperative hypovolaemia and hypotension, nephrotoxic drugs, and cardiovascular and renal comorbidities [3–6]. The avoidance of intraoperative hypotension is of great importance, as it is not only associated with an increased risk for acute renal failure, but also with other serious adverse events, such as mortality, stroke, and acute myocardial damage [7–11]. The optimum blood pressure target thresholds have not been established yet [11, 12]. The German Society for Anaesthesiology and Intensive Medicine (DGAI) has recently published a recommendation for intraoperative blood pressure thresholds. An intraoperative decrease of the absolute mean arterial blood pressure (MAP) to less than 55–65 mmHg or a relative systolic blood pressure decrease of more than 40–50% of the baseline value should be avoided [13]. Even a brief, 5-min MAP decrease to values less than 55–65 mmHg is associated with a significantly higher incidence of acute kidney injury and myocardial infarction [9, 14]. The haemodynamic management includes the use of fluids, inotropic drugs [3], and the optimised choice of anaesthetics. An ideal anaesthetic should preserve the cardiovascular stability and exhibit nephroprotective properties. Such properties were found in xenon in animal models [15–21]. Thus far, renal impairment has not been observed after a xenon anaesthesia in humans [22–24]. Our group recently conducted the PaNeX-study, wherein we hypothesised that the postoperative renal function after partial nephrectomy would differ between patients undergoing xenon and those undergoing isoflurane anaesthesia [25]. The primary endpoint was the maximum postoperative decrease of the glomerular filtration rate (GFR) until the seventh postoperative day. The results indicated that xenon has a potential nephroprotective effect. The underlying mechanism remained unclear. The direct nephroprotective effect, as well as the indirect effect via more stable intraoperative haemodynamics were discussed. However, the haemodynamic variables were not analysed in detail; only the mean systolic and diastolic blood pressures were described. Significantly more adverse events ($P = 0.001$), in particular, a higher incidence of intraoperative hypotension requiring catecholamine therapy ($P = 0.003$), were found in the isoflurane group. The intraoperative hypotension was not predefined in the PaNeX study; rather, it was based on the attending anaesthetist's judgement. Therefore, we have performed a predefined secondary analysis of the particular haemodynamic differences between the two study groups of the PaNeX study. We hypothesized that the patients undergoing xenon anaesthesia would exhibit significantly better haemodynamics during the surgery, as defined by the recommendation of the DGAI [13]. To the best of our knowledge, this is the first study that analysed in detail the haemodynamics of patients undergoing xenon anaesthesia.

Methods

Study design

This is a predefined secondary analysis of the prospective, single-blinded, single-centre, randomised controlled PaNeX trial [25], which was conducted between July 2013 and October 2015 in the University Hospital of the RWTH Aachen, in Aachen, Germany. The Ethics Committee of the Medical Faculty RWTH Aachen University approved the study in April 2013 (EK 012/13). Registration was performed with ClinicalTrials.gov (NCT01839084) and Eudra-CT (identifier: 2012–005698-30). The complete methodological details are presented elsewhere [25].

The objective of this analysis was to compare the haemodynamic stability under xenon anaesthesia with that under isoflurane anaesthesia and to explore its effects on the renal perfusion during partial nephrectomy. The potential indirect effects should be presented in greater detail.

Participants

All 46 patients of the PaNeX study [25] diagnosed with renal cell carcinoma and scheduled for a unilateral partial nephrectomy were included in this secondary analysis. The study groups included adult patients with an American Society of Anesthesiologists (ASA) status ≤II, without pre-existing severe cardiac, respiratory, or neurological diseases, allergies or contraindications to the study drugs, or stage 3 chronic renal insufficiency (GFR < 60 ml min^{-1} 1.73 m^{-2}).

Study conduction

A detailed description of the study is presented elsewhere [25]. In brief, the patients were randomly allocated 1:1 to receive xenon ($n = 23$) or isoflurane (n = 23) anaesthesia, following the placement of a thoracic epidural catheter and anaesthesia induction using propofol, sufentanil, and rocuronium. The target anaesthetic concentration was either 60% inspired xenon with 40% oxygen or 1.2% end-expiratory isoflurane with 40% oxygen. Further anaesthesia conduction was performed according to the clinical routine, at the discretion of the attending anaesthetist. Haemodynamic management was performed according to the standard operating procedure (SOP) for partial nephrectomy in our department; the goal was to maintain the MAP ≥65 mmHg by application of fluids and norepinephrine, as deemed clinically appropriate. Opioids were titrated according to the patients' need. A bolus dose of 6–7 ml of the mixture of 0.3% ropivacaine and 0.75 μg ml^{-1} sufentanil was applied into the epidural catheter before the skin incision, followed by a continuous application during the surgery. Only the patients were blinded during the study.

Outcome measures

All data used in this secondary analysis were prospectively collected. The blood pressure was measured every 5 min using non-invasive monitoring in all patients. Each measured value at these 5-min time-points was assumed to be representative for the preceding 5-min time span.

The primary outcome was the haemodynamic stability during anaesthesia, assessed by two analyses. First, the duration of a systolic blood pressure decrease by more than 40% from the baseline value, measured before anaesthesia induction. Second, the duration of an absolute MAP of < 65 mmHg during anaesthesia. The baseline blood pressure value was defined as the mean of two measurements at least 5 min apart after the patient's arrival in the operating room. The duration of the relative systolic blood pressure decrease and the absolute MAP decrease was calculated in each case as a cumulative time in minutes. The systolic and diastolic values were recorded every 5 min from the start of the monitoring in the operating room until the transfer to the post-anaesthesia care unit. The MAP was calculated as the diastolic blood pressure plus 1/3 of the systolic blood pressure minus the diastolic blood pressure.

The secondary outcomes comprised the analyses of the durations of the relative systolic blood pressure deviations (decrease and increase) by 20% from the baseline value and the absolute intraoperative MAP decrease to values < 60 mmHg. In addition, we assessed the proportions of the study treatment duration represented by all aforementioned blood pressure deviations.

Further, we assessed the intraoperative durations of bradycardia (defined as heart rate < 60 beats per minute [bpm]), tachycardia (defined as heart rate > 100 bpm), and the relative heart rate deviation (decrease and increase) by 20% from the baseline values. The heart rate was recorded every 5 min from the start of the monitoring in the operating room until the transfer to the post-anaesthesia care unit. The proportion of the study treatment duration represented by all aforementioned heart rate deviations was also analysed.

Other outcome measures included the analysis of the effect of the confounding variables on the patients' haemodynamics. These confounders comprised the anaesthetic concentrations (recorded every 5 min), the amount of administered norepinephrine and opioids, and anaesthesia depth (measured by bispectral index [BIS] monitoring). Furthermore, we analysed the influence of a pre-existent arterial hypertension on the need for a haemodynamic support with norepinephrine and the influence of the epidural anaesthesia on the applied opioid amount.

Statistical analysis

Statistical analysis was performed using SPSS software (Version 24, IBM Corporation, Amonk, New York, USA). After testing for normality using the Shapiro Wilk Test, the continuous data were explored using the Mann-Whitney U test and the dichotomous variables were analysed using Fisher's exact test. A p-value of < 0.05 was considered statistically significant. GraphPad PRISM® (Verson 7.0d, GraphPad Software Inc., La Jolla, California, USA) was used for figure creation.

Results

The results of the main PaNeX study are presented elsewhere [25]. For this secondary analysis, we analysed all the 46 enrolled patients (Fig. 1). Twenty-three patients underwent a xenon and 23 patients underwent an isoflurane anaesthesia. Thirty-two patients were male with a mean (standard deviation [SD]) age of 60 [14] years and mainly ASA II status ($n = 31$). Both study groups were comparable with regard to the sex, age, weight, and the pre-existing chronic diseases [25]. The baseline characteristics are presented in Additional file 1.

Analysis of the primary outcome

The cumulative duration of the relative systolic blood pressure decrease by > 40% did not significantly differ between the groups; the medians [interquartile range (IQR)] were 5.0 [0–35.0] and 2.5 [0–12.5] minutes for isoflurane and xenon, respectively, $P = 0.51$ (Table 1). In contrast, the cumulative duration of the absolute MAP of < 65 mmHg was significantly longer in the isoflurane than in the xenon group; the medians [IQR] were 25.0 [10.0–47.5] and 0 [0–10.0] minutes for isoflurane and xenon, respectively, $P < 0.01$ (Table 1).

Analysis of the secondary outcomes

Further blood pressure analyses (proportions, other thresholds, and sensitivity analyses)

The proportion analysis of the duration of cumulative relative blood pressure decrease by > 40% was similar in the two groups, $P = 0.55$. Nevertheless, the duration of MAP of < 65 mmHg was significantly longer in the isoflurane group, $P < 0.01$ (Table 1).

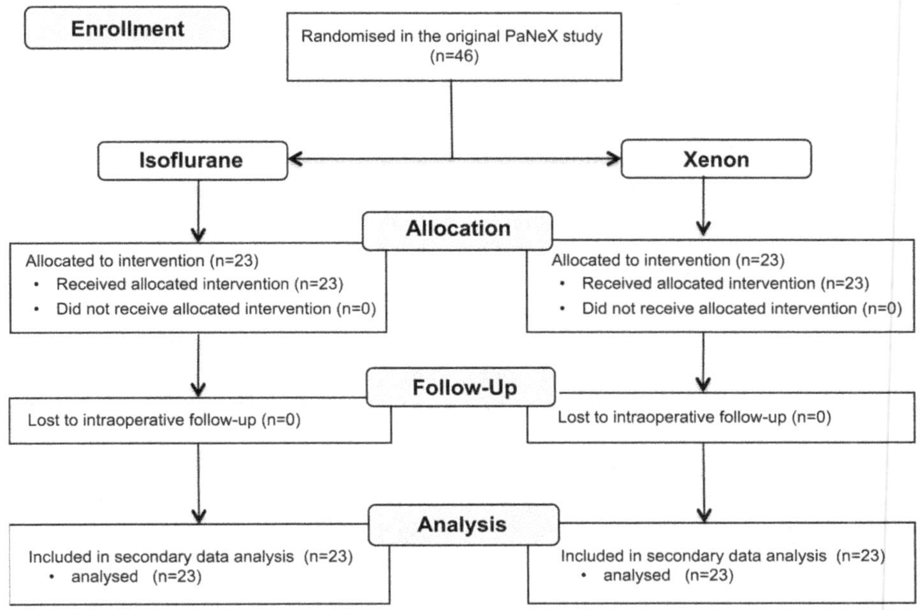

Fig. 1 The flowchart[a] of this secondary analysis [a]The flowchart was modified according to the PaNeX study for partial nephrectomy with xenon

When analysing the relative blood pressure drops > 20%, a significantly longer interval was found with isoflurane, $P = 0.018$. However, the proportion of the study treatment duration did not show a significant result ($P = 0.170$; Table 1).

The cumulative duration of the relative systolic blood pressure increase by > 20% was significantly longer and showed a higher proportion of the study treatment duration in the xenon group with $P = 0.049$ and $P = 0.036$, respectively (Table 1).

Table 1 Blood pressure analyses

	Isoflurane ($n = 23$)	Xenon ($n = 23$)	*P*-value
Blood pressure, median (IQR), mm Hg			
Systolic blood pressure	105.7 [100.9–113.0]	114.2 [104.4–131.3]	0.020*
Diastolic blood pressure	64.0 [56.9–68.5]	75.1 [63.9–83.2]	0.011*
Duration of systolic blood pressure deviation, median (IQR), minutes			
Decrease > 40% from baseline	5.0 [0–35.0]	2.5 [0–12.5]	0.510
Decrease > 20% from baseline	110.0 [47.5–162.5]	60.0 [12.5–120.0]	0.018*
Increase > 20% from baseline	0 [0–2.5]	0 [0–15.0]	0.049*
Proportion of the study treatment duration represented by the systolic blood pressure deviation duration, median (IQR), %			
Decrease > 40% from baseline	2 [0–18.0]	0 [0–7.7]	0.549
Decrease > 20% from baseline	76.9 [26.5–90.9]	33.3 [6.7–77.5]	0.170
Increase > 20% from baseline	0 [0–0.9]	0 [0–6.6]	0.036*
MAP, median (IQR), mmHg	77.2 [72.2–85.1]	84.2 [75.8–100.9]	0.029*
Duration of MAP decrease, median (IQR), minutes			
MAP < 65 mmHg	25.0 [10.0–47.5]	0 [0–10.0]	< 0.002**
MAP < 60 mmHg	5.0 [0–17.5]	0 [0–5.0]	0.041*
Proportion of the study treatment duration represented by the MAP decrease, median (IQR), %			
MAP < 65 mmHg	16.7 [4.2–22.8]	0 [0–5.8]	< 0.004**
MAP < 60 mmHg	3.9 [0–9.5]	0 [0–3.1]	0.048*

The *P*-values were derived using the Mann-Whitney *U* test. * indicates a significant *P*-value, ** indicates a highly significant *P*-value. *IQR* interquartile range, *MAP* mean arterial pressure, *n* number of patients

The duration of the MAP decrease to values < 60 mmHg was significantly longer in the isoflurane group for both analyses, the cumulative duration and the proportion of the study treatment duration, with $P = 0.041$ and $P = 0.048$, respectively (Table 1).

In an additional sensitivity analysis, we compared the group differences for both MAP and systolic blood pressure, using two mixed-models (repeated measurements ANOVA). For each model, the results showed a significant difference between the groups ($P < 0.001$ each). The overall time effect was also significant ($P < 0.001$ each) for both models (MAP and systolic blood pressure). In contrast, the group-by-time interaction effect was not significant for the MAP ($P = 0.546$), neither for the systolic blood pressure ($P = 0.183$).

Interestingly, though our institutional SOP demanded the maintenance of a MAP ≥65 mmHg during surgery, hypotensive periods were registered in both groups.

Heart rate analysis

The mean (SD) intraoperative heart rates were 65.2 (9.1) bpm and 61.6 (13.2) bpm in the isoflurane and xenon group, respectively [25]. Although the patients under xenon anaesthesia showed a lower intraoperative heart rate most of the time (Fig. 2), this difference was not significant ($P = 0.116$) (Table 2). The proportion of the study treatment duration represented by the duration of bradycardia (heart rate < 60 bpm) was also similar in both groups $P = 0.086$ (Table 2).

Moreover, the episodes of tachycardia, as well as the cumulative duration of a relative decrease or increase of the heart rate by > 20%, were similar in the two groups (Table 2).

An additional sensitivity analysis of the heart rate using a mixed-model repeated measures ANOVA did not show a statistically significant interaction between the time and groups ($P = 0.897$). Furthermore, there was neither a significant main effect for time nor for the group, with $P = 0.250$ and $P = 0.447$, respectively.

Norepinephrine and opioid analysis

The cumulative amount of administered norepinephrine was significantly higher in the isoflurane than in the xenon group, $P = 0.001$ (Table 3). The patients received a median [IQR] norepinephrine dose of 195.0 [17.5–538.5] μg and 0 [0–42.5] μg in the isoflurane and xenon group, respectively (Fig. 3). This significance was more pronounced in the patients with pre-existent arterial hypertension than in those without it, $P = 0.006$ and $P = 0.040$, respectively (Table 3). In addition, the treatment duration with norepinephrine was significantly longer in the isoflurane group (Table 3).

The cumulative amount of sufentanil did not differ between the two groups, $P = 0.912$. An additional epidural anaesthesia was performed in 15 (66%) and 19 (83%) patients, in the isoflurane and xenon group, respectively (Table 3). Epidural anaesthesia led to less opioid consumption, but without significant differences between the groups (Table 3).

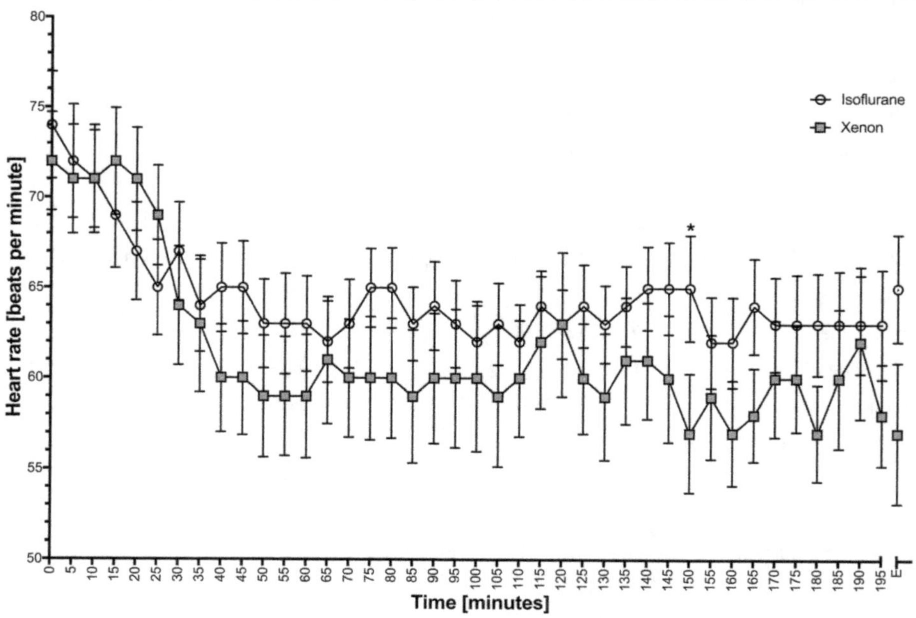

Fig. 2 Intraoperative heart rate Intraoperative heart rate in the xenon and isoflurane groups at different time points. The data were analysed using the Mann-Whitney *U* test and are presented as means ± standard deviation. *P-value < 0.05

Table 2 Heart rate analyses

	Isoflurane ($n = 23$)	Xenon ($n = 23$)	P-value
Heart rate			
Pre-existent bradycardia (heart rate < 60 min^{-1}) during study treatment, n (%)	3 (13)	3 (13)	
Heart rate, mean (SD), beats per minute	65.2 (9.1)	61.6 (13.2)	0.116
Duration of heart rate decrease > 20% from baseline, median (IQR), minutes	35.0 [2.5–77.5]	70.0 [7.5–157.5]	0.163
Proportion of the study treatment duration represented by the duration of a heart rate decrease > 20% from baseline, median (IQR), %	14.6 [0.9–46.0]	69.4 [5.7–88.9]	0.129
Duration of a heart rate increase > 20% from baseline, median (IQR), minutes	0 [0–7.5]	0 [0–12.5]	0.741
Proportion of the study treatment duration represented by the duration of a heart rate increase > 20% from baseline, median (IQR), %	0 [0–4.9]	0 [0–7.4]	0.694
Duration of bradycardia (heart rate < 60 min^{-1}), median (IQR), minutes	60.0 [10.0–145.0]	100.0 [47.5–155.0]	0.301
Proportion of the study treatment duration represented by the duration of bradycardia (heart rate < 60 min^{-1}), median (IQR), %	32.1 [6.5–79.3]	82.1 [35.4–94.9]	0.086
Pre-existent tachycardia (heart rate > 100 min^{-1}), n (%)	2 (9)	1 (4)	
Duration of tachycardia (heart rate > 100 min^{-1}) during study treatment, median (IQR), minutes	0 [0–0]	0 [0–0]	0.415
Proportion of the study treatment duration represented by the tachycardia (heart rate > 100 min^{-1}) duration, median (IQR), %	0 [0–0]	0 [0–0]	0.415

The P-values were derived using the Mann-Whitney U test. *IQR* interquartile range, *n* number of patients, *SD* standard deviation

Confounding factors on haemodynamics

This secondary analysis showed that the proportion of patients with pre-existent hypertension, bradycardia, and tachycardia did not differ between the groups (Tables 2 and 3). However, the analysis of concomitant preoperative antihypertensive medication in the patients with pre-existent hypertension revealed a difference with regard to the number of patients who received angiotensin-converting-enzyme (ACE) or AT_1 receptor (AR) antagonist before surgery (xenon (11 of 12), isoflurane (7 of 12)). The ACE/AR antagonist therapy was discontinued for all patients 24 h before the surgery in accordance with our SOP.

Furthermore, there were no differences with regard to the surgery duration, the surgical positioning, the duration of kidney manipulation and ischaemia time, and the histological and pathological analyses (resected tissue volume, weight, and tumour size) between the groups. Four patients in the isoflurane and one patient in the xenon group underwent a total nephrectomy due to an unforeseen intraoperative decision, based on the tumour extent and the urologic SOP. The mean (SD) study treatment duration was 197 (60) minutes in the isoflurane and 166 (59) minutes in the xenon group. The groups showed a similar fluid balance; crystalloid and colloid infusions, and total blood loss showed no significant differences with $P = 0.702$, $P = 0{,}248$, and $P = 0.361$, respectively. Volatile anaesthetics were administered according to the MAC values in the clinical routine and quantified by BIS. The patients received a mean (SD) of 0.8 (0.1) Vol.%, 0.7 MAC isoflurane, and 51.1 (2.5) Vol.%, 0.8 MAC xenon. The BIS values were comparable (Fig. 4). Both the systolic (Fig. 5) and the diastolic blood pressure were lower in the isoflurane group, $P = 0.02$ and $P = 0.01$, respectively (Table 1) [25]. The important outcomes are listed in the table in the Additional file 2.

Discussion

The present secondary analysis of the PaNeX study evaluated the haemodynamics during xenon anaesthesia in patients undergoing partial nephrectomy. The xenon group showed a significantly better intraoperative haemodynamic stability, with a lesser need for norepinephrine and no major differences in the heart rates, compared to the isoflurane group.

In contrast to our findings, previous studies have reported an absent or minimal negative impact of xenon on the peripheral vascular resistance or cardiac inotropy [26–28]. Isoflurane was found to exert a cardiodepressant effect [28] and peripheral vascular vasodilatation with consecutive hypotension [28, 29]. Haemodynamic stability was substantially preventing direct renal hypoperfusion and indirect vasoconstriction via neurohumoral responses to the intraoperative hypotension [3].

There is still no consensus regarding the lowest acceptable absolute or relative intraoperative blood pressure threshold and its tolerable maximum duration [8, 12]. The postulated associations of the intraoperative hypotension with adverse events have to be evaluated carefully regarding the thresholds and durations of hypotensive episodes [6, 12]. The common thresholds for systolic blood pressures are described as < 80 mmHg, a MAP < 60 mmHg, or a relative decrease by 30–50% [30]. Our analyses were based on the target blood

Table 3 Norepinephrine and opioid analyses

	Isoflurane ($n = 23$)	Xenon ($n = 23$)	P-value
Norepinephrine consumption			
Pre-existent arterial hypertension, n (%)	12 (52)	12 (52)	–
Total amount per group, µg	9945.5	934.5	–
- with pre-existent hypertension	7785.5	644.5	–
- without pre-existent hypertension	2160.0	290.0	–
Cumulative intraoperative consumption, median (IQR), µg	195.0 [17.5–538.5]	0 [0–42.5]	0.001**
- with pre-existent hypertension	422.8 [25.0–1415.5]	15 [0–77.5]	0.006**
- without pre-existent hypertension	20.0 [5.0–275.0]	0 [0–5.0]	0.040*
Duration of norepinephrine administration, median (IQR), min	95.0 [10–192.5]	0 [0–30.0]	0.002**
- with pre-existent hypertension	167.5 [15.0–260.0]	10.0 [0–42.5]	0.008**
- without pre-existent hypertension	20.0 [2.5–120.0]	0 [0–5.0]	0.065
Proportion of the study treatment duration represented by the norepinephrine administration duration, median (IQR), %	57.1 [6.2–91.7]	0 [0–13.2]	0.001**
- with pre-existent hypertension	68.6 [9.4–93.3]	6.7 [0–26.1]	0.008**
- without pre-existent hypertension	15.0 [1.0–88.0]	0 [0–2.6]	0.034*
Opioid (sufentanil) consumption			
Total intraoperative consumption per group, µg	905	1005	
Additional epidural anaesthesia, n (%)	15 (66)	19 (83)	
Cumulative intraoperative consumption, median (IQR), µg	40.0 [30.0–50.0]	30.0 [25.0–55.0]	0.912
- with epidural anaesthesia	30.0 [25.0–47.5]	30.0 [25.0–45.0]	0.891
- without epidural anaesthesia	47.5 [40.0–55.0]	62.5 [50.0–82.5]	0.109

The P-values were derived using the Mann-Whitney U test. * indicates a significant P-value, ** indicates a highly significant P-value. *IQR* interquartile range, *n* number of patients

pressure recommendations of the German DGAI guideline [13]. Although we could not determine a significant difference in the duration of a systolic blood pressure decrease of 40%, the results for a MAP decrease were unequivocal and favoured the xenon anaesthesia. This preservation of high MAP values under xenon anaesthesia might be a crucial factor for prevention of postoperative renal failure [4, 7, 9, 31]. Nevertheless, the thresholds have to be considered individually, since patients with chronic arterial hypertension and altered vascular autoregulation are susceptible to lower blood pressure limits [4, 8, 32]. The significantly larger need for norepinephrine in our patients with pre-existing arterial hypertension compared to those without arterial hypertension supports this assumption. It is remarkable that the patients with arterial hypertension in the isoflurane group needed a significantly higher and prolonged norepinephrine administration than those in the xenon group. One reason might be the vegetative property of xenon. It was shown that the endogen norepinephrine concentration is increased during xenon anaesthesia, without an alteration of the sympathetic activity and baroreflex gain [33]. A norepinephrine re-uptake inhibition in the neuronal cells was postulated [33]. Similar results were found in several large-scale studies [34, 35]. As we have not analysed the plasma concentrations of norepinephrine in our PaNeX study [25], a verification of this assumption is not possible. However, during cardiac surgery, iatrogenic-induced catecholamines were found to be independent predictors of postoperative morbidity and mortality [36] and they are also a risk for the renal function [3]. To the best of our knowledge, it is unknown whether this correlation also applies to the increased levels of the endogen catecholamines. Even though it is recommended to continue the ACE/AR antagonist therapy on the day of a non-cardiac surgery [37], the recent VISION study showed a lower risk for intraoperative hypotension in the patients who withheld their ACE/AR antagonists therapy 24 h before surgery [38]. In accordance with this publication and several other anaesthesia groups [38, 39], our policy was to discontinue the ACE/AR antagonists 24 h before surgery. Therefore, we assume that the different number of patients receiving ACE/AR antagonists more than 24 h before surgery did not have an effect on our results.

Several confounders on the patients' haemodynamics were analysed in detail and showed no difference in their appearance between the groups. Hypovolaemia is known to be an important additional cause for postoperative renal failure [3, 4]; however, the fluid management did

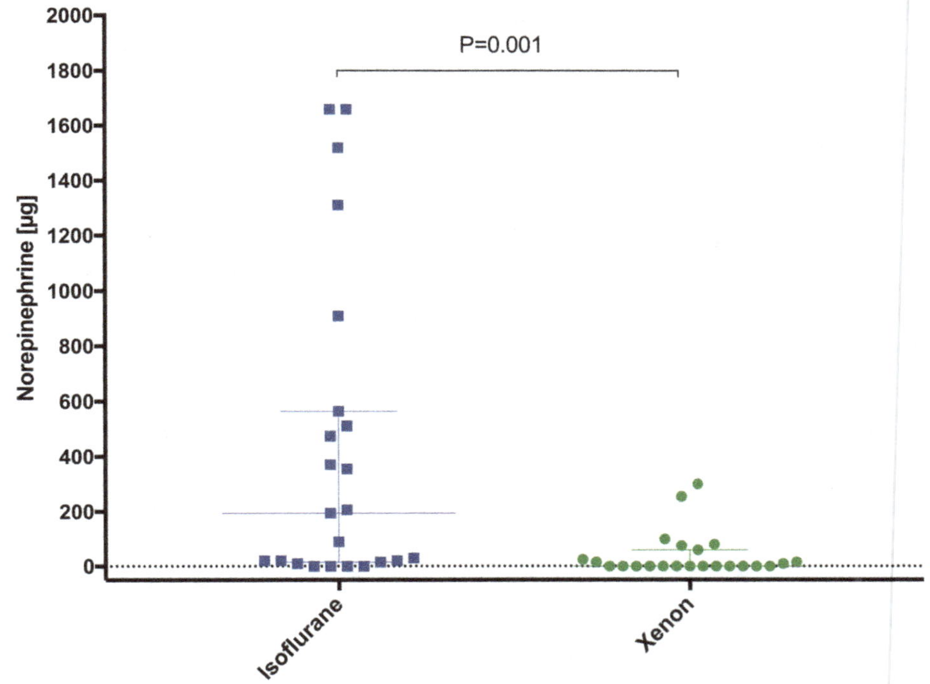

Fig. 3 Intraoperative norepinephrine consumption Cumulative intraoperative norepinephrine consumption in the xenon and isoflurane groups, presented as median with interquartile ranges. Individual data are presented as closed circles and squares. The data were analysed using the Mann-Whitney *U* test

not differ between the groups [25]. It is also unlikely that the similar demographic variables and pre-existent comorbidities may explain the different results.

The usually applied lateral position of the patient during open partial nephrectomy might induce haemodynamic and respiratory changes, but there were no differences regarding the positioning. The anaesthetics exposure times, and the surgical technique, duration and team were similar in our study.

Renal hypoperfusion is known to activate the renin-angiotensin-aldosterone system (RAAS) with a consecutive sympathetic response [2]. About half of the patients

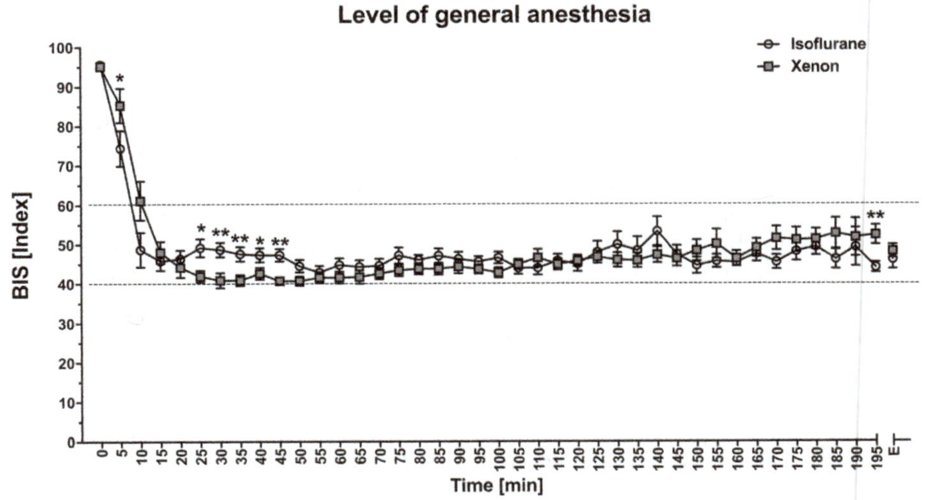

Fig. 4 Level of anaesthesia Level of anaesthesia measured by BIS monitoring in the xenon and isoflurane groups at different time points. BIS, bispectral index. The data were analysed using the Mann-Whitney *U* test and are presented as means ± standard deviation. *P-value < 0.05; **P-value < 0.01

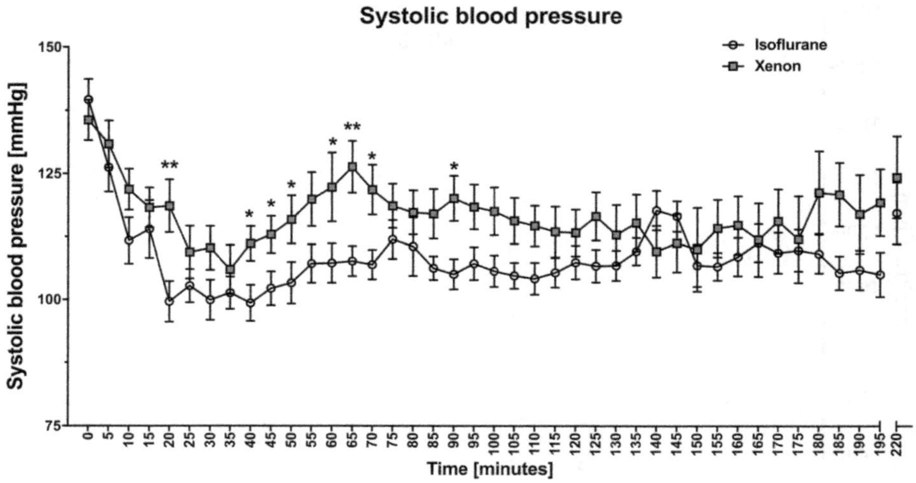

Fig. 5 Intraoperative systolic blood pressure Systolic blood pressure in the xenon and isoflurane groups at different time points. The data were analysed using the Mann-Whitney *U* test and are presented as means ± standard deviation. **P*-value < 0.05; ***P*-value < 0.01

in both groups (9 of the 23 in the isoflurane and 10 of the 23 in the xenon group) underwent an intraoperative hilar clamping of similar durations [25]. Thus, the activation of RAAS cannot be the main reason for the haemodynamic differences.

This secondary analysis included all enrolled patients, irrespective of a successful conduction of the partial nephrectomy. Even though there were no statistical differences between the groups regarding the pathological results, there was a difference in the number of patients with an unexpected total nephrectomy. The data on the effects of the unilateral nephrectomy on the levels of blood pressure and RAAS showed no difference before and after the nephrectomy [40]. Therefore, we assume that the blood pressure differences were not influenced by the cases of nephrectomy.

Since most of the anaesthetics are cardiodepressants, the anaesthesia depth might influence the intraoperative haemodynamics. In both groups, the anaesthesia was performed according to the SOPs. The MAC as well as the BIS values were in the recommended range, therefore a comparable anaesthesia depth could be expected. The higher blood pressure in the xenon group might indicate an insufficient analgesia, which induces sympathetic stimulation with tachycardia and hypertension. However, the tendency for lower heart rates argues against this postulation. The analgesic properties of xenon are controversial [41]. Xenon may induce a kind of pain tolerance, which clinically presents as reduced need for opioids [26, 28, 35, 42]. Beside the direct antinociceptive effects via inhibition of the N-methyl-D-aspartate receptors, indirect effects caused by an increased norepinephrine levels in cerebral cortex are considered as explanations [42]. However, the present analysis did not show significantly different consumption of sufentanil, even in combination with the similarly frequent applied epidural anaesthesia, which is known to increase the risk of hypotension [8].

The heart rate is one further important factor on the haemodynamic stability. Though not significant, we confirmed the observations of more pronounced intraoperative heart rate decrease with xenon [26, 33–35, 41, 43–45]. Xenon was described in this context to show a vagotonic effect [46]. In contrast, the heart rates under isoflurane anaesthesia are mainly reported as remaining unchanged [26, 27, 29, 46], whereas our analysis showed also a heart rate decrease. The reason for this observation remains unclear.

What renders our study novel, however, is that we used xenon in a partial nephrectomy setting and had already predefined this secondary analysis. Therefore, we could analyse the prospectively collected data for all patients and we possessed clearly documented baseline blood pressure values. This enabled us to quantify the haemodynamic stability directly via calculation of the cumulative times below different blood pressure thresholds as well as individual relative blood pressure drops from baseline. This is in contrast to other studies, which have only indirectly analysed the haemodynamics via the catecholamine consumption as a surrogate indicator [36, 47].

Limitations

We acknowledge several limitations in this secondary analysis:

First, the blood pressure was not measured by invasive methods but non-invasively every five minutes, which likely had an influence on our results [6].

Second, the attending anaesthetists could not be blinded for safety reasons. Due to the nature of our study, norepinephrine was applied for hypotensive therapy after an inadequate respond to fluid administration, according to the clinical routine in our hospital. The anaesthetists had to adhere to our SOPs for partial nephrectomy. Nevertheless, it might reflect a "real world" situation [48], that the required MAP ≥65 mmHg was not achieved throughout the surgeries.
Third, this study was a secondary analysis of a prospective trial with the primary outcome *maximum postoperative GFR decrease*. It was not powered to analyse the blood pressure differences.
Fourth, it may be questionable whether the reduced need for vasopressors and more stable intraoperative haemodynamic with xenon represents a better preservation of renal function apart from facilitating the haemodynamic management. The PaNeX study could only show a tendency to better postoperative renal function with xenon [25]. The underlying reason might be the drop-out of 5 patients from the per protocol analysis or the prevalence of mainly ASA II patients without pre-existent renal disease. It is known that patients with a higher ASA status and preoperatively impaired renal function have a greater risk for perioperative acute renal failure, in particular after an intraoperative hypotension [4, 7]. Nevertheless, we assume that xenon anaesthesia might have a significant impact on the renal outcome in these higher-risk patients. Of note, the enormous price difference between the xenon and isoflurane anaesthesia should always be weighed against the potential benefit of xenon anaesthesia. With approximately 20€ per litre xenon and 35€ per 250 ml isoflurane, we had mean (SD) costs in the xenon and isoflurane group of 196 [37] € and 0.77 (0.27) € per anaesthesia hour, respectively.

Conclusions

The patients undergoing partial nephrectomy under xenon anaesthesia presented a more stable haemodynamic profile, with a significantly lesser need for norepinephrine than those under isoflurane anaesthesia. The tendency of a better-preserved renal function after partial nephrectomy under xenon anaesthesia might be explained by a better renal perfusion.

Additional files

Additional file 1: Patients' baseline characteristics. Modified table according to [25]. [a]*P*-values were derived using Fisher's exact test (qualitative data) or the Mann-Whitney U-test (quantitative data). The data are presented as median (interquartile range) or number (proportion). ASA, American Society of Anesthesiologists; COPD, chronic obstructive pulmonary disease; GFR, glomerular filtration rate; IDDM, insulin dependent diabetes mellitus; n, number; NIDDM, non-insulin dependent diabetes mellitus; NYHA, New York Heart Association; PAOD, peripheral artery occlusive disease.

Additional file 2: Important outcomes. Modified previously published data [25]. [a]*P*-values were derived using Fisher's exact test (qualitative data) or the Mann-Whitney U-test (quantitative data). The data are presented as median (interquartile range) or number and percentage. AKIN, Acute Kidney Injury Network; GFR, Glomerular filtration rate; Min, minutes; n, number; PBRC, packed red blood cells; y/n, yes/ no.

Abbreviations

ACE: Angiotensin-converting-enzyme; AR: AT_1 receptor; ASA: American Society of Anesthesiologists; BIS: Bispectral index; bpm: Beats per minute; DGAI: German Society for Anaesthesiology and Intensive Medicine; GFR: Glomerular filtration rate; IQR: Interquartile range; MAP: Mean arterial pressure; n: Number of patients; SD: Standard deviation; SOP: Standard operating procedure

Acknowledgements

Not applicable.

Authors' contributions

PS designed this retrospective analysis with the help of AK. PS analysed the data and drafted the manuscript. AK, MC, AF and RR helped with the interpretation of data and revised the manuscript for important intellectual content. All authors read and approved the final manuscript.

Author details

[1]Department of Anaesthesiology, Medical Faculty RWTH Aachen University, Pauwelsstr. 30, 52074 Aachen, Germany. [2]Department of Anaesthesiology and Intensive Care Medicine, Campus Virchow-Klinikum, Charité–Universitätsmedizin Berlin, Berlin, Germany.

References

1. Doehn C, Grunwald V, Steiner T, Follmann M, Rexer H, Krege S. The diagnosis, treatment, and follow-up of renal cell carcinoma. Dtsch Arztebl Int. 2016;113(35–36):590–6.
2. Roggenbach. Postoperatives Nierenversagen. Nephrologe. 2009;4:118–27.
3. Brienza N, Giglio M, Marucci M, Fiore T. Does perioperative hemodynamic optimization protect renal function in surgical patients? A meta-analytic study. Crit Care Med. 2009;37(6):2079–90.
4. Agarwal R, Jain RK, Yadava A. Prevention of perioperative renal failure. Indian J Anaesth. 2008;52(1):38.
5. Bläser D, Weiler N. Acute kidney injury--prevention, risk stratification and biomarkers. Anasthesiol Intensivmed Notfallmed Schmerzther. 2013;48:2.
6. Lonjaret L, Lairez O, Minville V, Geeraerts T. Optimal perioperative management of arterial blood pressure. Integr Blood Press Control. 2014;7:49–59.
7. Hallqvist L, Granath F, Huldt E, Bell M. Intraoperative hypotension is associated with acute kidney injury in noncardiac surgery. Eur J Anaesthesiol. 2018;35(4):273–9.
8. Hallqvist L, Mårtensson J, Granath F, Sahlén A, Bell M. Intraoperative hypotension is associated with myocardial damage in noncardiac surgery: an observational study. Eur J Anaesthesiol. 2016;33(6):450–6.
9. Salmasi V, Maheshwari K, Yang D, Mascha EJ, Singh A, Sessler DI, et al. Relationship between intraoperative hypotension, defined by either reduction from baseline or absolute thresholds, and acute kidney and myocardial injury after noncardiac SurgeryA retrospective cohort analysis. Anesthesiology. 2017;126(1):47–65.
10. van Waes JA, Van Klei WA, Wijeysundera DN, Van Wolfswinkel L, Lindsay TF, Beattie WS. Association between intraoperative hypotension and myocardial injury after vascular surgery. Anesthesiology. 2016;124(1):35–44.
11. Wesselink E, Kappen T, Torn H, Slooter A, van Klei W. Intraoperative hypotension and the risk of postoperative adverse outcomes: a systematic review. Br J Anaesth. 2018;121(4):706–21.
12. Bijker J, van Klei W, Kappen T, van Wolfswinkel L, Moons K, Kalkman C. Incidence of intraoperative hypotension as a function of the chosen definition: literature definitions applied to a retrospective cohort using automated data collection. Anesthesiology. 2007;107(2):213–20.

13. Rossaint R, Coburn M. Choosing wisely in anesthesia : an important step in quality optimization. Anaesthesist. 2017;66:641–2.
14. Walsh M, Devereaux PJ, Garg AX, Kurz A, Turan A, Rodseth RN, et al. Relationship between intraoperative mean arterial pressure and clinical outcomes after noncardiac surgerytoward an empirical definition of hypotension. Anesthesiology. 2013;119(3):507–15.
15. De Deken J, Rex S, Monbaliu D, Pirenne J, Jochmans I. The efficacy of Noble gases in the attenuation of ischemia reperfusion injury: a systematic review and meta-analyses. Crit Care Med. 2016;44(9):e886–96.
16. Jia P, Teng J, Zou J, Fang Y, Zhang X, Bosnjak Z, et al. miR-21 contributes to xenon-conferred amelioration of renal ischemia-reperfusion injury in mice. Anesthesiology. 2013;119(3):621–30.
17. Ma D, Lim T, Xu J, Tang H, Wan Y, Zhao H, et al. Xenon preconditioning protects against renal ischemic-reperfusion injury via HIF-1alpha activation. J Am Soc Nephrol. 2009;20(4):713–20.
18. Rizvi M, Jawad N, Li Y, Vizcaychipi M, Maze M, Ma D. Effect of noble gases on oxygen and glucose deprived injury in human tubular kidney cells. Exp Biol Med (Maywood). 2010;235(7):886–91.
19. Smit K, Weber N, Hollmann M, Preckel B. Noble gases as cardioprotectants - translatability and mechanism. Br J Pharmacol. 2015;172(8):2062–73.
20. Zhao H, Rossaint R, Coburn M, Ma D. Argon Organo-protective network a. the renoprotective properties of xenon and argon in kidney transplantation. Eur J Anaesthesiol. 2017;34(10):637–40.
21. Zhao H, Watts H, Chong M, Huang H, Tralau-Stewart C, Maxwell P, et al. Xenon treatment protects against cold ischemia associated delayed graft function and prolongs graft survival in rats. Am J Transplant. 2013;13(8): 2006–18.
22. Bedi A, Murray J, Dingley J, Stevenson M, Fee J. Use of xenon as a sedative for patients receiving critical care. Crit Care Med. 2003;31(10):2470–7.
23. Esencan E, Yuksel S, Tosun Y, Robinot A, Solaroglu I, Zhang J. XENON in medical area: emphasis on neuroprotection in hypoxia and anesthesia. Med Gas Res. 2013;3(1):4.
24. Höcker J, Grünewald M, Bein B. Xenon anaesthesia--clinical characteristics, benefits and disadvantages and fields of application. Anasthesiol Intensivmed Notfallmed Schmerzther. 2012;47(6):374–80.
25. Stevanovic A, Schaefer P, Coburn M, Rossaint R, Stoppe C, Boor P, et al. Renal function following xenon anesthesia for partial nephrectomy-an explorative analysis of a randomized controlled study. PLoS One. 2017;12(7): e0181022.
26. Brücken A, Coburn M, Rex S, Rossaint R, Fries M. Current developments in xenon research. Importance for anesthesia and intensive care medicine. Anaesthesist. 2010;59(10):883–95.
27. Deile M, Damm M, Heller A. Inhaled anesthetics. Anaesthesist. 2013;62(6): 493–504.
28. Derwall M, Coburn M, Rex S, Hein M, Rossaint R, Fries M. Xenon: recent developments and future perspectives. Minerva Anestesiol. 2009;75(1–2): 37–45.
29. Torri G. Inhalation anesthetics: a review. Minerva Anestesiol. 2010;76(3): 215–28.
30. Futier E, Lefrant J-Y, Guinot P-G, Godet T, Lorne E, Cuvillon P, et al. Effect of individualized vs standard blood pressure management strategies on postoperative organ dysfunction among high-risk patients undergoing major surgery: a randomized clinical trial. Jama. 2017;318(14):1346–57.
31. Romagnoli S, Ricci Z, Ronco C. Perioperative acute kidney injury: prevention, early recognition, and supportive measures. Nephron. 2018;140(2):105–10.
32. Aronson S, Mythen MG. Perioperative Management of High-Risk Patients: going beyond "avoid hypoxia and hypotension". Jama. 2017; 318(14):1330–2.
33. Neukirchen M, Hipp J, Schaefer M, Brandenburger T, Bauer I, Winterhalter M, et al. Cardiovascular stability and unchanged muscle sympathetic activity during xenon anaesthesia: role of norepinephrine uptake inhibition. Br J Anaesth. 2012;109(6):887–96.
34. Hofland J, Ouattara A, Fellahi J-L, Gruenewald M, Hazebroucq J, Ecoffey C, et al. Effect of xenon anesthesia compared to sevoflurane and Total intravenous anesthesia for coronary artery bypass graft surgery on postoperative cardiac troponin ReleaseAn international, multicenter, phase 3, single-blinded, randomized noninferiority trial. Anesthesiology. 2017; 127(6):918–33.
35. Rossaint R, Reyle-Hahn M, am Esch JS, Scholz J, Scherpereel P, Vallet B, et al. Multicenter randomized comparison of the efficacy and safety of xenon and isoflurane in patients undergoing elective surgery. Anesthesiology. 2003; 98(1):6–13.
36. Al Tmimi L, Devroe S, Dewinter G, Van de Velde M, Poortmans G, Meyns B, et al. Xenon as an adjuvant to Propofol anesthesia in patients undergoing off-pump coronary artery bypass graft surgery: a pragmatic randomized controlled clinical trial. Anesth Analg. 2017;125(4):1118–28.
37. Fleisher L, Fleischmann K, Auerbach A, Barnason S, Beckman J, Bozkurt B, et al. 2014 ACC/AHA guideline on perioperative cardiovascular evaluation and management of patients undergoing noncardiac surgery: a report of the American College of Cardiology/American Heart Association task force on practice guidelines. Circulation. 2014;130(24):e278–333.
38. Roshanov P, Rochwerg B, Patel A, Salehian O, Duceppe E, Belley-Côté E, et al. Withholding versus continuing angiotensin-converting enzyme inhibitors or angiotensin II receptor blockers before noncardiac surgery: an analysis of the vascular events in noncardiac surgery patients cOhort evaluatioN prospective cohort. Anesthesiology. 2017;126(1):16–27.
39. Walker S, Abbott T, Brown K, Pearse R, Ackland G. Perioperative management of angiotensin-converting enzyme inhibitors and/or angiotensin receptor blockers: a survey of perioperative medicine practitioners. PeerJ. 2018;6:e5061.
40. Ohashi N, Isobe S, Ishigaki S, Suzuki T, Motoyama D, Sugiyama T, et al. The effects of unilateral nephrectomy on blood pressure and its circadian rhythm. Intern Med. 2016;55(23):3427–33.
41. Baumert J-H. Xenon-based anesthesia: theory and practice. Open Access Surgery. 2009;2:5–13.
42. Giacalone M, Abramo A, Giunta F, Forfori F. Xenon-related analgesia: a new target for pain treatment. Clin J Pain. 2013;29(7):639–43.
43. Coburn M, Kunitz O, Baumert J-H, Hecker K, Haaf S, Zühlsdorff A, et al. Randomized controlled trial of the haemodynamic and recovery effects of xenon or propofol anaesthesia. Br J Anaesth. 2004;94(2):198–202.
44. Devroe S, Lemiere J, Van de Velde M, Gewillig M, Boshoff D, Rex S. Safety and feasibility of xenon as an adjuvant to sevoflurane anaesthesia in children undergoing interventional or diagnostic cardiac catheterization: study protocol for a randomised controlled trial. Trials. 2015;16(1):74.
45. Wappler F, Rossaint R, Baumert J, Scholz J, Tonner PH, van Aken H, et al. Multicenter randomized comparison of xenon and isoflurane on left ventricular function in patients undergoing elective surgery. Anesthesiology. 2007;106(3):463–71.
46. Kirkland LL. Protecting both heart and brain: a noble goal for a noble gas. Crit Care Med. 2013;41(9):2228–9.
47. Al Tmimi L, Van Hemelrijck J, Van De Velde M, Sergeant P, Meyns B, Missant C, et al. Xenon anaesthesia for patients undergoing off-pump coronary artery bypass graft surgery: a prospective randomized controlled pilot trial. BJA: Br J Anaesth. 2015;115(4):550–9.
48. Stapelfeldt WH, Yuan H, Dryden JK, Strehl KE, Cywinski JB, Ehrenfeld JM, et al. The SLUScore: a novel method for detecting hazardous hypotension in adult patients undergoing noncardiac surgical procedures. Anesth Analg. 2017;124(4):1135.

18

Anesthetics and long-term survival after cancer surgery—Total intravenous versus volatile anesthesia

Boohwi Hong[1,2†], Sunyeul Lee[1,2†], Yeojung Kim[1], Minhee Lee[3], Ann Misun Youn[1], Hyun Rhim[1], Seok-Hwan Hong[1], Yoon-Hee Kim[1,2], Seok-Hwa Yoon[1,2] and Chaeseong Lim[1,2*]

Abstract

Background: Intravenous anesthesia has been reported to have a favorable effect on the prognosis of cancer patients. This study was performed to analyze data regarding the relation between anesthetics and the prognosis of cancer patients in our hospital.

Methods: The medical records of patients who underwent surgical resection for gastric, lung, liver, colon, and breast cancer between January 2006 and December 2009 were reviewed. Depending on the type of anesthetic, it was divided into total intravenous anesthesia (TIVA) or volatile inhaled anesthesia (VIA) group. The 5-year overall survival outcomes were analyzed by log-rank test. Cox proportional hazards modeling was used for sensitivity.

Results: The number of patients finally included in the comparison after propensity matching came to 729 in each group. The number of surviving patients at 5 years came to 660 (90.5%) in the TIVA and 673 (92.3%) in the VIA. The type of anesthetic did not affect the 5-year survival rate according to the log-rank test ($P = 0.21$). Variables associated with a significant increase in the hazard of death after multivariable analysis were male sex and metastasis at surgery.

Conclusions: There were no differences in 5-year overall survival between two groups in the cancer surgery.

Keywords: Anesthesia, Cancer, Propofol, Surgery, Survival

Background

In Korea, more than 200,000 new cancer patients are diagnosed each year and one in four deaths is due to cancer [1]. Although considerable progress has been made in chemotherapy and radiation therapy, excision of cancerous lesions remains a preferred treatment option for patients with solid tumors [2]. However, the cancer may metastasize or proliferate during surgery [3]; moreover, surgery can spread cancer cells throughout the body [4], so both doctors and patients are keenly aware of the postoperative prognosis. Cancer recurrence and metastasis are influenced by cancer propagation, patient immunity, and related factors [5].

Methods of general anesthesia for tumor resection of malignant tumors include the use of volatile anesthetics and the use of intravenous anesthetics. Several in vitro studies have investigated the use of volatile inhaled anesthetics (VIA) to increase the activation of hypoxia-inducible factor (HIF) and insulin-like growth factor, which are factors involved in tumor growth [6, 7]. There is a possibility of adverse effects on the prognosis of surgical patients. On the other hand, propofol, an intravenous anesthetic, has been reported to reduce the expression of HIF-1α and inhibit tumor growth [8].

In 2016, Wigmore et al. [9] revealed that total intravenous anesthesia (TIVA) has a favorable effect on the

* Correspondence: limtwo2@gmail.com
†Boohwi Hong and Sunyeul Lee contributed equally to this work.
[1]Department of Anesthesiology and Pain Medicine, Chungnam National University Hospital, 282 Munhwa-ro, Jung-gu, Daejeon 35015, Republic of Korea
[2]Department of Anesthesiology and Pain Medicine, Chungnam National University College of Medicine, 266 Munhwa-ro, Jung-gu, Daejeon 35015, Republic of Korea

prognosis of cancer patients. Subsequently, many similar studies have been described in the literature. In 2017, a retrospective study showed that the use of inhalation anesthetics in 191 esophageal cancer patients had a negative effect on prognosis [10]. In a study published in 2018 regarding 1158 patients with colorectal cancer, patients who received TIVA had a better prognosis than those who received desflurane anesthesia [11]. However, other recent studies have shown that cancer prognosis is not related to the type of anesthesia [12, 13]. So far, there have been no reports that propofol-based TIVA is significantly more harmful to patient survival.

This study investigated whether 5-year overall mortality differed between patients who received propofol-based TIVA and those who received VIA during major cancer surgeries in our hospital. Based on the findings reported by Wigmore et al. [9], we hypothesized that patients who received TIVA would show a high 5-year survival rate after cancer surgery (i.e., resection for gastric, lung, liver, colon, or breast cancer), compared to patients who received VIA.

Methods

Setting

The study was approved by the institutional review board of Chungnam National University Hospital (approval number CNUH 2017–08-018). The requirement for informed consent was waived in view of the retrospective nature of the study. This clinical trial has been registered at Clinical Research Information Service (registration number KCT0004101).

Participants

We reviewed the medical records of patients who underwent surgical resection for gastric, lung, liver, colon, or breast cancer from January 2006 to December 2009 in our hospital. Surgeries during the investigation period in which patients received TIVA included general and thoracic surgeries, such as thyroid, breast, colon, hepatobiliary, gastric, and lung cancer surgery. Although a high number of patients had thyroid cancer, the survival rate was sufficiently high that a comparison was not meaningful. In our hospital, thyroidectomy is rapid and it is difficult to manage intravenous catheters for affected patients; accordingly, these patients have received inhalational anesthesia for many years. Therefore, the five major cancers selected for this study were gastric, colon, liver, breast, and lung cancers.

Patients who had undergone emergency surgery, with no follow-up after surgery, patients whose medical records could not be confirmed, patients whose anesthesia was changed during surgery, and patients who died during or immediately after surgery were excluded from the study. Patients who did not fulfill any of the variables examined in the medical record were excluded. Remifentanil with 2% propofol was used via target-controlled infusion for the induction and maintenance of anesthesia in the TIVA group, while remifentanil or nitrous oxide with a volatile anesthetic agent (desflurane, sevoflurane, or isoflurane) was used for the maintenance of anesthesia in the VIA group. At the induction of anesthesia in the VIA group, propofol or etomidate was used, depending on the condition of the patient and the anesthesiologist's preference. Because the benefits of restrictive fluid therapy were not clearly established, liberal fluid therapy was used. The type of anesthesia selected was entirely based on the anesthesiologist's preference.

Variables

Patient factors were age at the time of surgery, sex, body mass index (BMI), and American Society of Anesthesiologists (ASA) class. Surgical and anesthetic factors were the presence of hypertension and diabetes mellitus (DM), total anesthesia time, operation time, type of anesthesia (volatile inhalational anesthesia vs. total intravenous anesthesia), use of nitrous oxide, application of remifentanil infusion, and presence of metastasis at the time of surgery. We also investigated the patient's total length of hospital stay. We investigated the correlations between each of the factors and 5-year survival. Patients were followed-up only with regard to the primary outcome, i.e., overall survival.

Data sources

All data related to the surgery were obtained from the hospital statistical records. Data related to anesthesia, metastasis, and deaths were obtained from the hospital electronic medical records. If we could not find an electronic medical record of the patient's survival at 5 years after surgery, the patient or caregiver was contacted by phone. In such instances, we briefly explained the study and received verbal consent. In addition, the contact information used at this time was not recorded on the case record sheet. If the contact information was unknown, the case was classified as a missed medical record.

Sample size

Based on the results of a previous study [9], to achieve a power of 80% and a two-tailed type I error rate of $\alpha = 0.05$, G*Power 3.1 calculations revealed that at least 495 patients were needed in each matched group. The total number of surgeries per year in our hospital is approximately 10,000; of these surgeries, approximately 600 involve surgical treatments for the five major cancers. Because the ratio between inhalation anesthesia and TIVA was approximately 2:1 during the test period, a 4-year study period was chosen. Patients who underwent surgery between 2006 and 2009 were included because 5 years had already passed at the beginning of the study. After propensity score matching, there were 729 patients in each group, which exceeded the minimum of 495 patients per group.

Statistics

The sample consisted of all subjects during the study period. All available patients were considered. To adjust for possible selection bias and confounding factors [14], 1: 1 ratio propensity score matching was performed using the MatchIt package in R [15]. The dependent variable was set as a binary response of 0 or 1, and logistic regression analysis was performed by designating the covariate (age, sex, height, weight, BMI, ASA class, hypertension, DM, anesthesia time, operation time, metastasis, transfusion) to be corrected as an independent variable. The survival rate was different for each cancer, and the numbers of anesthetic methods used were different for each cancer. Therefore, we matched for each type of cancer.

Nearest neighbor matching was performed, which matches the absolute differences of the estimated propensity scores of all subjects in both groups from the smallest to the largest difference. Absolute standardized difference (ASD) was calculated to validate the suitability of propensity score matching balance diagnostics between the two groups, with ASD < 0.1 for the covariate indicating that the two groups were sufficiently balanced.

After validating the balance of the matched data, the normality of continuous data was assessed using the Shapiro–Wilk test. If normality was satisfied, comparisons between groups were performed by independent t tests, with the results expressed as means ± standard deviations. If normality was not satisfied, groups were compared using the Mann–Whitney U test, with the results expressed as medians (interquartile ranges). Categorical data were compared using the chi-squared test or Fisher's exact test, as appropriate, with the results expressed as numbers (%).

Survival outcomes were analyzed by the log-rank test and expressed by the Kaplan–Meier plot. Cox proportional hazards modeling was used for univariate and multivariable analysis of demographic and clinical variables influencing the survival outcomes. The cut points of the continuous variables were obtained using the maxstst package; survival analysis was performed by separating the patients into two categories based on the following cut points: age, 65 years; height, 165 cm; weight, 57 kg; BMI, 19.7; and anesthesia time, 210 min. Only the meaningful variables ($P < 0.2$) from univariate analysis were included in multivariable analysis. Akaike's Information Criterion was considered for final model selection by backward elimination. Associations with $P < 0.05$ were considered statistically significant. All Data were analyzed using R software version 3.5.2 (R Project for Statistical Computing, Vienna, Austria).

Results

We reviewed the following items in the anesthesia and operation records of patients who underwent surgery. From January 2006 to December 2009, 2496 patients underwent resection of five major malignant tumors. After exclusion of 289 patients according to the exclusion criteria, the analysis included a total of 2207 patients (Fig. 1). All patient information is shown in Table 1. Anesthesia was maintained by inhalation anesthesia in 1304 patients and TIVA in 903 patients undergoing surgery. The numbers of patients finally included in the comparison after propensity score matching were 729 in each group.

Anesthesia

In the TIVA group, all patients used propofol, and all patients were treated with remifentanil, except one patient treated with alfentanil. One patient in the TIVA group was treated with nitrous oxide, which was administered within 5 min after induction of anesthesia because the anesthesia machine was set up to automatically administer nitrous oxide when the fraction of inspired oxygen was reduced. Among the 1304 patients in the VIA group, remifentanil was administered to 701 and nitrous oxide was administered to 550; fentanyl was continuously or intermittently administered to the remaining 53 patients. No patients received epidural pain control or regional block.

Five-year survival: TIVA vs. VIA

The numbers of surviving patients at 5 years were 829/903 (91.8%) in the TIVA group and 1214/1304 (93.1%) in the VIA group; after propensity score matching, these numbers were 660/729 (90.5%) and 673/729 (92.3%), respectively. The type of anesthetic did not affect the 5-year survival rate, according to log-rank analysis, as shown in the Kaplan–Meier plot in Fig. 2 ($P = 0.21$). The type of anesthetic showed no correlation with survival, even in univariate analysis (HR = 1.26, CI = 0.88 to 1.79, $P = 0.21$).

Sensitivity analysis: multivariable cox regression analysis

The hazard ratios of the groups in the univariate model for the propensity score-matched groups are shown in Table 2. Male sex, high BMI, long anesthesia time, and metastasis affected risk of death in the univariate model. The hazard ratios of the groups in the multivariable model for the propensity score-matched groups are shown in Table 3. Variables associated with significant increases in the risk of death after multivariable analysis were male sex and the presence of metastasis at surgery. Only five variables were included in multivariable analysis, based on the selection of meaningful variables ($P < 0.2$) from univariate analysis.

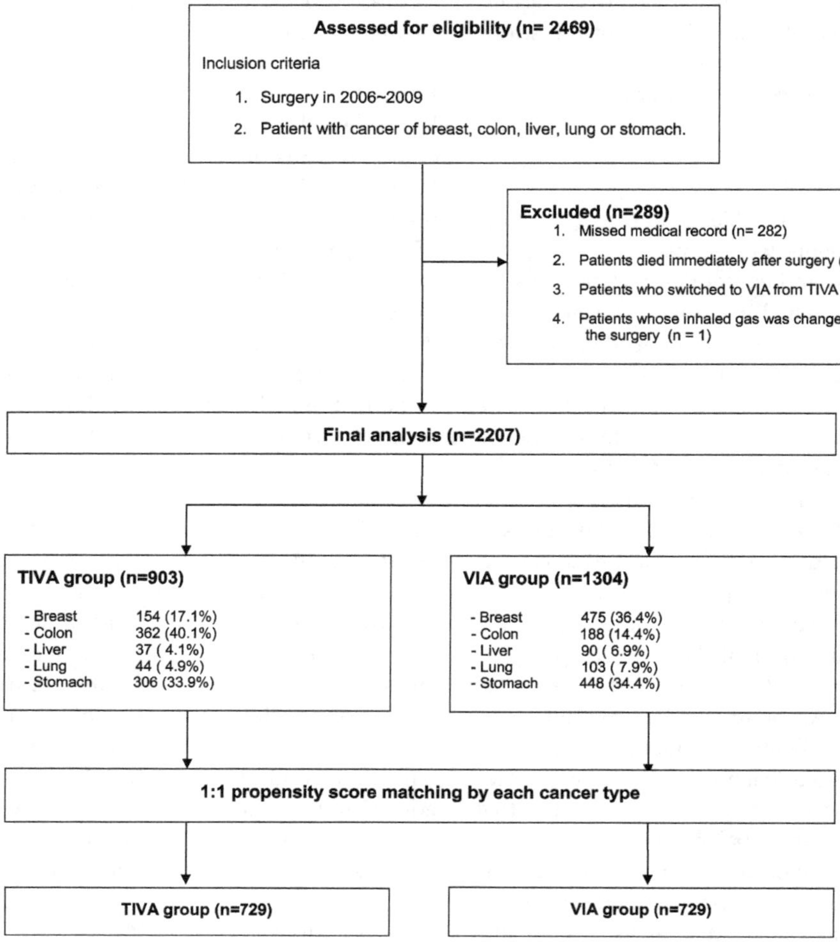

Fig. 1 Flow diagram. TIVA = total intravenous anesthesia; VIA = volatile inhaled anesthesia

Survival rates of each cancer

Survival was highest in patients with breast cancer, followed by patients with colon and stomach cancers; similar mortalities were observed in patients with lung and liver cancers (Fig. 3). We divided the patients based on the types of cancer and analyzed whether the factors from multivariable analysis influenced survival differently among the groups. The results of this subgroup analysis were similar to those of all cancers combined, with the exception of stomach cancer patients without hypertension, who had a low survival rate according to the log-rank test; this is shown in the Kaplan–Meier plot in Fig. 4 ($P = 0.01$).

Discussion

In this study, there was no effect of TIVA or VIA on the survival rate of the overall population of patients undergoing surgery for the five major types of cancer. There was no significant association between the type of anesthetic used and prognosis following cancer surgery.

Each anesthetic has a unique effect on immune regulation and cancer growth factor production [16–19]. It has been reported that propofol exhibits better immunomodulatory properties than volatile anesthetics [20–22]. Some studies have shown that survival rates after cancer surgery are better for patients who receive TIVA than for those who receive VIA [9, 10, 23, 24]. After matching, postoperative survival was investigated in 1158 patients with colon cancer [11]; the propofol-treated group had better survival (189 deaths, 32.6%, in the desflurane group vs. 87, 15.0%, in the propofol group). A recent study showed that propofol was associated with better survival after surgery in 670 patients with hepatocellular carcinoma [25]. For patients with breast cancer, propofol may reduce the relapse rate within 5 years, but a study of patients in the Korea Cancer Center showed no difference in 5-year survival based on the type of anesthetic used during surgery [26]. A comparison of 3532 patients with breast cancer at Seoul National University Hospital revealed no differences in recurrence-free survival and

Table 1 Data for Patients Overall and Matched Patients after Propensity Scoring

	Overall Patients				Matched Patients			
Variables	TIVA (*n* = 903)	VIA (*n* = 1304)	ASD	*P*	TIVA (*n* = 729)	VIA (*n* = 729)	ASD	*P*
Age, yr	58.0 [49.0;67.0]	57.0 [48.0;67.0]	0.098	0.018	58.0 [49.0;67.0]	57.0 [48.0;67.0]	0.003	0.861
Sex			0.233	< 0.001			0.019	0.753
Female	404 (44.7%)	734 (56.3%)			337 (46.2%)	344 (47.2%)		
Male	499 (55.3%)	570 (43.7%)			392 (53.8%)	385 (52.8%)		
Height, cm	161.0 [154.0;166.0]	159.0 [154.0;165.0]	0.118	0.007	161.0 [154.0;166.0]	161.0 [155.0;166.0]	0.015	0.610
Weight, kg	60.0 [54.0;67.0]	60.0 [54.0;67.0]	0.002	0.368	60.0 [54.0;67.0]	60.0 [53.0;67.0]	0.023	0.527
BMI, kg m^{-2}	23.6 [21.8;25.8]	23.8 [21.8;26.1]	0.062	0.210	23.6 [21.7;25.8]	23.5 [21.5;25.8]	0.039	0.577
ASA class			0.098	0.067			0.053	0.605
I	399 (44.2%)	633 (48.5%)			311 (42.7%)	310 (42.5%)		
II	503 (55.7%)	671 (51.5%)			417 (57.2%)	419 (57.5%)		
III	1 (0.1%)	0 (0.0%)			1 (0.1%)	0 (0.0%)		
Hypertension			0.008	0.894			< 0.001	1.000
Yes	233 (25.8%)	341 (26.2%)			188 (25.8%)	188 (25.8%)		
No	670 (74.2%)	963 (73.8%)			541 (74.2%)	541 (74.2%)		
DM			0.057	0.204			0.032	0.593
Yes	121 (13.4%)	150 (11.5%)			95 (13.0%)	103 (14.1%)		
No	782 (86.6%)	1154 (88.5%)			634 (87.0%)	626 (85.9%)		
Anesthesia time, min	230.0 [185.0;285.0]	210.0 [170.0;260.0]	0.166	< 0.001	215.0 [180.0;260.0]	220.0 [180.0;265.0]	0.017	0.696
Operation time, min	190.0 [150.0;240.0]	175.0 [135.0;220.0]	0.146	< 0.001	180.0 [149.0;220.0]	180.0 [149.0;225.0]	0.012	0.787
Remifentanil infusion				< 0.001				< 0.001
Yes	902 (99.9%)	701 (53.8%)			728 (99.9%)	395 (54.2%)		
No	1 (0.1%)	603 (46.2%)			1 (0.1%)	334 (45.8%)		
Gas type				< 0.001				< 0.001
Des	0 (0.0%)	345 (26.5%)			0 (0.0%)	193 (26.5%)		
Iso	0 (0.0%)	31 (2.4%)			0 (0.0%)	25 (3.5%)		
Sevo	0 (0.0%)	927 (71.1%)			0 (0.0%)	511 (70%)		
Nitrous oxide				< 0.001				< 0.001
Yes	1 (0.1%)	550 (42.2%)			1 (0.1%)	302 (41.4%)		
No	902 (99.9%)	754 (57.8%)			728 (99.9%)	427 (58.6%)		
Metastasis at surgery			0.006	0.947			0.014	0.855
Yes	68 (7.5%)	96 (7.4%)			64 (8.8%)	67 (9.2%)		
No	835 (92.5%)	1208 (92.6%)			665 (91.2%)	662 (90.8%)		
Transfusion			0.056	0.252			0.038	0.626
Yes	19 (2.1%)	39 (3.0%)			10 (1.4%)	7 (1.0%)		
No	884 (97.9%)	1265 (97.0%)			719 (98.6%)	722 (99.0%)		
Hospital stay, day	13.0 [11.0;18.0]	13.0 [10.0;18.0]	0.014	0.238	13.0 [11.0;18.0]	13.0 [10.0;18.0]	0.023	0.355
Survival, month	60.0 [44.0;60.0]	60.0 [45.0;60.0]		0.945	60.0 [40.0;60.0]	60.0 [47.0;60.0]		0.523
5 years survival				0.291				0.262
Yes	829 (91.8%)	1214 (93.1%)			660 (90.5%)	673 (92.3%)		
No	74 (8.2%)	90 (6.9%)			69 (9.5%)	56 (7.7%)		
Cancer type				< 0.001				1.000
Breast	154 (17.1%)	475 (36.4%)			154 (21.1%)	154 (21.1%)		
Colon	362 (40.1%)	188 (14.4%)			188 (25.8%)	188 (25.8%)		

Table 1 Data for Patients Overall and Matched Patients after Propensity Scoring *(Continued)*

	Overall Patients				Matched Patients			
Variables	TIVA ($n = 903$)	VIA ($n = 1304$)	ASD	*P*	TIVA ($n = 729$)	VIA ($n = 729$)	ASD	*P*
Liver	37 (4.1%)	90 (6.9%)			37 (5.1%)	37 (5.1%)		
Lung	44 (4.9%)	103 (7.9%)			44 (6.0%)	44 (6.0%)		
Stomach	306 (33.9%)	448 (34.4%)			306 (42.0%)	306 (42.0%)		

Number (%): chi-square test, median [interquartile range]: Mann–Whitney U test
ASD Absolute standardized mean difference, *BMI* Body mass index, *ASA* American Society of Anesthesiologists, *TIVA* Total intravenous anesthesia, *VIA* Volatile inhalational anesthesia, *DM* Diabetes mellitus, *Des* Desflurane, *Iso* Isoflurane, *Sevo* Sevoflurane

overall survival, based on the type of anesthetic used during surgery [13]. An analysis of 1794 patients with gastric cancer demonstrated that TIVA was associated with better survival after surgery [27]. Depending on the time of gastric cancer resection surgery, some patients had a long-term survival of 80–90 months. Another study of 1538 patients with gastric cancer found that propofol-based TIVA had no significant effect on 1-year overall survival or cancer-related mortality after surgery, but this could have been related to the short 1-year study period [12]. Finally, a study of 392 patients with non-small cell carcinoma showed no benefit for long-term prognosis when TIVA was used during surgery [28].

Thus far, the findings have differed among studies depending on the type of cancer, the research institute involved, the duration of the investigation, and whether overall survival or recurrence-free survival is assessed. However, there have been no reports that propofol-based TIVA is significantly more harmful to patient survival. Although it did not include the most recent reports, a meta-analysis of 21,000 patients showed that both recurrence-free survival and overall survival rates were higher in the TIVA group than in the volatile anesthesia group [29]. Despite these data, one survey revealed that most anesthesiologists preferred inhalation anesthesia [30]. As many as 43% of respondents presumed that TIVA could reduce cancer recurrence; however, only 29% of them used TIVA for cancer surgery. Factors affecting cancer prognosis are very diverse and complex; therefore, they may not differ simply because of the anesthetic used. In our hospital, regardless of whether the surgery involves cancer treatment, most anesthesiologists use sevoflurane or desflurane for general anesthesia. Notably, the proportion of patients who received TIVA for general anesthesia in 2018 at Chungnam National University Hospital was 1575 of 12,659 (12%). This is likely because the benefits of the TIVA are not yet clear and a syringe infuser is not available.

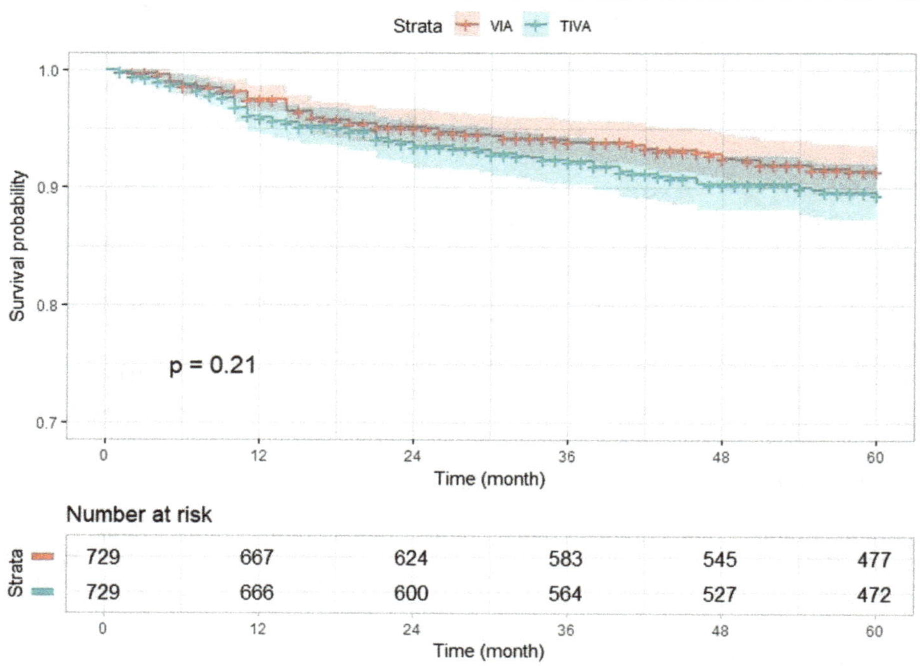

Fig. 2 Comparison of survival rate by Kaplan–Meier survival curves after propensity matching. VIA = volatile inhaled anesthesia group; TIVA = total intravenous anesthesia group

Table 2 Hazard Ratios by Univariate Model

	HR	95% CI	*P*-value
Anesthesia type: TIVA vs VIA	1.255	0.882 to 1.785	0.206
Age, yr: > 65 vs ≤ 65	1.000	0.988 to 1.019	0.616
Sex: male vs female	1.602	0.990 to 1.034	0.011*
Height, cm: > 166 vs ≤ 166	1.012	0.990 to 1.004	0.283
Weight, kg: > 57 vs ≤ 57	0.932	0.883 to 0.983	0.117
BMI, kg m^{-2}: > 19.7 vs ≤ 19.7	0.932	0.883 to 0.983	0.010*
ASA class: II vs I	1.248	0.870 to 1.790	0.228
Hypertension: no vs yes	1.200	0.788 to 1.828	0.394
DM: no vs yes	0.903	0.548 to 1.489	0.690
Anesthesia time, min: > 210 vs ≤ 210	1.003	1.001 to 1.005	0.002**
Metastasis: no vs yes	0.123	0.085 to 0.179	< 0.001**
Transfusion: no vs yes	0.684	0.169 to 2.769	0.595

BMI Body mass index, *ASA* American Society of Anesthesiologists, *HR* Hazard ratio, *TIVA* Total intravenous anesthesia, *VIA* Volatile inhaled anesthesia, *DM* Diabetes mellitus; *$P < 0.05$; **$P < 0.01$

There have been several reports that neither TIVA nor volatile anesthesia affected the prognosis of cancer patients [13, 28, 31], and the present study was consistent with these results. In this study, hypertension was shown to be associated with 5-year survival only in gastric cancer patients on univariate analysis. As the effect of medication taken daily by hypertensive patients has not been investigated, it will be difficult to estimate accurately the mechanism underlying this observation. As observed in patients with gastric cancer in this study, hypertension may provide a survival advantage, as indicated in a study of women with ovarian cancer [32]. New research from epidemiologists at Roswell Park Cancer Institute provided evidence that hypertension and diabetes as well as the use of medications to treat these common conditions may influence the survival of ovarian cancer patients. Hypertension was reported to be associated with lower risk of disease progression among patients with endometrioid tumors ($n = 339$, HR = 0.54; 95% CI = 0.35 to 0.84). In Korea, hypertension is treated indiscriminately by combination therapy with aspirin or statins, which may be another explanation for these observations. Aspirin use may have only a small effect on gastric carcinoma [33]. One meta-analysis [34] showed that statins were inversely related to the risk of gastric cancer (RR = 0.56; 95% CI = 0.35 to 0.90). Thus far, there is no clear explanation for the good prognosis we observed in patients who take medications for hypertension control, especially among patients with stomach cancer. To explain this observation, further studies are required to determine which medications were taken daily by patients with hypertension who underwent surgery for stomach cancer.

This study had some limitations, primarily due to its retrospective nature. The size of the study population was also small, although this was partially addressed by propensity score matching. Furthermore, overall survival was used as the primary outcome. Thus, we did not distinguish among deaths from cancer recurrences, deaths from other diseases, or sudden accidents. However, considering the very long average life span of Koreans [35], we considered this unlikely to be a problem. This use of overall survival may be why multivariable Cox regression analysis showed that age was not a significant covariate. The final limitation was that no special fluid therapy, mechanical ventilation, or postoperative management was included.

Table 3 Hazard Ratios by Multivariable Analysis

	Cancer type included			Cancer type excluded		
	HR	95% CI	*P*-value	HR	95% CI	*P*-value
Sex: male vs female	1.031	0.625 to 1.700	0.905	1.731	1.078 to 2.781	0.023*
Weight, kg: > 57 vs ≤ 57	0.990	0.956 to 1.026	0.591	0.980	0.946 to 1.016	0.275
BMI, kg m^{-2}: > 19.7 vs ≤ 19.7	0.983	0.889 to 1.087	0.743	1.015	0.917 to 1.122	0.777
Anesthesia time, min: > 210 vs ≤ 210	1.001	0.998 to 1.003	0.573	1.000	0.998 to 1.002	0.911
Metastasis: no vs yes	0.119	0.078 to 0.180	< 0.001**	0.132	0.088 to 0.199	< 0.001**
Cancer type						
Breast (reference)						
Colon	2.594	0.917 to 7.341	0.072			
Liver	8.168	2.556 to 26.104	< 0.001**			
Lung	7.235	2.295 to 22.810	< 0.001**			
Stomach	6.576	2.533 to 17.069	< 0.001**			

Only variables with a significance level of $P < 0.2$ in univariable analysis were included in the multivariable model. *BMI* Body mass index, *ASA* American Society of Anesthesiologists, *HR* Hazard ratio, *TIVA* Total intravenous anesthesia, DM Diabetes mellitus; *$P < 0.05$; **$P < 0.01$

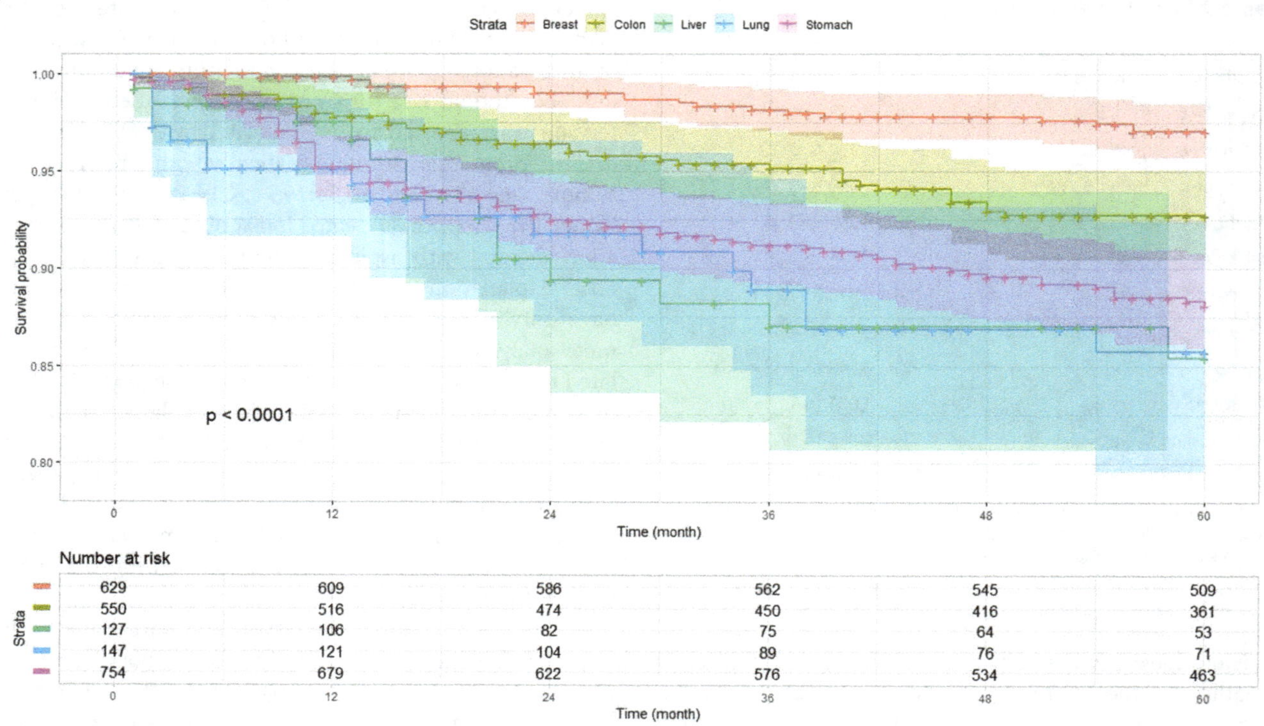

Fig. 3 Kaplan–Meier survival curves grouped by cancer type

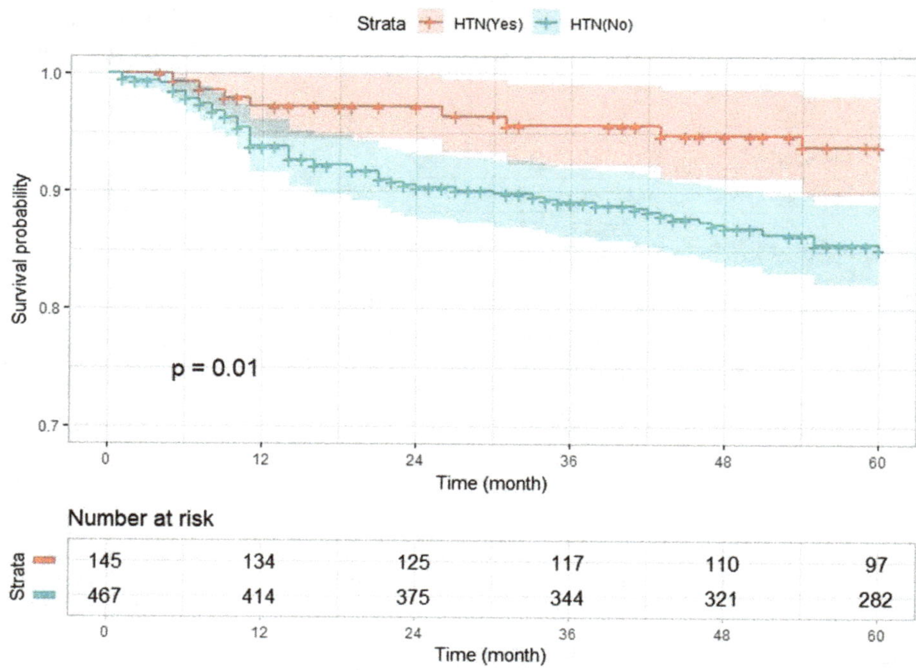

Fig. 4 Kaplan–Meier survival curves according to hypertension after propensity matching in stomach cancer patients. HTN = hypertension history

Conclusions

There were no differences in 5-year overall survival between the TIVA and VIA groups in patients who underwent major cancer surgeries in our hospital. Therefore, we cannot conclude that propofol-based TIVA is more suitable than VIA for use in cancer surgery. Unexpectedly, patients with stomach cancer showed better survival when they had hypertension than when they did not have hypertension. To increase the objectivity of these results, further studies with a larger number of patients are needed.

Abbreviations

ASA: American society of anesthesiologists; ASD: Absolute standardized difference; BMI: Body mass index; CRIS: Clinical research information service; DM: Diabetes mellitus HIF: Hypoxia-inducible factors; PSM: Propensity score matching; TIVA: Total ntravenous anesthesia; VIA: Volatile inhaled anesthesia

Acknowledgements

These results were presented at the Euroanaesthesia 2019 (Vienna, Austria, 01/06/2019 - 03/06/2019) in electronic poster format.

Authors' contributions

Conceptualization, S.L., C.L., Y.K.; methodology, B.H. and S.-H.Y.; software, B.H.; validation, A.M.Y.,H.R.; formal analysis, B.H.; investigation, Y.-H.K.; resources, M.L.; data curation, H.R., Y.K.; writing-original draft preparation, B.H.; writing-review and editing, C.L., S.L., S.-H.H.; visualization, B.H.; supervision, C.L.; project administration, S.-H.H.; funding acquisition, C.L. All authors have read and approved the manuscript.

Author details

[1]Department of Anesthesiology and Pain Medicine, Chungnam National University Hospital, 282 Munhwa-ro, Jung-gu, Daejeon 35015, Republic of Korea. [2]Department of Anesthesiology and Pain Medicine, Chungnam National University College of Medicine, 266 Munhwa-ro, Jung-gu, Daejeon 35015, Republic of Korea. [3]MediRedox (Biomedical convergence Research Center), 266 Munhwa-ro, Jung-gu, Daejeon 35015, Republic of Korea.

References

1. Jung K-W, Won Y-J, Kong H-J, Lee ES. Cancer statistics in Korea: incidence, mortality, survival, and prevalence in 2015. Cancer Res Treat: Official J Korean Cancer Assoc. 2018;50(2):303.
2. Miller KD, Siegel RL, Lin CC, Mariotto AB, Kramer JL, Rowland JH, Stein KD, Alteri R, Jemal A. Cancer treatment and survivorship statistics, 2016. CA Cancer J Clin. 2016;66(4):271–89.
3. Ceelen W, Pattyn P, Mareel M. Surgery, wound healing, and metastasis: recent insights and clinical implications. Crit Rev Oncol Hematol. 2014;89(1):16–26.
4. Xu Y, Li S, Cheng Q, Chen W,W Wang S, Ren Y, Miao C: Effects of anaesthesia on proliferation, invasion and apoptosis of LoVo colon cancer cells in vitro. Anaesth 2016, 71(2):147–154.
5. Vogelaar FJ, Lips DJ, van Dorsten FR, Lemmens VE, Bosscha K. Impact of anaesthetic technique on survival in colon cancer: a review of the literature. Gastroenterol Rep. 2015;4(1):30–4.
6. Shi QY, Zhang SJ, Liu L, Chen QS, Yu LN, Zhang FJ, Yan M. Sevoflurane promotes the expansion of glioma stem cells through activation of hypoxia-inducible factors in vitro. Br J Anaesth. 2015;114(5):825–30.
7. Benzonana LL, Perry NJ, Watts HR, Yang B, Perry IA, Coombes C, Takata M, Ma D. Isoflurane, a commonly used volatile anesthetic, enhances renal cancer growth and malignant potential via the hypoxia-inducible factor cellular signaling pathway in vitro. Anesthesiol. 2013;119(3):593–605.
8. Li R, Liu H, Dilger JP, Lin J. Effect of Propofol on breast Cancer cell, the immune system, and patient outcome. BMC Anesthesiol. 2018;18(1):77.
9. Wigmore TJ, Mohammed K, Jhanji S. Long-term survival for patients undergoing volatile versus IV anesthesia for Cancer SurgeryA retrospective analysis. Anesthesiol: J Am Soc Anesthesiol. 2016;124(1):69–79.
10. Jun IJ, Jo JY, Kim JI, Chin JH, Kim WJ, Kim HR, Lee EH, Choi IC. Impact of anesthetic agents on overall and recurrence-free survival in patients undergoing esophageal cancer surgery: a retrospective observational study. Sci Rep. 2017;7(1):14020.
11. Wu ZF, Lee MS, Wong CS, Lu CH, Huang YS, Lin KT, Lou YS, Lin C, Chang YC, Lai HC. Propofol-based Total intravenous anesthesia is associated with better survival than Desflurane anesthesia in Colon Cancer surgery. Anesthesiol. 2018;129(5):932–41.
12. Oh TK, Kim HH, Jeon YT. Retrospective analysis of 1-year mortality after gastric cancer surgery: Total intravenous anesthesia versus volatile anesthesia. Acta Anaesthesiol Scand. 2019;63(9):1169–77.
13. Yoo S, Lee HB, Han W, Noh DY, Park SK, Kim WH, Kim JT. Total intravenous anesthesia versus inhalation anesthesia for breast Cancer surgery: a retrospective cohort study. Anesthesiology. 2019;130(1):31–40.
14. Dong Kyu L. An introduction to propensity score matching methods. Anesth Pain Med. 2016;11(2):130–48.
15. Stevens RA, Chester WL, Artuso JD, Bray JG, Nellestein JA. Back pain after epidural anesthesia with chloroprocaine in volunteers: preliminary report. Reg Anesth. 1991;16(4):199–203.
16. Luo X, Zhao H, Hennah L, Ning J, Liu J, Tu H, Ma D. Impact of isoflurane on malignant capability of ovarian cancer in vitro. Br J Anaesth. 2015;114(5):831–9.
17. Rohwer N, Lobitz S, Daskalow K, Jons T, Vieth M, Schlag PM, Kemmner W, Wiedenmann B, Cramer T, Hocker M. HIF-1alpha determines the metastatic potential of gastric cancer cells. Br J Cancer. 2009;100(5):772–81.
18. Buckley A, McQuaid S, Johnson P, Buggy DJ. Effect of anaesthetic technique on the natural killer cell anti-tumour activity of serum from women undergoing breast cancer surgery: a pilot study. Br J Anaesth. 2014; 113(Suppl 1):i56–62.
19. Huang H, Benzonana LL, Zhao H, Watts HR, Perry NJ, Bevan C, Brown R, Ma D. Prostate cancer cell malignancy via modulation of HIF-1alpha pathway with isoflurane and propofol alone and in combination. Br J Cancer. 2014; 111(7):1338–49.
20. Melamed R, Bar-Yosef S, Shakhar G, Shakhar K, Ben-Eliyahu S. Suppression of natural killer cell activity and promotion of tumor metastasis by ketamine, thiopental, and halothane, but not by propofol: mediating mechanisms and prophylactic measures. Anesth Analg. 2003;97(5):1331–9.
21. Ke JJ, Zhan J, Feng XB, Wu Y, Rao Y, Wang YL. A comparison of the effect of total intravenous anaesthesia with propofol and remifentanil and inhalational anaesthesia with isoflurane on the release of pro- and anti-inflammatory cytokines in patients undergoing open cholecystectomy. Anaesth Intensive Care. 2008;36(1):74–8.
22. Dubowitz JA, Sloan EK, Riedel BJ. Implicating anaesthesia and the perioperative period in cancer recurrence and metastasis. Clin Exp Metastasis. 2018;35(4):347–58.
23. Enlund M, Berglund A, Andreasson K, Cicek C, Enlund A, Bergkvist L. The choice of anaesthetic—sevoflurane or propofol—and outcome from cancer surgery: a retrospective analysis. Ups J Med Sci. 2014;119(3):251–61.
24. Soltanizadeh S, Degett TH, Gogenur I. Outcomes of cancer surgery after inhalational and intravenous anesthesia: a systematic review. J Clin Anesth. 2017;42:19–25.
25. Lai HC, Lee MS, Lin C, Lin KT, Huang YH, Wong CS, Chan SM, Wu ZF. Propofol-based total intravenous anaesthesia is associated with better survival than desflurane anaesthesia in hepatectomy for hepatocellular carcinoma: a retrospective cohort study. Br J Anaesth. 2019;123(2):151–60.
26. Lee JH, Kang SH, Kim Y, Kim HA, Kim BS. Effects of propofol-based total intravenous anesthesia on recurrence and overall survival in patients after modified radical mastectomy: a retrospective study. Korean J Anesthesiol. 2016;69(2):126–32.
27. Zheng X, Wang Y, Dong L, Zhao S, Wang L, Chen H, Xu Y, Wang G. Effects of propofol-based total intravenous anesthesia on gastric cancer: a retrospective study. Onco Targets Ther. 2018;11:1141–8.
28. Oh TK, Kim K, Jheon S, Lee J, Do SH, Hwang JW, Song IA. Long-term oncologic outcomes for patients undergoing volatile versus intravenous anesthesia for non-small cell lung Cancer surgery: a retrospective propensity matching analysis. Cancer Control. 2018;25(1):1073274818775360.
29. Yap A, Lopez-Olivo MA, Dubowitz J, Hiller J, Riedel B: Anesthetic technique and cancer outcomes: a meta-analysis of total intravenous versus volatile anesthesia. Canadian journal of anaesthesia = J Canadien d'anesthesie 2019, 66(5):546–561.
30. Lim A, Braat S, Hiller J, Riedel B. Inhalational versus propofol-based total intravenous anaesthesia: practice patterns and perspectives among Australasian anaesthetists. Anaesth Intensive Care. 2018;46(5):480–7.

31. Yan T, Zhang GH, Wang BN, Sun L, Zheng H. Effects of propofol/remifentanil-based total intravenous anesthesia versus sevoflurane-based inhalational anesthesia on the release of VEGF-C and TGF-beta and prognosis after breast cancer surgery: a prospective, randomized and controlled study. BMC Anesthesiol. 2018;18(1):131.
32. Minlikeeva AN, Freudenheim JL, Cannioto RA, Szender JB, Eng KH, Modugno F, Ness RB, LaMonte MJ, Friel G, Segal BH, et al. History of hypertension, heart disease, and diabetes and ovarian cancer patient survival: evidence from the ovarian cancer association consortium. Cancer Causes Control : CCC. 2017;28(5):469–86.
33. Yang L, Zhu H, Liu D, Liang S, Xu H, Chen J, Wang X, Xu Z. Aspirin suppresses growth of human gastric carcinoma cell by inhibiting survivin expression. J Biomed Res. 2011;25(4):246–53.
34. Ma Z, Wang W, Jin G, Chu P, Li H. Effect of statins on gastric cancer incidence: a meta-analysis of case control studies. J Cancer Res Ther. 2014; 10(4):859–65.
35. Kontis V, Bennett JE, Mathers CD, Li G, Foreman K, Ezzati M. Future life expectancy in 35 industrialised countries: projections with a Bayesian model ensemble. Lancet (London, England). 2017;389(10076):1323–35.

19

Comparison of volume-controlled ventilation mode and pressure-controlled ventilation with volume-guaranteed mode in the prone position during lumbar spine surgery

Jung Min Lee, Soo Kyung Lee, Kyung Mi Kim, You Jung Kim and Eun Young Park*

Abstract

Background: During lumbar spine surgery, patients are placed in the prone position for surgical access. The prone position has various effects on cardiac and pulmonary function, including a decreased cardiac index (CI), decreased dynamic lung compliance (Cdyn), and increased peak inspiratory pressure (Ppeak). In this study, we compared the volume-controlled ventilation mode (VCV) and pressure-controlled ventilation with volume guaranteed mode (PCV-VG) based on hemodynamic and pulmonary variables in the prone position during lumbar spine surgery.

Methods: Thirty-six patients scheduled for lumbar spine surgery in the prone position were enrolled in this prospective, randomized clinical trial. The patients were randomly assigned to receive VCV or PCV-VG. Hemodynamic variables, respiratory variables, and arterial blood gases were measured in the supine position 15 min after the induction of anesthesia, 15 min after placement in the prone position, 30 min after placement in the prone position, and 15 min after placement in the supine position at the end of anesthesia.

Results: The hemodynamic variables and arterial blood gas results did not differ significantly between the two groups. Lower Ppeak values were observed in the PCV-VG group than in the VCV group ($p = 0.045$). The Cdyn values in the VCV group were lower than those in the PCV-VG group ($p = 0.040$).

Conclusion: PCV-VG led to lower Ppeak and improved Cdyn values compared with VCV, showing that it may be a favorable alternative mode of mechanical ventilation for patients in the prone position during lumbar spine surgery.

Keywords: Mechanical ventilation, General anesthesia, Spine surgery, Cardiac output

Background

The prone position is commonly required to enable surgical access during lumbar spine surgery. When a patient moves into the prone position, inferior vena cava obstruction causes reduced venous return and increased thoracic pressure results in reduced left ventricular compliance, leading to a decreased cardiac index (CI) [1]. Pulmonary physiology is also influenced in the prone position. Although the V/Q mismatch is reduced and arterial oxygenation is improved in the prone position [2], lung compliance is reduced and the peak inspiratory pressure (Ppeak) increases to achieve the set tidal volume [3].

The volume-controlled ventilation mode (VCV) is commonly used during general anesthesia: the minute ventilation is fixed and airway pressure is influenced by pulmonary resistance or compliance [4]. The pressure-controlled ventilation with volume guaranteed mode

* Correspondence: parkey00@hanmail.net
Department of Anesthesiology and Pain Medicine, Hallym University Sacred Heart Hospital, College of Medicine, Hallym University, 22, Gwanpyeong-ro 170beon-gil, Dongan-gu, Gyeonggi-do, 14068 Anyang-si, Republic of Korea

(PCV-VG) has recently been introduced in the field of anesthesiology. In this mode, the ventilator compares the tidal volume of the previous breath and automatically regulates the pressure limits to achieve a set tidal volume with the lowest airway pressure [5, 6].

In this randomized study, we tested the null hypothesis that VCV or PCV-VG does not affect hemodynamic or pulmonary variables during lumbar spine surgery in the prone position. The primary outcome of this study was Ppeak. The secondary outcomes were lung compliance and hemodynamic variables including cardiac output (CO), CI, stroke volume (SV), and stroke volume variation (SVV).

Methods

This study was approved by the Institutional Review Board of Hallym University Sacred Heart Hospital. After written informed consent was obtained from all participants, 36 patients who were scheduled for lumbar spine surgery in the prone position were enrolled. Patients with morbid obesity (body mass index > 30 kg/m^2), hypotension (systolic blood pressure < 100 mmHg), bradycardia (heart rate < 60 bpm), uncompensated cardiologic disease (heart failure, history of myocardial infarction, or heart block), hypoxia (PaO_2 < 60 mmHg or SpO_2 < 90%), uncontrolled asthma, or chronic obstructive pulmonary disease (forced expiratory volume in 1 s < 60%) were excluded. Patients who were younger than 20 years or older than 70 years were also excluded. This study was registered at ClinicalTrials.gov (NCT 03571854). The study was conducted in accordance with the Consolidated Standards of Reporting Trials (CONSORT) 2010 statement [7].

All patients fasted for 8 h before surgery and were premedicated with intramuscular glycopyrrolate (0.2 mg). In the operating room, patients were monitored by non-invasive blood pressure, electrocardiography, and pulse oximetry (SpO_2) before the induction of anesthesia. Anesthesia was induced with remifentanil (0.1–0.2 μg/kg/min), propofol (1.5–2 mg/kg), and rocuronium (0.6 mg/kg), and maintained at a fractional inspired oxygen concentration of 0.5 with sevoflurane (2.0–2.5 vol%), remifentanil (0.05–0.3 μg/kg/min), and vecuronium (0.03–0.05 mg/kg/h). The patients were ventilated with a Datex-Ohmeda Ventilator (S/S AVANCE) and randomly assigned to receive either VCV (n = 18) or PCV-VG (n = 18) using a computer-generated randomization method. The tidal volume in both groups was set to deliver 8 mL/kg of ideal body weight. The respiratory rate (RR) was adjusted to maintain an end tidal CO_2 ($ETCO_2$) level of 33–38 mmHg, and the inspiratory to expiratory time (I:E) ratio was 0.5. After the induction of anesthesia, a 20 G catheter was inserted into the radial artery to monitor continuous arterial pressure and connected to the FloTrac®/Vigileo system (Edwards Lifesciences Corp., Irvine, CA) for the continuous monitoring of variables, including CO, CI, SV, stroke volume index (SVI), and SVV.

Hemodynamic variables, respiratory variables, and arterial blood gases were measured in the supine position 15 min after the induction of anesthesia, 15 min after placement in the prone position, 30 min after placement in the prone position, and 15 min after placement in the supine position at the end of anesthesia. The measured hemodynamic variables included mean arterial pressure (MAP), heart rate (HR), CO, CI, SV, SVI, and SVV. Respiratory variables included RR, Ppeak, mean inspiratory pressure (Pmean), SpO_2, $ETCO_2$, and dynamic lung compliance (Cdyn).

As there have been no previous studies comparing the effects of PCV-VG and VCV during surgery in the prone position, the sample size for this study was determined in a pilot study. The results indicated a mean difference in Ppeak between the two modes of 10% (α = 0.05, power = 80%, effect size = 1.007). Assuming a 20% dropout rate, 18 patients were included in each group in this study.

All data are presented as the median (interquartile range) or number of patients. Hemodynamic and respiratory data were analyzed with a repeated-measures analysis of variance, and differences between groups at the same time point were analyzed with the two-sample t-test or Mann-Whitney U test; p-values < 0.05 were considered statistically significant. Statistical analyses were performed using the Statistical Package for the Social Sciences version 24.0 (IBM Corp., Armonk, NY).

Results

A total of 36 patients were enrolled in this study and a CONSORT flow diagram is shown in Fig. 1. There were no significant differences between the groups in patient characteristics (Table 1). Among the respiratory variables, Ppeak increased after placement in the prone position during surgery and in the supine position at the end of anesthesia in both groups, and there were lower Ppeak values in the PCV-VG group than in the VCV group throughout the study period ($p = 0.045$, Fig. 2). The Cdyn values at the later three time points were lower than the initial values in both groups, and Cdyn was lower in the VCV group than in the PCV-VG group throughout the study period ($p = 0.040$, Fig. 3). Pmean increased after placement in the prone position in both groups, and there was no significant intergroup difference in Pmean over time during surgery (Table 2).

HR decreased after placement in the prone position in both groups, but no significant intergroup

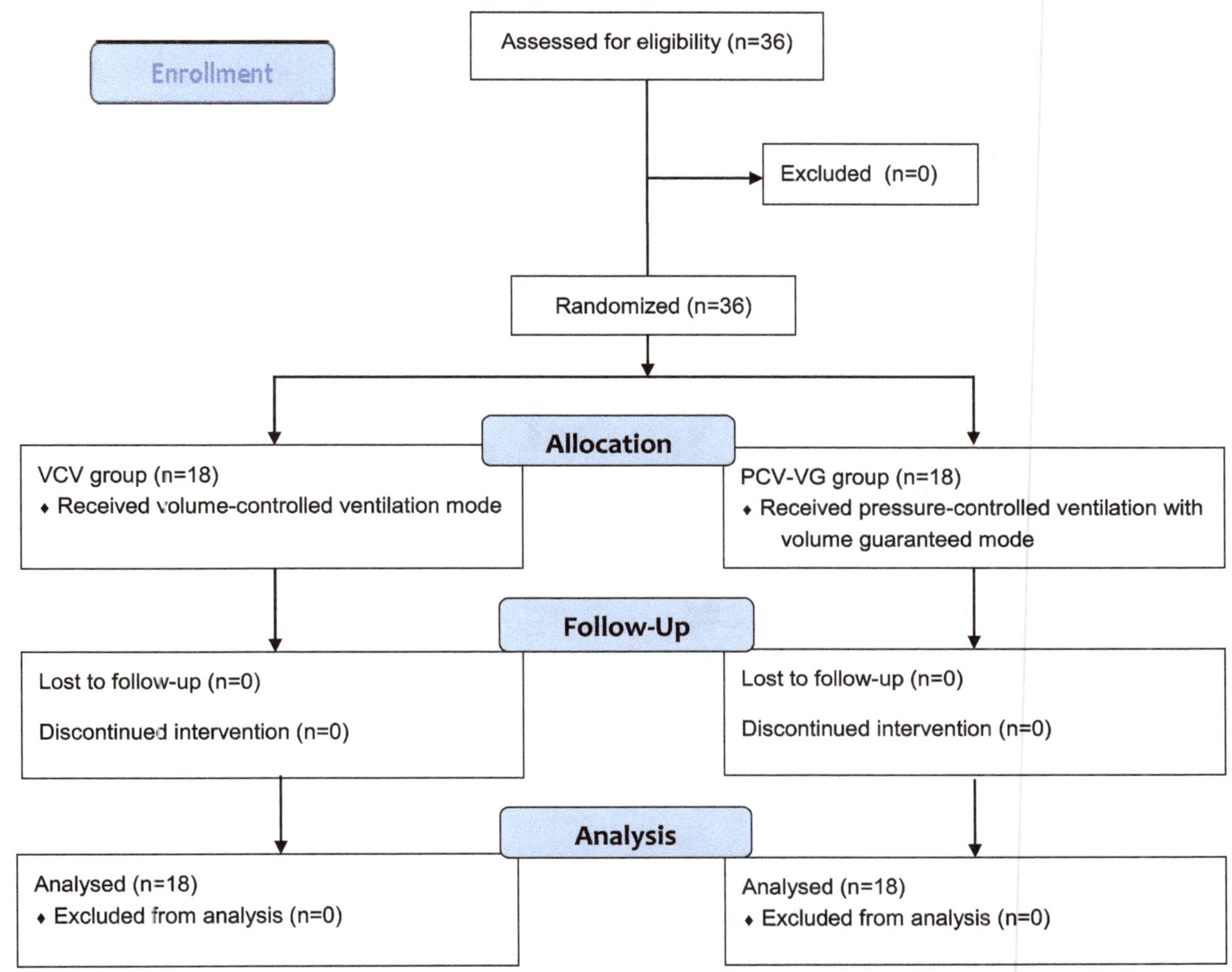

Fig. 1 The CONSORT flow diagram

difference was present. CO and CI did not differ significantly between groups, while the CO and CI values decreased 15 min after placement in the prone position (Table 3). The blood gas results did not differ between groups (Table 4).

Table 1 Patient characteristics

	VCV (*n* = 18)	PCV-VG (*n* = 18)
Age (years)	50.0 (41–60)	56 (52–61)
Male/female	11/7	11/7
BMI (kg/m^2)	24.1 (22.4–26.8)	24.5 (22.6–27.4)
ASA PS classification (I/II/III)	5/9/4	2/13/3
Duration of anesthesia (min)	240 (176–280)	295 (204–341)
Duration of surgery (min)	163 (108–196)	223 (115–244)

BMI body mass index, *ASA PS* classification, American Society of Anesthesiologists physical status classification, *VCV* volume-controlled ventilation, *PCV-VG* pressure-controlled ventilation with volume guaranteed
Data are listed as the median (interquartile range) or number of patients

Discussion

In the present study, we compared the effects of the VCV and PCV-VG on hemodynamic and pulmonary variables in the prone position. In VCV, the ventilator delivers a target volume with a constant flow and the airway pressure increases in a linear manner. This approach ensures minute ventilation regardless of airway compliance but cannot control airway pressure [8]. Compared with VCV, the pressure-controlled ventilation mode (PCV) provides the tidal volume at a preset pressure with decelerating flow, and the tidal volume can be varied depending on lung compliance [9]. PCV-VG delivers a target tidal volume with a decelerating flow and calculates lung compliance to adjust the inspiratory pressure based on the previous breath [6, 8]. It reaches the target volume with the lowest inspiratory pressure and has the benefits of both VCV and PCV [9].

Several studies have examined the effects of the PCV-VG compared with conventional modes (VCV or PCV).

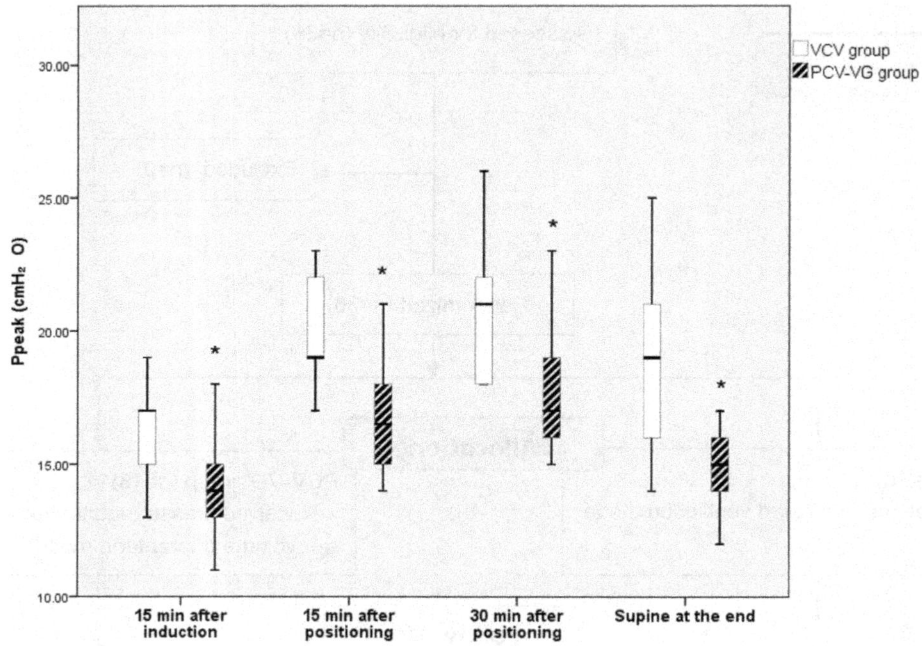

Fig. 2 Peak airway pressure at each measurement timepoint in each groupData are displayed as ranges, medians, and interquartile ranges. VCV, volume controlled ventilation; PCV-VG, pressure-controlled ventilation with volume guaranteed mode. *$p < 0.05$ compared with the VCV group at the same time point

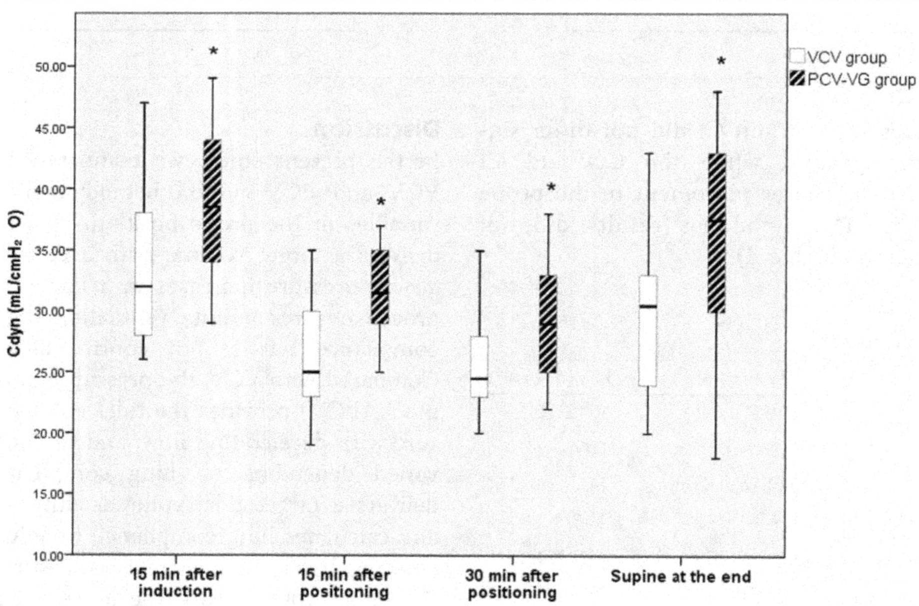

Fig. 3 Dynamic lung compliance at each measurement timepoint in each group. Data are displayed as ranges, medians, and interquartile ranges. VCV, volume-controlled ventilation, PCV-VG, pressure-controlled ventilation with volume guaranteed. *$p < 0.05$ compared with the VCV group at the same time point

Table 2 Respiratory variables

	Group	15 min after induction	15 min after positioning	30 min after positioning	Supine at the end
Ppeak (cmH_2O)	VCV	17 (15–17)	19 (19–22)†	21 (18–22)†	19 (16–22)†
	PCV-VG	14 (13–15)*	17 (15–18)*†	17 (16–19)*†	15 (14–16)*
Pmean (cmH_2O)	VCV	7 (6–7)	7 (7–8)†	8 (7–8)†	7 (6–8)
	PCV-VG	7 (6–7)	7 (7–8)†	8 (7–9)†	7 (7–8)
RR (breaths/min)	VCV	12 (12–14)	11 (10–12)	12 (10–12)	12 (10–13)
	PCV-VG	12 (11–13)	12 (10–12)	12 (10–12)	11 (10–13)
Cdyn (mL/cmH_2O)	VCV	32 (28–39)	25 (23–30)†	25 (23–28)†	31 (24–33)†
	PCV-VG	39 (34–44)*	32 (29–35)*†	29 (25–33)*†	38 (30–43)*†
$ETCO_2$ (mmHg)	VCV	33 (31–34)	32 (30–33)	32 (30–35)	34 (31–35)
	PCV-VG	31 (30–33)	32 (31–34)	32 (30–34)	33 (31–35)
SaO_2 (%)	VCV	99 (98–100)	99 (98–99)	99 (98–100)	99 (99–100)
	PCV-VG	99 (98–100)	99 (98–100)	99 (98–100)	99 (99–100)

Ppeak peak inspiratory pressure, *Pmean* mean inspiratory pressure, *RR* respiratory rate, *Cdyn* dynamic compliance, *$ETCO_2$* end tidal CO_2, *VCV* volume-controlled ventilation, *PCV-VG* pressure-controlled ventilation with volume guaranteed
Data are listed as the median (interquartile range)
*$p < 0.05$ compared with the VCV group at the same time point
†$p < 0.05$ compared with 15 min after induction in each group

In thoracic surgery with one-lung ventilation, PCV-VG led to lower Ppeak, peak plateau pressure, and Pmean values compared with VCV [10, 11]. Similar results were obtained in a laparoscopic surgery study that showed lower Ppeak values with PCV-VG than with VCV [6, 9, 12].

Spine surgery is commonly performed with patients in the prone position. In respiratory physiology, Ppeak increases and Cdyn decreases as increased intra-thoracic pressure and abdominal pressure compromise diaphragm movement when a patient is turned to the prone position [3, 4, 13, 14]. To our knowledge, no previous study has compared VCV and PCV-VG in the prone position. However, several studies have compared PCV and VCV for patients undergoing posterior lumbar surgery and found that PCV is associated with lower Ppeak values compared with VCV [13, 14].

Pmean correlates with alveolar ventilation and improved oxygenation [15]. Although the values for patients in the prone position were higher than for patients in the supine position in both groups, placement in the prone position

Table 3 Hemodynamic variables

	Group	15 min after induction	15 min after positioning	30 min after positioning	Supine at the end
MAP (mmHg)	VCV	89 (80–100)	86 (77–98)	82 (75–90)	106 (88–109)
	PCV-VG	92 (71–102)	83 (72–93)	82 (73–94)	91 (80–98)
HR (beats/min)	VCV	78 (65–82)	68 (56–71)†	66 (61–69)†	71 (65–89)
	PCV-VG	70 (63–73)	63 (58–69)†	61 (56–67)†	73 (63–93)†
CO (L/min)	VCV	4.7 (3.8–5.7)	4.0 (3.2–4.7)†	4.1 (3.2–4.8)	5.4 (3.7–7.3)
	PCV-VG	4.2 (3.7–4.4)	3.6 (3.3–4.0)†	3.7 (3.3–4.2)	4.6 (4.0–5.7)†
CI ($L/min/m^2$)	VCV	2.8 (2.2–3.1)	2.3 (1.9–2.7)†	2.4 (1.7–2.9)	3.2 (2.4–3.3)
	PCV-VG	2.4 (2.2–2.6)	2.3 (1.8–2.4)†	2.2 (1.9–2.6)	2.8 (2.4–3.3)†
SV (mL/beat)	VCV	63 (54–75)	56 (46–74)	57 (47–71)	67 (56–84)
	PCV-VG	57 (55–65)	59 (51–66)	59 (53–65)	66 (54–78)
SVI ($mL/m^2/beat$)	VCV	37 (32–41)	33 (29–39)	34 (26–40)	38 (32–51)
	PCV-VG	34 (32–39)	34 (31–40)	36 (32–40)	39 (32–44)
SVV (%)	VCV	11 (9–14)	12 (10–16)	11 (9–17)	10 (6–13)
	PCV-VG	12 (8–14)	13 (10–15)	13 (10–15)	9 (8–15)

MAP mean arterial pressure, *HR* heart rate, *CO* cardiac output, *CI* cardiac index, *SV* stroke volume, *SVI* stroke volume index, *SVV* stroke volume variation, *VCV* volume controlled ventilation, *PCV-VG*, pressure controlled ventilation with volume guaranteed
Data are listed as the median (interquartile range)
†$p < 0.05$ compared with 15 min after induction in each group

Table 4 Arterial blood gas analyses

	Group	15 min after induction	15 min after positioning	30 min after positioning	Supine at the end
pH	VCV	7.44 (7.42–7.45)	7.44 (7.41–7.47)	7.44 (7.42–7.46)	7.42 (7.38–7.45)
	PCV-VG	7.43 (7.41–7.48)	7.43 (7.42–7.45)	7.42 (7.40–7.47)	7.41 (7.39–7.45)
PaO_2 (mmHg)	VCV	242 (209–285)	252 (237–271)	258 (234–272)	216 (192–255)
	PCV-VG	209 (177–248)	234 (215–260)	233 (218–259)	230 (215–262)
$PaCO_2$ (mmHg)	VCV	32 (30–34)	31 (30–33)	31 (30–33)	34 (31–36)
	PCV-VG	34 (31–35)	33 (31–35)	34 (31–35)	35 (32–38)
SaO_2 (%)	VCV	99.9 (99.8–99.9)	99.9 (99.8–99.9)	99.9 (99.8–99.9)	99.8 (99.7–99.9)
	PCV-VG	99.8 (99.6–99.9)	99.9 (99.8–99.9)	99.8 (99.8–99.9)	99.8 (99.8–99.9)

PaO_2 partial arterial oxygen tension, *$PaCO_2$* partial arterial carbon dioxide tension, *VCV* volume-controlled ventilation, *PCV-VG* pressure-controlled ventilation with volume guaranteed
Data are listed as the median (interquartile range)

did not significantly improve oxygenation. One previous study found similar results; the authors attributed them to a lack of positive end-expiratory pressure [14].

It is known that the CI decreases when a patient moves in the prone position. This is caused by reduced venous return and increased intra-thoracic pressure, which results in decreased arterial filling and reduced ventricular compliance [1]. Dharmavaram et al. [16] compared the effects of prone positioners on hemodynamic values using transesophageal echocardiography (TEE). They found that decreases in CI in the prone position resulted from a decreased SV. This effect seemed to be caused by increased afterload rather than decreased preload because the left ventricle end-diastolic area was not significantly altered. Blood flow through the mitral valve was reduced on TEE, suggesting that reduced chest wall compliance diminished diastolic function and increased afterload. The Jackson table had less effect on cardiac function than the Wilson frame.

In the present study, the CO and CI values measured 15 min after placement in the prone position were lower compared with the same values measured in the supine position. The SV values did not significantly change as patients were positioned on the Jackson table, so it is thought that the decreased CO and CI in the prone position may have been caused by a decreased HR, rather than decreased preload or increased afterload.

It can be expected that differences in Ppeak between VCV and PCV-VG will affect pleural pressure, inducing changes in the cardiovascular response [17]. However, we noted no significant hemodynamic change between VCV and PCV-VG. An animal study comparing the effects of VCV and PCV on anesthetized dogs showed that hemodynamic functions such as CO, CI, and SVI did not differ significantly between VCV and PCV, although the Ppeak was higher in VCV than in PCV [18]. Balick-Weber et al. [19] used TEE to compare the effects of VCV and PCV on cardiac function and found that there was no echocardiographic change in right ventricular SV, left ventricular preload, or left ventricle end-systolic wall stress. They concluded that Ppeak was not associated with cardiac function and that the main determinant of right ventricle afterload was transpulmonary pressure rather than Ppeak.

The present study has several limitations. First, although the FloTrac®/Vigileo system is widely used in anesthesia, it is an uncalibrated pulse contour analysis and may be less accurate under conditions such as sepsis or reduced systemic vascular resistance [20]. Grensemann et al. [21] reported that the FloTrac®/Vigileo system had a clinically unacceptable high degree of error in the prone position compared with transpulmonary thermodilution techniques and calibrated pulse contour CO analysis. We believed that the transpulmonary thermodilution technique using a pulmonary catheter would be more invasive than pulse contour analysis. As a calibrated pulse contour analysis device was not available in our center, we used an uncalibrated pulse contour analysis device as a less invasive means of measuring hemodynamic variables. Since patients in the previous study were mechanically ventilated with acute respiratory distress syndrome or acute lung injury and expected to be in a septic condition or undergoing vasopressor treatment, the effect of placement in the prone position on uncalibrated CO analysis in healthy volunteers warrants further evaluation. Second, patients with compromised cardiac or pulmonary diseases, as well as those with morbid obesity, were excluded from the study. Respiratory mechanics or hemodynamics may be affected by various lung conditions and we wanted to standardize lung function among the patients. Although there were statistically significant differences between VCV and PCV-VG for Ppeak and Cdyn, these differences were quite small and may have been more prominent for patients with pulmonary disease or morbid obesity. Additional studies are therefore needed to compare the hemodynamic and respiratory effects of VCV and PCV-VG in patients with uncompensated cardiac and pulmonary function or morbid obesity. Third, we measured Cdyn rather than static lung compliance. Static lung compliance does not depend on inspiratory flow and is influenced by the elastic properties of the lung [22]. However, the inspiratory hold maneuver was not available in the ventilator we used, and there may have been detrimental effects on oxygenation while disconnecting the circuit to measure the plateau pressure.

Conclusion

In conclusion, PCV-VG provided a lower Ppeak and improved Cdyn compared with VCV, and was not associated with significant differences in CO, CI, SV, SVV, and oxygenation. These results show that PCV-VG may be an effective alternative mode of mechanical ventilation for patients in the prone position during lumbar spine surgery. Additional studies are required to evaluate the effects of Ppeak on postoperative patient outcome.

Abbreviations

Cdyn: Dynamic lung compliance; CI: Cardiac index; CO: Cardiac output; $ETCO_2$: End tidal carbon dioxide; PaO_2: Arterial oxygen partial pressure; PCV: Pressure-controlled ventilation; PCV-VG: Pressure-controlled ventilation with volume guaranteed mode; Pmean: Mean inspiratory pressure; Ppeak: Peak inspiratory pressure; RR: Respiratory rate; SV: Stroke volume; SVI: Stroke volume index; SVV: Stroke volume variation; VCV: Volume-controlled ventilation mode

Acknowledgments

Not applicable.

Authors' contributions

LJM participated in the study design, and data analysis, and drafted the manuscript. LSK and KKM performed the study and collected data. KYJ participated in patient recruitment and data collection. PEY participated in the study design and drafted the manuscript. All authors have read and approved the final manuscript.

References

1. Edgcombe H, Carter K, Yarrow S. Anaesthesia in the prone position. Br J Anaesth. 2008;100:165–83.
2. Chui J, Craen RA. An update on the prone position: continuing professional development. Can J Anaesth. 2016;63:737–67.
3. Palmon SC, Kirsch JR, Depper JA, Toung TJ. The effect of the prone position on pulmonary mechanics is frame-dependent. Anesth Analg. 1998;87:1175–80.
4. Şenay H, Sıvacı R, Kokulu S, Koca B, Bakı ED, Ela Y. The effect of pressure-controlled ventilation and volume-controlled ventilation in prone position on pulmonary mechanics and inflammatory markers. Inflammation. 2016;39: 1469–74.
5. Keszler M. Volume-targeted ventilation. Early Hum Dev. 2006;82:811–8.
6. Dion JM, McKee C, Tobias JD, Sohner P, Herz D, Teich S, et al. Ventilation during laparoscopic-assisted bariatric surgery: volume-controlled, pressure-controlled or volume-guaranteed pressure-regulated modes. Int J Clin Exp Med. 2014;7:2242–7.
7. Schulz KF, Altman DG, Moher D, group C. CONSORT 2010 statement: updated guidelines for reporting parallel group randomized trials. Ann Intern Med. 2010;152:726–32.
8. Ball L, Dameri M, Pelosi P. Modes of mechanical ventilation for the operating room. Best Pract Res Clin Anaesthesiol. 2015;29:285–99.
9. Kothari A, Baskaran D. Pressure-controlled volume guaranteed mode improves respiratory dynamics during laparoscopic cholecystectomy: a comparison with conventional modes. Anesth Essasys Res. 2018;12:206–12.
10. Pu J, Liu Z, Yang L, Wang Y, Jiang J. Applications of pressure control ventilation volume guaranteed during one-lung ventilation in thoracic surgery. Int J Clin Exp Med. 2014;7:1094–8.
11. Song SY, Jung JY, Cho MS, Kim JH, Ryu TH, Kim BI. Volume-controlled versus pressure-controlled ventilation-volume guaranteed mode during one-lung ventilation. Korean J Anesthesiol. 2014;67:258–63.
12. Assad OM, El Sayed AA, Khalil MA. Comparison of volume-controlled ventilation and pressure-controlled ventilation volume guaranteed during laparoscopic surgery in Trendelenburg position. J Clin Anesth. 2016;34:55–61.
13. Kang WS, Oh CS, Kwon WK, Rhee KY, Lee YG, Kim TH, et al. Effect of mechanical ventilation mode type on intra- and postoperative blood loss in patients undergoing posterior lumbar interbody fusion surgery: a randomized controlled trial. Anesthesiology. 2016;125:115–23.
14. Jo YY, Kim JY, Kwak YL, Kim YB, Kwak HJ. The effect of pressure-controlled ventilation on pulmonary mechanics in the prone position during posterior lumbar spine surgery: a comparison with volume-controlled ventilation. J Neurosurg Anesthesiol. 2012;24:14–8.
15. Marini JJ, Ravenscraft SA. Mean airway pressure: physiologic determinants and clinical importance-part 1: physiologic determinants and measurements. Crit Care Med. 1992;20:1461–72.
16. Dharmavaram S, Jellish WS, Nockels RP, Shea J, Mehmood R, Ghanayem A, et al. Effect of prone positioning systems on hemodynamic and cardiac function during lumbar spine surgery: an echocardiographic study. Spine. 2006;31:1388–93.
17. Pinsky MR. Recent advances in the clinical application of heart-lung interactions. Curr Opin Crit Care. 2002;8:26–31.
18. Fantoni DT, Ida KK, Lopes TF, Otsuki DA, Auler JO Jr, Ambrósio AM. A comparison of the cardiopulmonary effects of pressure controlled ventilation and volume controlled ventilation in healthy anesthetized dogs. J Vet Emerg Crit Care. 2016;26:524–30.
19. Balick-Weber CC, Nicolas P, Hedreville-Montout M, Blanchet P, Stéphan F. Respiratory and haeomdynamic effects of volume-controlled vs pressure-controlled ventilation during laparoscopy: a cross-over study with echocardiographic assessment. Br J Anaesth. 2007;99:429–35.
20. Argueta E, Berdine G, Pena C, Nugent KM. FloTrac® monitoring system: what are its uses in critically ill medical patients? Am J Med Sci. 2015;349:352–6.
21. Grensemann J, Bruecken U, Treszl A, Wappler F, Sakka SG. The influence of prone positioning on the accuracy of calibrated and uncalibrated pulse contour derived cardiac index measurements. Anesth Analg. 2013;116:820–6.
22. Manna EM, Ibraheim OA, Samarkandi AH, Alotaibi WM, Elwatidy SM. The effect of prone position on respiratory mechanics during spinal surgery. Middle East J Anaesthesiol. 2005;18:623–30.

20

Transversus abdominis plane block with general anesthesia blunts the perioperative stress response in patients undergoing radical gastrectomy

Ruizhu Liu[1], Haiyan Qin[2], Meng Wang[3], Kai Li[1*] and Guoqing Zhao[1*]

Abstract

Background: Surgical stress induces the release of neuroendocrine mediators and cytokines during perioperative period, which may have adverse effects on cancer patients. While the surgical stress responsse can be affected by anesthetic technique. Therefore, we designed this study to assess whether subcostal transversus abdominis plane (TAP) block can affect perioperative neuroendocrine stress response, postoperative analgesia and postoperative recovery in patients undergoing radical gastrectomy under general anesthesia.

Methods: Sixty-five patients were recruited. Patients randomly received general anesthesia (control group), or general anesthesia combined with TAP block (40 mL of 0.375% ropivacaine) (TAP group). The primary outcome was neuroendocrine levels including norepinephrine (NE), epinephrine (E), cortisol (Cor), glucose (Glu), interleukin (IL)-6 and IL-10 during 48 h after surgery. Secondary outcomes included pain score, hemodynamic variables and recovery characteristics.

Results: Data from 61 of 65 patients were analyzed. The levels of NE, E, Cor, and Glu were blunt by TAP block during perioperative period. The levels of IL-6 and IL-10 were significantly lower in TAP group than in control group. TAP block efficiently relieved postoperative acute pain up to 12 h postoperatively with more stable perioperative hemodynamics compared with control group.

Conclusions: Subcostal TAP block blunts perioperative stress response and provides efficient analgesia, with good hemodynamic stability and minimal adverse effects.

Keywords: Gastric cancer, Nerve block, Analgesia, Stress

Background

Gastric cancer is one of the most commonly diagnosed cancers around the world. Surgical resection is currently the mainstay of curative treatment for this cancer, which is recommended to maximize the probability of complete tumor clearance, reduce loco-regional recurrence, and improve long-term survival [1]. Transabdominal radical gastrectomy is an effective therapeutic strategy for malignant gastric disease. However, open gastrectomy causes severe pain in the incision of abdominal wall. Surgical trauma accompanied with considerable surgical pain is a key variable affecting the surgical stress response and prognosis [2]. The responses of patients towards surgical pain may result in unstable hemodynamics, and this excessive stress action is adverse for postoperative rehabilitation and long-term prognosis for patients with malignant tumor [3]. Thus, effective modulation of stress response may reduce the incidence of complications [4, 5].

Transversus abdominis plane (TAP) block, as an emerging regional anesthetic technique, can provide efficient analgesia by blocking the regulation of sensory nerve at the anterior abdominal wall [6], which can reduce opioid consumption, and lessen opioid-related side effects [7–9]. TAP block is given before the occurrence of noxious

* Correspondence: likai82@126.com; zhaogq65@126.com
[1]Department of Anesthesiology, China-Japan Union Hospital of Jilin University, No. 126 Xiantai Road, Changchun 130000, Jilin Province, China

stimulation, which could relieve the postoperative pain by alleviating the pain of peripheral and central sensitization [10]. Recently, analgesic effect of TAP block has been widely studied, but the study associated with its efficiency on stress response that compared with general anesthesia is limited.

Subcostal, mid-axillary and lumbar triangle of Petit approaches are widely used in TAP block [11]. The bi-subcostal approach is associated with wide block area of spread (T7-L1) [12, 13], and could provide a satisfactory analgesic plane for transabdominal gastrectomy. The current study was aimed to investigate the effects of subcostal TAP block on stress response and analgesic effect in patients undergoing open radial gastrectomy under general anesthesia.

Methods

Patients and grouping

Our study was approved by the Ethics Committee of China-Japan Union Hospital of Jilin University (2016ks008) and was in accordance with good clinical practice and the guiding principles of the Helsinki Declaration. The written informed consents were obtained from all patients. The trial was registered prior to patient enrollment at clinicaltrials.gov (NCT03035916, principal investigator: Guoqing Zhao, Ruizhu Liu, Kai Li, date of registration: 01/27/2017).

Patients meeting the following inclusion criteria were enrolled: patients who were scheduled for open radical gastrectomy; patients who had no contraindication to local anesthetic, and patients whose American Society of Anesthesiologists' (ASA) physical status I, II or III. Emergency patients and patients with preoperative infection, or patients with a history of immune disease, endocrine system disease, blood transfusion, or chemotherapy were excluded from this study.

Patients were randomly divided into two groups by a computerized random-number generator with 1:1 ratio for TAP group and control group. The pre-anesthetic interview was carried out by a single investigator to assess the eligibility of participants and to record the baseline data. Another anesthesiologist (not involved in study) who took the corresponding opaque envelope in the operating room performed the block and anesthesia induction, so he was unblinded to group allocation. A resident anesthetist who was blinded to randomization was responsible for collection of intraoperative data and blood. Postoperative data and blood were collected by another investigator who visited the participants at 1, 6, 12, 24, 48 h after surgery. All patients underwent surgery from the same operative team. The patients allocated to respective groups were administered as follows: TAP group: general anesthesia and ultrasonography-guided TAP block with 40 ml of 0.375% ropivacaine; Control group: standard general anesthesia (no sham intervention for TAP block).

Operation process

No preoperative sedatives or analgesics were administered before the operation. Routine monitoring including electrocardiogram, invasive arterial blood pressure, pulse oximetry, and end-tidal carbon dioxide was established before anesthetic induction. All patients underwent standard general anesthesia induced by midazolam 0.02 mg/kg (Enhua Pharmaceutical Co., Ltd., Jiangsu, China), propofol 2.0–2.5 mg/kg (Fresenius Kabi Deutschland, Germany), sufentanil 0.3 μg/kg (Yichang Humanwell Pharmaceutical Co., Ltd., Yichang, China), and cis-Atracurium 0.15 mg/kg (Hengrui Pharmaceutical Co., Ltd., Jiangsu, China). In order to maintain general anesthesia, intravenous and inhaled volatile anaesthetics of nitrous oxide, sevoflurane (Maruishi Pharmaceutical Co., Ltd., Japan), sufentanil, and cis-Atracurium were used. During the operation, the MAC value was maintained within 1.2–1.5% by regulating the inhalation concentration of nitrous oxide and sevoflurane. Tidal volume and rate were adjusted to maintain an end-tidal PCO2 of 30–40 mmHg. When hemodynamic values increased more than 15% above pre-induction baseline values, an appropriate dose (0–10 μg) of sufentanil was used to intervene. Heart rate (HR) < 40 beats/min (bradycardia) was intervened with 0.5 mg atropine, and mean arterial blood pressure (MAP) < 60 mmHg (hypotension) was treated with 5 mg ephedrine. The body temperature was maintained between 36 °C and 37 °C during the operation.

TAP block was administered after anesthesia induction. In the TAP group, TAP block was performed bilaterally under ultrasound (SonoSite Portable M-Turbo, Sonosite Inc., Bothwell, UT, USA) guidance at 30 min before the surgical incision. The probe was placed in the midline of abdomen below the xiphoid and moved right laterally along the subcostal margin to the anterior axillary line. After the probe identified the plane between the rectus and transverse abdominal muscles, a 100-mm, 20-G Stimuplex block needle was guided within the plane to the point just inferior to the right costal margin such that the tip laid between the obliquus internus abdominis and transversus abdominis within the neurovascular fascial plane. After aspiration, to exclude vascular puncture, 1 mL test dose was injected to determine the flow resistance and confirm needle tip placement within the fascial plane. Then, 10 mL 0.375% ropivacaine was multi-point injected in this plane laterally along the subcostal margin. The probe was moved back to the anterior axillary line, and another 10 mL 0.375% ropivacaine was injected through the needle inferior to the costal margin within the TAP using an identical technique, making this two injected drug a continuous plane under the costal margin, from the medial margin of the rectus abdominis muscle to anterior axillary line. The left side of TAP block was conducted with the identical technique.

After extubation, patients were transferred to the post-anesthesia care unit (PACU), and all of them received morphine patient-controlled analgesia (PCA) with a standard dosing regimen: 2 mL/h continuous infusion (a bolus of 1 mL with a lock-time of 15 min) by using the electronics pump (Shanghai Bochuang, China).

Postoperative detection

The primary outcome was neuroendocrine mediators and cytokines at different time points of 48 h after operation. Venous blood samples were collected before anesthesia (baseline), immediately after surgery, and at 6, 24, and 48 h after surgery, and stored in pre-chilled tubes on ice and then centrifuged within 90 min. The separated plasma was stored at − 80 °C. Glucose (Glu) level was measured immediately after venous blood was collected using glucometer (ACCU- CHEK Active, Inc.). Plasma levels of norepinephrine (NE), epinephrine (E), C-reactive protein (CRP), cortisol (Cor), interleukin (IL)-6, and IL-10 were measured by micro enzyme-linked immunosorbent assays kits (R&D system, Inc.,USA).

The second outcomes included pain scores, hemodynamic variables and recovery characteristics during the first 2 postoperative days. Pain scores included VAS scores at rest and during movement (cough or rotating the body) in the first 2 postoperative days. The MAP and HR were continuously measured and recorded before anesthesia, during induction, tracheal intubation, incision, immediately after tracheal extubation, as well as at 6, 24, and 48 h postoperatively. The other recorded observations included additional sufentanil consumption, postoperative opioid requirement, and recovery profiles (duration of PACU, side effects such as nausea, sedation, and vomiting, time of first flatus, and hospital stays). Sedation was assessed by Ramsay score (2–4: satisfactory sedation, > 4: excessive sedation). Additionally, discontinuing PACU was determined by a standard score test (= 10: PACU should be discontinued). The study processes are shown in Additional file 1: Figure S1.

The minimum detectable difference of plasma cortisol concentration was estimated immediately after surgery between two groups. The mean and SD values of plasma cortisol were as follows: MTAP = 410 nmol/L, MControl = 521 nmol/L, STAP = 142 nmol/L, and SControl = 16.4 nmol/L. Based on sample size analysis performed using PASS 11.0 (NCSS Statistical Software, Kaysville, UT), with $\alpha = 0.05$ and $\beta = 0.2$, a minimum sample of 25 cases in each group was required, respectively.

Statistical analysis

Statistical analyses were performed using SPSS 18.0 (Chicago, IL, USA). The normal distribution of data was evaluated using Shapiro-Wilk test. Data were expressed as mean (± SD) or percentages of the total number of patients (%). Comparisons of NE, E, Cor, Glu, cytokines, hemodynamic data, and VAS scores between groups were performed by repeated-measures analysis of variance. The differences for opioid consumption, time to first flatus, and time in PACU were analyzed using Student's t test followed by 2-tailed Dunnett test. Categorical data were analyzed by using χ^2 or Fisher exact test. *P* value < 0.05 was considered significant.

Results

Total 65 patients were enrolled from February 2017 to August 2017. According to the exclusion criteria, 4 patients were excluded, and data from 61 patients (30 in TAP group, 31 in control group) were finally analyzed. Baseline characteristics showed no significant difference between two groups (Table 1).

There were no significant differences for NE, E, and Cor values on baseline. Compared with control group, the NE and E values were significantly lower in the TAP group at 6 h ($P_{NE} = 0.001$, $P_E = 0.010$), 24 h ($P_{NE} = 0.022$, $P_E < 0.001$) and 48 h postoperatively ($P_{NE} = 0.001$, $P_E < 0.001$) (Fig. 1a, b). The Cor levels were significantly higher in the control group than in TAP at all time points postoperatively (Fig. 1c). Additionally, the levels of NE, E, and Cor were more stable in TAP group compared with that in control group. Moreover, in TAP group, levels of the three hormones returned to baseline values by 24 h, whereas in the control group these parameters were significantly higher than the baseline values (Fig. 1). Glu levels did not differ between the two groups at baseline, but their levels were higher in the control group than in TAP group immediately after surgery, and at 6 h and 24 h postoperatively ($P < 0.001$) (Fig. 1d).

Plasma levels of IL-6 and IL-10 were not different at baseline. In the control group, IL-6 and IL-10 continued to increase even at 48 h postoperatively, whereas in TAP

Table 1 Demographic and perioperative characteristics by study group

Parameters	Control group (*n* = 31)	TAP group (*n* = 30)	*P*-value
Age (yr)	60.20 ± 8.93	58.95 ± 8.24	0.31
Gender (M/F)	23/8	21/9	0.75
Weight (kg)	65.90 ± 8.63	67.33 ± 11.62	0.42
Height (cm)	165.40 ± 12.10	168.90 ± 12.37	0.49
ASA physical status (I/II/III)	4/20/7	5/19/6	0.56
Duration of anesthesia (min)	235.25 ± 42.14	238.50 ± 43.66	0.79
Duration of surgery (min)	207.00 ± 34.01	195.83 ± 34.76	0.18

Values are mean ± SD or number
ASA American Society of Anesthesiologists

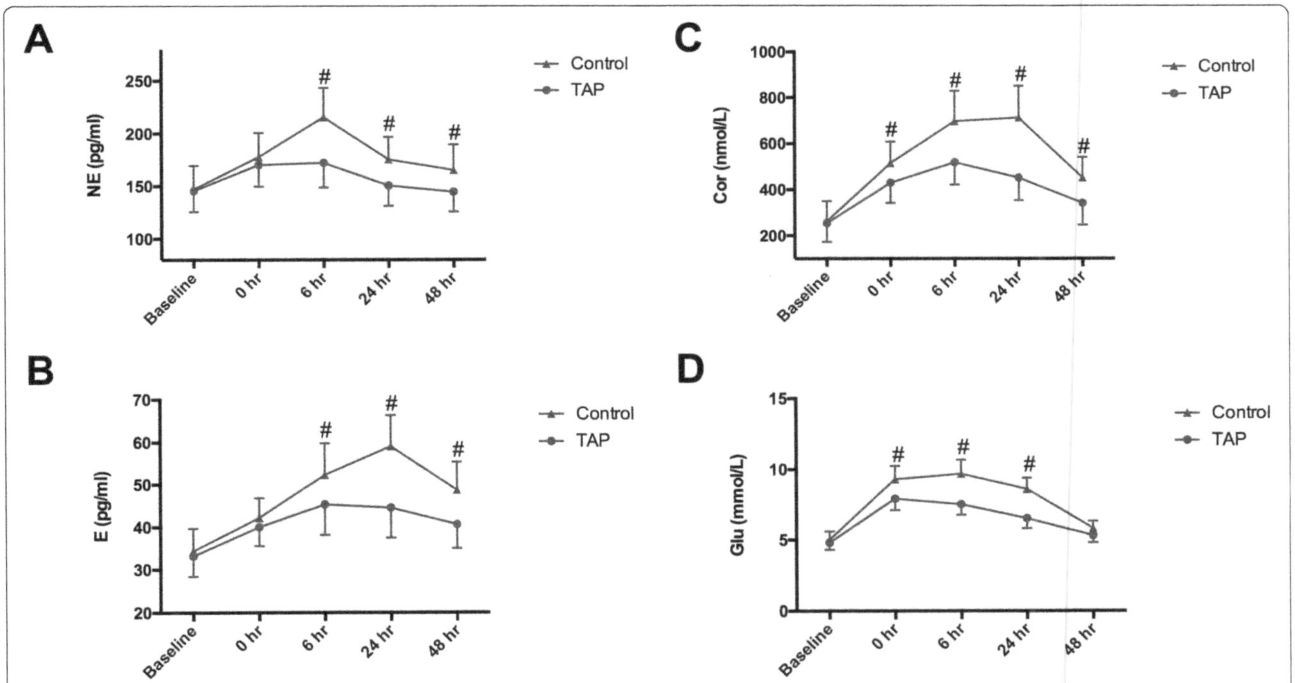

Fig. 1 Plasma concentration of norepinephrine (NE) (**a**), epinephrine (E) (**b**), cortisol (Cor) (**c**), and glucose (Glu) (**d**). TAP: transversus abdominis plane. Time interval is defined as time between baseline and postoperative time. Data are expressed as mean ± SD. #: $P < 0.05$ compared with TAP group; *: $P < 0.05$ compared with baseline

groups they peaked at 24 h postoperatively and then decreased (Fig. 2a, b). The IL-6 level was significantly lower in TAP group compared with in control group at 6 h ($P = 0.0040$), 24 h ($P < 0.0001$), and 48 h postoperatively ($P < 0.001$) (Fig. 2a). The IL-10 level was higher in the control group than in TAP group at 48 h postoperatively ($P < 0.001$) (Fig. 2b). Ratio of IL-6/IL-10 markedly greater in control group than in TAP group at postoperative 6 h, 24 h, and 48 h (all P < 0.001) (Fig. 2c).

Pain scores for different time points are presented in Table 2. TAP group showed lower VAS scores at postoperative 1 h, 6 h, and 12 h whether the patients at rest or on movement. Whereas, no significant difference of VAS scores was found between TAP and control groups at postoperative 24 h and 48 h at rest. Hemodynamic data are shown in Fig. 3. In the control group, HR and MAP were higher at the incision time point relative to baseline and the TAP group ($P_{HR} = 0.003$, $P_{HR} = 0.001$; $P_{MAP} = 0.002$, $P_{MAP} = 0.001$). In TAP group, HR and MAP showed no significant difference relative to baseline except for induction and intubation time point.

Consumption of intraoperative sufentanil and postoperative morphine in TAP was significantly less compared with that in the control group (all $P < 0.001$) (Table 3). In control group 16 patients experienced sedation while in TAP group eight cases experienced. Additionally, patients in control group showed longer PACU stays, and hospital stays compared with TAP group. For time to first flatus, nausea, and vomit, no significant difference was identified between the two groups (Table 3).

Discussion

In this prospective, randomized trial, we found that the levels of NE, E, Cor, and Glu were blunt by TAP block during the perioperative period. Additionally, the levels of IL-6 and IL-10 were lower in TAP group significantly. Moreover, TAP block could efficiently relieve postoperative acute pain up to 12 h postoperatively with more stable perioperative hemodynamics compared with control group. Thus, TAP block can be used as an adjunct to general anesthesia to suppress stress responses and control pain in open radical gastrectomy surgery.

Perioperative stress response could be accurately indicated by changes of neuroendocrine mediators and cytokines via direct activation of the somatic and sympathetic nervous systems. It is well known that epidural block could block the sympathetic response and efficiently block the plasma levels of cortisol and relevant cytokines in patients [14–16]. TAP block is another method of pre-analgesic techniques. The anterior branches of spinal nerves T7-L1, running through the transversus abdominis plane, dominate the sensation of skin, muscle and parietal peritoneum [6, 17], which could be interdicted by wide-range TAP block. Subcostal TAP blocks afferent neural input and reduces central sensitization, which is consistent with the fact that local anesthetics inhibit both non-nociceptive and

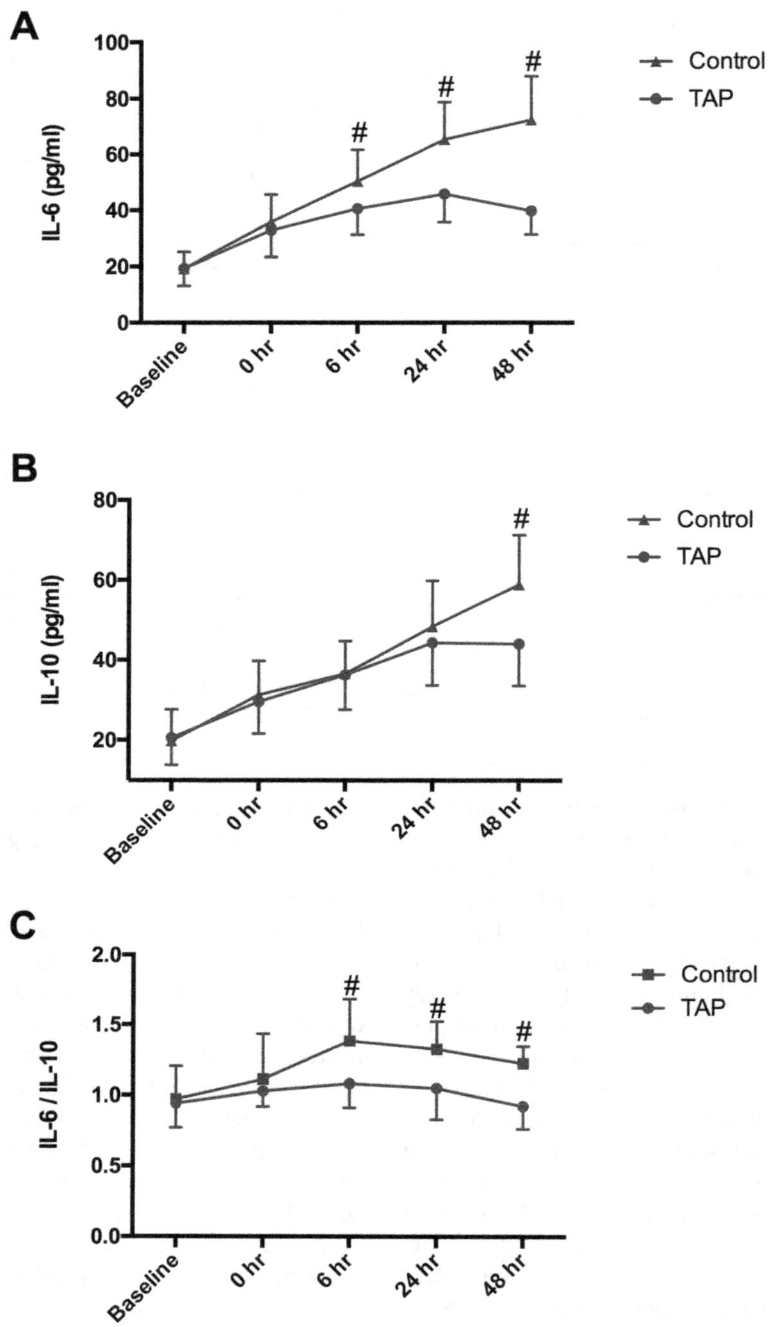

Fig. 2 Serum concentration of interleukin (IL)-6 (**a**), IL-10 (**b**), and ratio of IL-6/IL-10 (**c**). TAP: transversus abdominis plane. Time interval is defined as time between baseline and postoperative time. Data are expressed as mean ± SD. #: P < 0.05 compared with TAP group; *: $P < 0.05$ compared with baseline

nociceptive stimuli. It has been reported that reported that there is a more stable level of cortisol in patients undergoing laparoscopic hysterectomy combined with TAP block than without TAP block [18]. Moreover, a case report indicated that TAP block efficiently ameliorated the stress response of a six-year-old boy who suffered from Wolf-Hirschhorn syndrome [19]. Mohamed et al. [20] reported that TAP block was effective to decrease blood glucose level in children. In this study, TAP block reduced the levels of NE, E, Cor, and glucose significantly.

Surgical trauma and perioperative pain initiate neuroendocrine response, and stimulate the release of cytokines.

Table 2 Visual Analog Scale Pain scores by study group

	TAP group *n* = 30	Control group *N* = 31	*P*-value
At rest			
1 h	2.2 ± 0.9	2.9 ± 0.9	0.017
6 h	2.2 ± 1.0	2.9 ± 1.0	0.045
12 h	2.1 ± 0.9	2.7 ± 1.2	0.008
24 h	2.2 ± 1.0	2.7 ± 1.0	0.175
48 h	1.0 ± 0.8	1.2 ± 0.8	0.417
On movement			
1 h	2.7 ± 1.2	4.3 ± 0.8	< 0.001
6 h	2.9 ± 0.7	4.2 ± 0.7	< 0.001
12 h	3.3 ± 0.5	4.3 ± 1.0	0.001
24 h	4.1 ± 0.6	4.6 ± 0.8	0.016
48 h	4.2 ± 0.8	4.5 ± 0.9	0.008

Data are presented as mean ± SD

The pro- and anti-inflammatory cytokines are crucial for acute-phase immune response after surgery. Wind et al. [21] have showed that the concentration of circulating tumor cells is the highest after the onset of surgery. Thus, the stability of immune function is essential for patients with malignant disease. IL-6, as a pro-inflammatory cytokine, induces the synthesis of CRP and other acute phase proteins within adult stem cells. Plasma level of IL-6 is reportedly related to the severity of surgical trauma [22] and closely associated with immune status. In contrast, IL-10 is involved in immunomodulation and acts as an anti-inflammatory cytokine, which could cause systemic suppression of antitumor immunity [23]. Over the past years, the anti-inflammatory effects of local anesthetic have been extensively studied [24]. The regional anesthetic technique has been reported to reduce the cytokines and attenuate perioperative immunosuppression [25, 26]. Importantly, some retrospective studies have showed that local anesthetic had a potential benefit in patients undergoing cancer surgery [27, 28]. In our study, TAP block significantly inhibited the release of IL-6 and IL-10, whereas the levels of IL-6 and IL-10 continued increasing in the control group. Additionally, study has reported that IL-6/IL-10 is potentially related to an inflammatory poor prognosis [29]. Our results showed that the ratio (IL-6/IL-10) in control group was greater than that in TAP group during

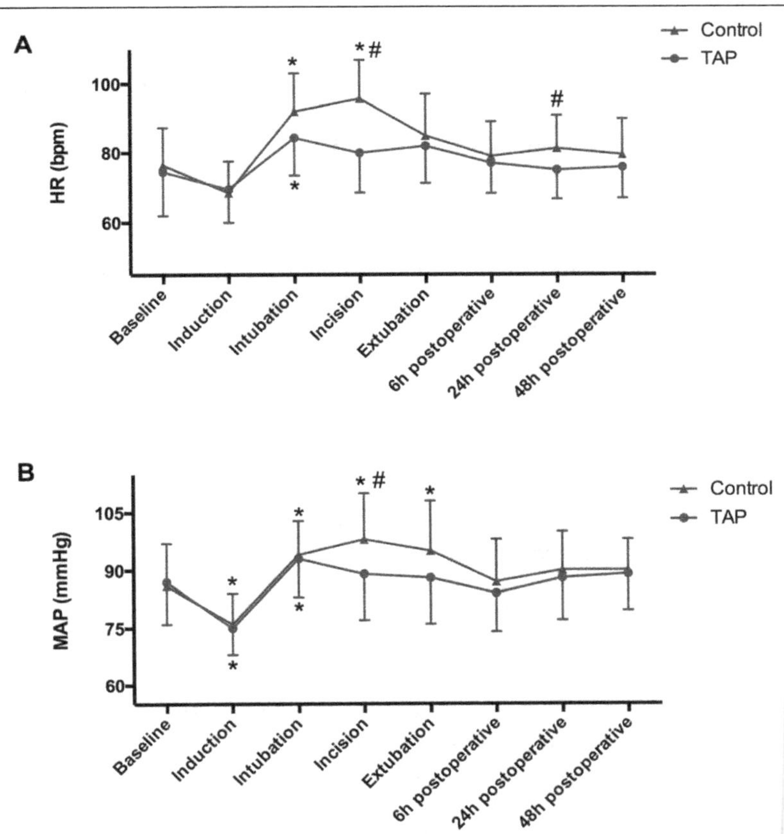

Fig. 3 Hemocynamic changes during operation and 2 days postoperatively. **a** heart rate (HR); **b** mean arterial blood pressure (MAP). TAP: transversus abdominis plane. Data are expressed as mean ± SD. #: $P < 0.05$ compared with TAP group; *$P < 0.05$ compared with baseline

Table 3 Doses of sufentanil, ephedrine, and nicardipine and recovery time

	Group TAP $n = 30$	Group Control $N = 31$	P-value
Opium consumption			
Intraoperative superaddition of sufentanil (μg)	4.3 ± 1.5	10.2 ± 2.8	< 0.001
Postoperative morphine consumption (mg)	46.6 ± 8.4	66.8 ± 10.9	< 0.001
Patients requiring ephedrine, n (%)	2, (6.7%)	1, (3.2%)	0.976
Time to first flatus (h)	77.6 ± 10.4	81.6 ± 10.4	0.131
PACU stay, (min)	44.2 ± 7.9	54.5 ± 8.2	< 0.001
Incidence of opium-related side effects, n(%)			
Sedation	8, (26.7%)	16, (51.6%)	0.046
Nausea	5, (16.7%)	6, (19.4%)	0.785
Vomiting	0, (0%)	1, (3.2%)	0.987
Long hospitalization, n(%)	5, (16.7%)	13, (41.9%)	0.031

Data are presented as mean ± SD or number;
Criteria for out of PACU: Aldrete scores ≥9;
Long hospitalization is defined as postoperative time ≥ 7 days

postoperative 48 h. Therefore, TAP block partially attenuated surgical trauma and maintained stable cytokine levels among patients who underwent open radical gastrectomy.

Efficient analgesia of TAP block has been well documented in human studies. Recent Meta-analyses have suggested that TAP block improves postoperative pain at both rest and movement up to 24 h postoperatively independent of the surgery types [30, 31]. In a prospective study, Niraj et al. [7] revealed that continuous TAP block could provide efficient analgesia for 8 to 72 h comparable to epidural block. In consistent with that study, our results showed that the analgesic efficacy of single-injection subcostal TAP block lasted for 12 to 16 h. Previous study reported that TAP block has more advantages for high-risk patients with cardiovascular systemic disease due to its better intraoperative hemodynamic stability [32]. Currently, the concept of the enhanced recovery after surgery has been widely addressed. Zafar et al. [33] reported that TAP block allowed an accelerated recovery before a 48 h scheduled removal of the epidural catheter. Joanne et al. [34] reported that using TAP block, a 23 h hospital stay became a realistic goal after laparoscopic colorectal resection. Similarly, our study revealed that the hospital stays significantly decreased in TAP group, which supported a trend towards decreasing hospital stay with regional blockade.

Limitations

There were some limitations in our study. First, we only enrolled patients who underwent elective open radical gastrectomy and met the inclusion criteria, which limited the external generalizability of our results. Second, we used sufentanil for analgesia, known to affect the neuroimmunoendocrine network, which may influence our results. Third, patients in control group were not given subcostal TAP block with placebo, thus our study may be an open randomized controlled trial. Fourth, different anesthetic and antalgic medications may have complex effects on the prognosis of patient, in terms of postoperative recuperation, cancer migration, invasion, and interference with immune system, but we did not evaluate the long-term clinical effects on these individuals. Therefore, our findings are preliminary and a more comprehensive trial that assesses the long-term functional outcomes is necessary.

Conclusions

In conclusion, subcostal TAP block could inhibit the undesirable stress response and provide efficient analgesia without increasing the adverse reactions for open radical gastrectomy. For patients with malignant tumor, the relationship between reduction in stress response and long-term clinical outcomes needs to be further studied.

Abbreviations
ASA: American Society of Anesthesiologists; Cor: Cortisol; E: Epinephrine; Glu: Glucose; HR: Heart rate; IL: Interleukin; NE: Norepinephrine; PACU: Post-anesthesia care unit; PCA: Patient-controlled analgesia; TAP: Transversus abdominis plane

Acknowledgements
None.

Authors' contributions
Conception and design of the research: RL Acquisition of data: HQ Analysis and interpretation of data: MW Statistical analysis: MW Obtaining funding: GZ Drafting the manuscript: RL Revision of manuscript for important intellectual content: KL, GZ. All authors have read and approved the manuscript.

Author details
[1]Department of Anesthesiology, China-Japan Union Hospital of Jilin University, No. 126 Xiantai Road, Changchun 130000, Jilin Province, China. [2]Department of Plastic Surgery, China-Japan Union Hospital of Jilin University, Changchun 130000, Jilin Province, China. [3]Department of Cardiology, No. 965 Hospital of PLA, Jilin 132000, Jilin Province, China.

References
1. Long AJ, Burton PR, De Veer MJ, Ooi GJ, Laurie CP, Nottle PD, Watt MJ, Brown WA. Radical gastric cancer surgery results in widespread upregulation of pro-tumourigenic intraperitoneal cytokines. ANZ J Surg. 2018;88(5):E370–6.
2. Desborough JP. The stress response to trauma and surgery. Br J Anaesth. 2000;85(1):109–17.
3. Li K, Li L, Gao M, Zhu Z, Chen P, Yang L, Zhao G. Application of ultrasound-guided subcostal transversus abdominis plane block in gastric cancer patients undergoing open gastrectomy. Int J Clin Exp Med. 2015;8(8):13976.
4. Brodner G, Van Aken H, Hertle L, Fobker M, Von Eckardstein A, Goeters C, Buerkle H, Harks A, Kehlet H. Multimodal perioperative management--combining thoracic epidural analgesia, forced mobilization, and oral nutrition--reduces hormonal and metabolic stress and improves convalescence after major urologic surgery. Anesth Analg. 2001;92(6):1594–600.
5. Holte K, Kehlet H. Epidural anaesthesia and analgesia - effects on surgical stress responses and implications for postoperative nutrition, Clinical nutrition (Edinburgh, Scotland). 2002;21(3):199–206.
6. Rafi AN. Abdominal field block: a new approach via the lumbar triangle. Anaesthesia. 2001;56(10):1024–6.
7. Niraj G, Kelkar A, Jeyapalan I, Graff-Baker P, Williams O, Darbar A, Maheshwaran A, Powell R. Comparison of analgesic efficacy of subcostal transversus abdominis plane blocks with epidural analgesia following upper abdominal surgery. Anaesthesia. 2011;66(6):465–71.
8. Tolchard S, Davies R, Martindale S. Efficacy of the subcostal transversus abdominis plane block in laparoscopic cholecystectomy: comparison with conventional port-site infiltration. J Anaesthesiol Clin Pharmacol. 2012;28(3):339–43.
9. Wu Y, Liu F, Tang H, Wang Q, Chen L, Wu H, Zhang X, Miao J, Zhu M, Hu C, et al. The analgesic efficacy of subcostal transversus abdominis plane block compared with thoracic epidural analgesia and intravenous opioid analgesia after radical gastrectomy. Anesth Analg. 2013;117(2):507–13.
10. Kissin I. Preemptive analgesia. Anesthesiology. 2000;93(4):1138–43.
11. Milan Z, Tabor D, McConnell P, Pickering J, Kocarev M, du Feu F, Barton S. Three different approaches to transversus abdominis planeblock: a cadaveric study. Med Glas. 2011;8(2):181–4.
12. Hebbard PD, Barrington MJ, Vasey C. Ultrasound-guided continuous oblique subcostal transversus abdominis plane blockade: description of anatomy and clinical technique. Reg Anesth Pain Med. 2010;35(5):436–41.
13. Lee TH, Barrington MJ, Tran TM, Wong D, Hebbard PD. Comparison of extent of sensory block following posterior and subcostal approaches to ultrasound-guided transversus abdominis plane block. Anaesth Intensive Care. 2010;38(3):452–60.
14. Aono H, Takeda A, Tarver SD, Goto H. Stress responses in three different anesthetic techniques for carbon dioxide laparoscopic cholecystectomy. J Clin Anesth. 1998;10(7):546–50.
15. Li Y, Wang B, Zhang LL, He SF, Hu XW, Wong GT, Zhang Y. Dexmedetomidine combined with general anesthesia provides similar intraoperative stress response reduction when compared with a combined general and epidural anesthetic technique. Anesth Analg. 2016;122(4):1202–10.
16. Li Y, Zhu S, Yan M: Combined general/epidural anesthesia (ropivacaine 0. 375%) versus general anesthesia for upper abdominal surgery. Anesthesia and analgesia 2008, 106(5):1562–1565, table of contents.
17. Findlay JM, Ashraf SQ, Congahan P. Transversus abdominis plane (TAP) blocks-a review. Surgeon. 2012;10(6):361–7.
18. Yuanc W, Aij Y: Effect of transversus abdominis plane block on cortisol after laparoscopic hysterectomy (in Chinese with English abstract). J Qiqijaer medical college 2014, 35:945–950.
19. Kondo S, Okuyama K, Ikemoto K, Furuya A, Matsukawa T: [General anesthesia for a boy with wolf-Hirschhorn syndrome]. Masui 2013, 62(12): 1466–1468.
20. Abu Elyazed MM, Mostafa SF, Abdullah MA, Eid GM. The effect of ultrasound-guided transversus abdominis plane (TAP) block on postoperative analgesia and neuroendocrine stress response in pediatric patients undergoing elective open inguinal hernia repair. Paediatr Anaesth. 2016;26(12):1165–71.
21. Wind J, Tuynman JB, Tibbe AG, Swennenhuis JF, Richel DJ, van Berge Henegouwen MI, Bemelman WA. Circulating tumour cells during laparoscopic and open surgery for primary colonic cancer in portal and peripheral blood. Eur J Surg Oncol. 2009;35(9):942–50.
22. Cruickshank AM, Fraser WD, Burns HJ, Van Damme J, Shenkin A. Response of serum interleukin-6 in patients undergoing elective surgery of varying severity. Clinical science (London, England: 1979). 1990;79(2):161–5.
23. Seo N, Hayakawa S, Takigawa M, Tokura Y. Interleukin-10 expressed at early tumour sites induces subsequent generation of CD4(+) T-regulatory cells and systemic collapse of antitumour immunity. Immunology. 2001;103(4):449–57.
24. Hollmann MW, Durieux ME. Local anesthetics and the inflammatory response: a new therapeutic indication? Anesthesiology. 2000;93(3):858–75.
25. Deegan CA, Murray D, Doran P, Moriarty DC, Sessler DI, Mascha E, Kavanagh BP, Buggy DJ. Anesthetic technique and the cytokine and matrix metalloproteinase response to primary breast cancer surgery. Reg Anesth Pain Med. 2010;35(6):490–5.
26. Sultan SS. Paravertebral block can attenuate cytokine response when it replaces general anesthesia for cancer breast surgeries. Saudi J Anaesth. 2013;7(4):373–7.
27. Biki B, Mascha E, Moriarty DC, Fitzpatrick JM, Sessler DI, Buggy DJ. Anesthetic technique for radical prostatectomy surgery affects cancer recurrence: a retrospective analysis. Anesthesiology. 2008;109(2):180–7.
28. Christopherson R, James KE, Tableman M, Marshall P, Johnson FE. Long-term survival after colon cancer surgery: a variation associated with choice of anesthesia. Anesth Analg. 2008;107(1):325–32.
29. Weis F, Beiras-Fernandez A, Schelling G, Briegel J, Lang P, Hauer D, Kreth S, Kaufmann I, Lamm P, Kilger E. Stress doses of hydrocortisone in high-risk patients undergoing cardiac surgery: effects on interleukin-6 to interleukin-10 ratio and early outcome. Crit Care Med. 2009;37(5):1685–90.
30. Baeriswyl M, Kirkham KR, Kern C, Albrecht E. The analgesic efficacy of ultrasound-guided transversus abdominis plane block in adult patients: a meta-analysis. Anesth Analg. 2015;121(6):1640–54.
31. Champaneria R, Shah L, Geoghegan J, Gupta JK, Daniels JP. Analgesic effectiveness of transversus abdominis plane blocks after hysterectomy: a meta-analysis. Eur J Obstet Gynecol Reprod Biol. 2013;166(1):1–9.
32. Tsuchiya M, Takahashi R, Furukawa A, Suehiro K, Mizutani K, Nishikawa K. Transversus abdominis plane block in combination with general anesthesia provides better intraoperative hemodynamic control and quicker recovery than general anesthesia alone in high-risk abdominal surgery patients. Minerva Anestesiol. 2012;78(11):1241–7.
33. Zafar N, Davies R, Greenslade GL, Dixon AR. The evolution of analgesia in an 'accelerated' recovery programme for resectional laparoscopic colorectal surgery with anastomosis. Colorectal Dis. 2010;12(2):119–24.
34. Favuzza J, Brady K, Delaney CP. Transversus abdominis plane blocks and enhanced recovery pathways: making the 23-h hospital stay a realistic goal after laparoscopic colorectal surgery. Surg Endosc. 2013;27(7):2481–6.

21

Combined ultrasound and nerve stimulator-guided deep nerve block may decrease the rate of local anesthetics systemic toxicity

Xu-hao Zhang[†], Yu-jie Li[†], Wen-quan He, Chun-yong Yang, Jian-teng Gu, Kai-zhi Lu and Bin Yi[*]

Abstract

Background: Ultrasound guidance might decrease the incidence of local anesthetics systemic toxicity (LAST) for many peripheral nerve blocks compared with nerve stimulator guidance. However, it remains uncertain whether ultrasound guidance is superior to nerve stimulator guidance for deep nerve block of the lower extremity. This study was designed to investigate whether deep nerve block with ultrasound guidance would decrease the incidence of LAST compared with that with nerve stimulator guidance, and to identify associated risk factors of LAST.

Methods: Three hundred patients undergoing elective lower limb surgery and desiring lumbar plexus blocks (LPBs) and sciatic nerve blocks (SNBs) were enrolled in this study. The patients were randomly assigned to receive LPBs and SNBs with ultrasound guidance (group U), nerve stimulator guidance (group N) or dual guidance (group M). The primary outcome was the incidence of LAST. The secondary outcomes were the number of needle redirection, motor and sensory block onset and nerve distribution restoration time, as well as associated risk factors.

Results: There were 18 patients with LAST, including 12 in group U, 4 in group N and 2 in group M. By multiple comparisons among the three groups, we found that the incidence of LAST in group U (12%) was significantly higher than that in group N (4%)($P = 0.037$) and group M(2%)($P = 0.006$). The OR of LAST with hepatitis B (HBV) infection and the female sex was 3.352 (95% CI,1.233–9.108, $P = 0.013$) and 9.488 (95% CI,2.142–42.093, $P = 0.0004$), respectively.

Conclusions: Ultrasound guidance, HBV infection and the female sex were risk factors of LAST with LPBs and SNBs. For patients infected with HBV or female patients receiving LPBs and SNBs, we recommended that combined ultrasound and nerve stimulator guidance should be used to improve the safety.

Keywords: Ultrasound, Nerve stimulation, Nerve block, Female, HBV, LAST

* Correspondence: yibin1974@163.com
[†]Xu-hao Zhang and Yu-jie Li contributed equally to this work.
Department of Anesthesia, Southwest Hospital, Army Medical University, Chongqing 400038, China

Background

Although peripheral nerve blocks have been a safe and effective way to provide analgesia for procedures in a variety of settings, using this type of anesthesia does have risks that should not be overlooked. The incidence of Local Anesthetics Systemic Toxicity (LAST) was reported to be 0.04/1000 to 1.8/1000 in a recent summary [1]. LAST, a life-threatening and sometimes fatal condition, was reported to be related to patient characteristics (such as advanced age, low muscle mass, liver disease, cardiac disease, renal disease or diabetes), local anesthetic characteristics and practice settings [1].

Lumbar plexus blocks (LPBs) combined with sciatic nerve blocks (SNBs) for lower extremity surgery are becoming increasingly popular. Due to the depth of the lumbar plexus and sciatic nerves, LPBs and SNBs were advanced regional anesthesia techniques and may be more likely to lead to LAST [2]. LPBs and SNBs are traditionally performed using surface anatomical landmarks and nerve stimulation guidance. Ultrasound could offer direct visualization of the nerve structures, needle pathway and local anesthetics (LAs) spread in real time and is thus widely used in peripheral nerve blocks. Accumulating published data suggests higher efficacy and safety of nerve blocks with ultrasound guidance (US) [3, 4], specifically for interscalene [5], supraclavicular [6], infraclavicular [7], and axillary [8] blocks. Michael et al. [9] reported that the use of ultrasound reduced the risk of LAST throughout its continuum by 60 to 65% compared to without ultrasound. However, most studies have focused on upper extremity blocks. Due to the deep location of the lumbar plexus and sciatic nerves, whether the use of ultrasound in LPBs and SNBs would be beneficial in terms of efficacy and safety remains a matter of debate. Most relevant published studies have suggested that ultrasound guidance would shorten both the time required to perform the block and the onset time [10–12]. However, there are limited studies comparing the incidence of LAST for LPBs and SNBs with ultrasound and nerve stimulator.

We designed this study to determine whether ultrasound guidance deep nerve blocks would decrease the incidence of LAST compare with nerve stimulation guidance and to identify associated risk factors of LAST.

Methods

This study was approved by the Ethical Committee of the First Affiliated Hospital of Army Medical University (previous name: Southwest Hospital of the Third Military Medical University). The protocol was registered prospectively with the Chinese Clinical Trial Registry (ChiCTR-IOR-16008099) on March 15, 2016. The principal investigator was Bin Yi. The study took place at the Department of Anesthesia, the First Affiliated Hospital, Army Medical University, Chongqing, from August 25, 2016, to August 14, 2017.

Patients scheduled for elective lower limb surgery in the Southwest Hospital and desiring LPBs and SNBs were offered enrolment. Written informed consent was obtained from the participants for publication of this article and any accompanying Tables. A copy of the written consent is available for review by the Editor of this journal. The inclusion criteria were as follows: willingness to participate in the study (written informed consent); ASA classification of I to III; older than 18 years old. The exclusion criteria were as follows: refusal to participate; history of neurological diseases; coagulopathy or infection at the site of the block, allergy to local anesthetics (LAs), and any contraindication to peripheral nerve blockade noted by the attending anesthesiologist. All patients were randomly allocated to group U (ultrasound guidance), group N (nerve stimulator guidance) or group M (combined guidance) by a random number table.

Blinding

The anesthesiologist who performed the LPBs and SNBs was strictly blinded to the patient's group assignment before the procedure. Only when the anesthesiologist commenced with the block was a prepared sealed opaque envelope containing the patient's group assignment opened. Then the anesthesiologist completed the block with the indicated technique. There were two investigators in the study. One investigator blinded to the technique used was present in the block area to assess the procedure-related outcomes. To ensure blindness of the patient to the method, all procedures performed behind an opaque screen and investigators were required not to say anything about the technique in use. Another investigator assessing the block quality was blinded to the group allocation and remained outside the block area until completion of the procedure. Finally, a statistician blinded to the entire process performed the statistical analysis, with group data labelled only as numbers until all analyses were completed.

Block preparation

LPBs and SNBs were performed preoperatively by 1 of 3 attending anesthesiologists who were skilled in peripheral nerve blocks with both ultrasound guidance (US) and nerve stimulator guidance (NS). All of them had been in clinical practice with a focus on regional anesthesia for at least 5 years. After arriving in the operating room, the patient was placed in the lateral decubitus position with the surgical limb uppermost and monitored continuously via electrocardiography, SpO_2 measurements, and non-invasive blood pressure monitoring during the nerve blockade and surgery. Both the ultrasound and nerve stimulation systems were prepared and positioned conventionally in each group. The ultrasound machine and nerve stimulator were turned on, and a grounding lead was placed on the lateral aspect of the leg being blocked for each group. The patient's group allocation was given to the anesthesiologist only after the preparation of both systems and just before the block procedure. The patient was pretreated with 0.05 mg/kg midazolam and 1.5 μg/kg fentanyl. The injection site was prepared with chlorhexidine gluconate. Five millilitres of 0.5% lidocaine was injected subcutaneously at the site of needle insertion. The LA mixture was composed of 200 mg of ropivacaine, 200 mg of lidocaine and 20 ml of 0.9% sodium chloride solution. The concentration of ropivacaine and lidocaine was 0.4%. The total amount of LAs used was determined by the dosage of ropivacaine needed, namely, 3 mg/kg. The patient and investigators assessing the block quality prevented from seeing both the block procedure itself and the sonographic image displayed by an opaque screen. According to the group allocation, the patient received the nerve blocks under one of the following three techniques.

Nerve stimulation technique

In the operating room, LPB was performed using Chayen's approach [13, 14]. The puncture site was located 4–5 cm lateral to the posterior midline along the intercristal line. A 110-mm, 22-G stimulating needle connected to a nerve stimulator (Stimuplex HNS 11, B. Braun) was advanced perpendicular to the skin. The nerve stimulator was set to a pulse duration of 0.1 ms, current intensity of 1.0 mA, and frequency of 2 Hz. The stimulating intensity was progressively reduced to 0.4 mA or less while maintaining the twitch in the quadriceps distribution. The total volume of LAs was determined by the amount of the LA mixture calculated according to the patient's weight, as mentioned above. Each point was given half of the total calculated volume of the LA mixture. When the correct needle position was achieved based on evoking the desired motor response, the amounts of LAs described above were injected. SNB was performed with the classic Labat approach [15]. The needle was inserted 5 cm below the midpoint of a line connecting the posterior superior iliac spine and the greater trochanter. After an appropriate stimulus was localized in the sciatic distribution, the LAs described above were injected.

Ultrasound-guided technique

We chose the "Shamrock Method" for the LPBs [16]. A sterile cover was placed on a 3-MHz low-frequency ultrasound probe (LOGIQe 4C-RS, GE Inc., USA). The ultrasound transducer was positioned on the line connecting the subcostal margin and iliac spine and adjusted until a clear view of the psoas, erector muscle and quadratus lumborum appeared. The hyperechoic structure located in the posterior internal quadrant of the psoas was the lumbar plexus. The puncture site was beneath the probe and 4–5 cm lateral to the vertebral body. We chose a subgluteal approach for the SNBs [17]. The ultrasound transducer was positioned perpendicular to the skin on the line connecting the ischial tuberosity and greater trochanter, and a clear transverse image of the hyperechoic sciatic nerve between the ischial tuberosity and greater trochanter was obtained. For the LPBs and SNBs, the needle placement and LA spread were confirmed by ultrasound visualization. After the proper needle placement was confirmed, incremental injection of the same LA solution in the same volume was performed as previously described until circumferential spread around the nerve was obtained. The needle was redirected, when required, to achieve this goal. In group M, initially, needle-to-nerve guidance was applied as in group U. Maintaining the needle nerve position, the nerve stimulator was set as described for group N. When the correct needle position was achieved based on evoking the desired motor response, the LAs described above were injected.

Block evaluation

Evaluation of the nerve blocks was performed by an investigator blinded to those who administered the LPBs and SNBs. The motor and sensory responses in the nerve distribution area were assessed every 5 min until complete motor and sensory effects were achieved. If it took more than 30 min to achieve sensory loss in both distributions after the end of the LAs injection, the block was considered to have failed. The attending anesthesiologist had the right to perform general anesthesia, rescue block, or supplementation with a local field block in case of a failed block. The motor block was assessed with a modified Bromage scale: 2, full motor strength; 1, decreased strength; and 0, no strength. Similarly, the sensory block was evaluated with ice: 2, full sensation (no change); 1, decreased sensation; and 0, no sensation.

Postoperative follow-ups were performed in the post-anesthesia care unit and by telephone within 72 h after the procedure by clinical personnel in addition to study-related procedures.

Outcomes

The primary outcome was the incidence of LAST. LAST can present with clinical manifestations related to both the central nervous system (CNS) and the cardiovascular system (CVS). CNS symptoms include tongue numbness, tinnitus, light-headedness, metallic taste, nystagmus, confusion, tremors, agitation, seizures, coma, and respiratory arrest [18]. CVS symptoms include tachycardia, arrhythmias, hypertension, and later toxic symptoms, such as bradycardia, cardiac depression, cardiovascular collapse, and asystole [18]. The secondary outcomes were the quality of the nerve block and associated risk factors. The quality of the block included the number of needle redirections, motor and sensory block onset and restoration times in the lumbar and sciatic nerve distributions. The associated risk factors included age, sex and comorbidities. The number of needle redirections was counted as the number of times the needle was withdrawn by at least 10 mm with subsequent forward movement. The upper limit of redirections was 20, but if necessary, the needle was allowed to be redirected as many times as possible to achieve proper placement, as previously described. The onset of motor and sensory block was assessed using the modified Bromage scale as mentioned above for the distributions of both the lumbar plexus and sciatic nerves. The onset time was measured between the final LA injection and the first observation of a 0 score. During the phone follow-up interviews, the patient provided the time of first return of sensation and any block-related complications on postoperative day 1. The block duration time was defined as the interval between block completion and the first return of sensation. Any reported complications were recorded.

Statistical analysis

The statistical analyses were performed using Statistical Package for the Social Sciences (Windows Software, version 19.0; SPSS Inc., Chicago, IL) and Power Analysis and Sample Size (Windows Software, version 11.0; NCSS Inc., Utah).

Demographic and perioperative data are expressed as the mean and standard deviation. Parametric and non-parametric Kolmogorov–Smirnov tests were applied to assess normality. The primary outcome (incidence of LAST) and potential risk factors were compared by χ^2 test or Fisher exact test when appropriate ($n < 5$ in any field). In the χ^2 test, we tested whether there were differences in the incidence of LAST and the odds ratios of potential risk factors among different groups. The demographics and secondary outcomes were compared among the three groups by one-way ANOVA, followed by multiple comparisons using the LSD test or Welch and Dunnett's T3 test for unequal variances. Using one-way ANOVA, we tested whether there were differences in the patient characteristics and block quality among the three groups. This analysis was followed by the determination of 95% CIs with Bonferroni's correction to adjust for multiple comparisons (three different methods for nerve block for motor and sensory onset, restoration time and demographics) to minimize the chance of a type I error (0.05). For all comparisons, 2-tailed P values < 0.05 were considered statistically significant.

The incidence of LAST is low according to published data. Therefore, we performed a test to determine the power of the analysis regarding the incidence of LAST in the three groups after the experiment. In the current study, 319 patients were randomly allocated to the three groups. Finally, data from 100 patients for each group were analysed. We performed a test to determine the power of the analysis regarding the primary outcome after the experiment. We calculated the effect size (0.182) using PASS software. Then, we set the significance level to 0.05. We found that when the total sample size was 300, the power(1-β) of the test was 0.81.

Results

The study flow diagram is presented in Fig. 1. A total of 319 patients were evaluated for eligibility and offered enrolment in this study. Eighteen were excluded; 3 did not meet the inclusion criteria, 13 declined to participate, and 2 were excluded for other reasons. There were no failed or aborted blocks in either group. One patient in group U was lost to follow-up.

The patient characteristics are presented in Tab 1. There was no statistically significant difference in age, sex, weight or height among the three groups. Only one patient in group M had an ASA III status. Most of the operations were performed on the knee or ankle. There was a statistically significant difference in the operative time between group U (41.0 ± 24.21 min) and in group M (51.5 ± 30.8 min).

The primary and secondary outcomes are shown in Tab 2. The incidence of LAST in all three groups was 6%. Moreover, there was a statistically significant difference in the incidence of LAST among the three groups. By multiple comparisons among the three groups, we found that the incidence of LAST in group U (12%) was significantly higher than that in group N (4%)($P = 0.037$) and group M (2%)($P = 0.006$). (shown in Tab 4). Regarding the LPBs, the motor onset time was significantly shorter in group N (9.5 ± 3.55 s) than in group U (11.30 ± 4.94 s) and group M (11.10 ± 4.38 s) (shown in Tab 2). There was no statistically significant difference in the sensory onset time or sensory and motor restoration time among the three groups. Regarding the SNBs, the motor and sensory onset time was significantly shorter in group N than in groups U and M. Meanwhile, the sensory and motor restoration time in group N was statistically significantly longer than that in groups U and M.

Detailed information of the 18 patients who developed LAST is summarized in Tab 3. There were 12 patients from group U (66.7%), 4 from group N (22.2%) and 2 from group M (11.1%) who experienced LAST during the process. Most of the symptoms were CNS symptoms. None of the 18 patients developed permanent complications after correct and timely treatment. To our

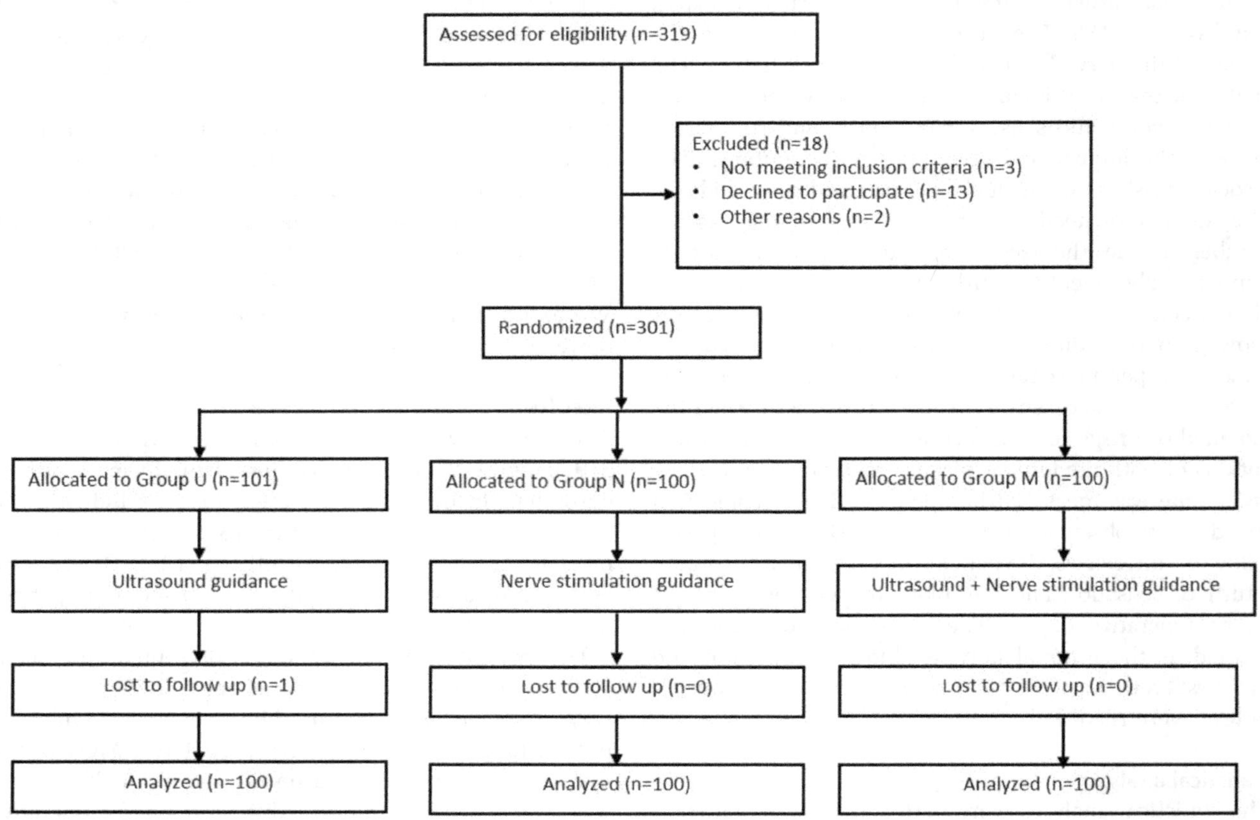

Fig. 1 CONSORT flow diagram of the study. CONSORT indicates Consolidated Standards of Reporting Trials. Group U was short for nerve block with ultrasound guidance, group N was short for nerve block with nerve stimulation guidance, group M was for nerve block with combined guidance

interest, 16 of the 18 patients were female. The age of the 18 patients ranged from 19 to 81. The shortest occurrence time was 1 min after finishing the block, and the longest occurrence time was 22 min. The shortest duration time was 3 min without any treatment. The longest duration time was 100 min due to the use of propofol.

We analysed risk factors such as age, sex, liver disease, and diabetes according to *The Third American Society of Regional Anesthesia and Pain Medicine Practice Advisory on Local Anesthetic Systemic Toxicity* [1]. In the current study, 52 patients were infected with HBV, and 7 of these patients experienced LAST. As shown in Tab 4, the OR of LAST for HBV infection and the female sex was 3.352(95% CI,1.233–9.108, $P = 0.013$) and 9.488(95% CI,2.142–42.093, $P = 0.0004$), respectively. However, age, needle passes, renal disease and diabetes did not increase the risk of LAST in the current study. Overall, the use of ultrasound, HBV infection and the female sex may be related to the increased incidence of LAST in the current study.

Table 1 Patients characteristics

	group U(100)	group N(100)	group M(100)	*F*	*P*
Age (yr) (SD)	41.7(12.85)	39.9 (14.71)	42.0 (19.94)	0.6222	0.53745
Gender (F/M)	55/45	47/53	43/57		(N vs U)0.51/(M vs U)0.49
Weight (kg) (SD)	63.8 (11.92)	64.7(11.06)	64.7(11.20)	0.2185	0.8038
Height (cm) (SD)	163.0 (8.07)	165.0 (9.68)	164.9 (9.3)	1.5282	0.2186
Surgical duration (min)	41.0(24.21)	46.9 (32.26)	51.5(30.8)	3.1996	0.04219
Surgical site(knee/ankle/other)	89/10/1	78/21/1	84/16/0		
ASA I/II/III	53/47/0	48/52/0	49/50/1		

Data are expressed as mean ± SD

Abbreviations: *group U* nerve block with ultrasound guidance, *group N* nerve block with nerve stimulation-guidance, *group M* nerve block with combined guidance, *F* female, *M* male, *ASA* American Society of Anesthesiologists

Table 2 Outcomes

Outcomes	group U(100)	group N(100)	group M(100)	*P*
Incidence of LAST(%)	4%	12%	2%	0.007
Motor onset, Lumbar plexus, min (SD)	11.3(4.94)	9.5 (3.55)	11.1 (4.38)	0.00729
Motor onset, Sciatica, min (SD)	15.1 (4.04)	13.4 (3.03)	15.0 (3.20)	0.00041
Sensory onset, Lumbar plexus, min (SD)	8.5(3.64)	7.8 (2.52)	8.8 (2.88)	0.07676
Sensory onset, Sciatica, min (SD)	9.6 (2.62)	8.8 (1.59)	9.5 (1.79)	0.02399
Sensory restoration, Lumbar plexus, h (SD)	8.0 (1.90)	8.4 (1.71)	8.1 (1.63)	0.19313
Sensory restoration, Sciatica, h (SD)	7.1 (1.73)	7.7 (1.63)	7.0 (1.57)	0.00329
Motor restoration, Lumbar plexus, h (SD)	8.9 (2.11)	9.3 (1.78)	9.0 (1.59)	0.18912
Motor restoration, Sciatica, h (SD)	7.9(1.87)	8.5 (1.72)	7.8 (1.44)	0.00760

Data are expressed as mean ± SD or number with %
Abbreviations: *group U* nerve block with ultrasound guidance, *group N* nerve block with nerve stimulation-guidance, *group M* nerve block with combined guidance

Discussion

There were three main findings in the current study. First, the use of ultrasound did not improve the quality of deep nerve block. Second, the use of ultrasound increased the incidence of LAST. Third, the use of ultrasound, HBV infection and the female sex may be risk factors of LAST.

In the present study, we found that LPBs and SNBs with US were not superior to those with NS in terms of the onset or restoration time. Spencer S. Liu et al. [19] found that 8 of 10 RCTs reported that the use of ultrasound would shorten the onset time of lower extremity blocks, 2 of 10 reported no difference, and no RCTs reported slower onset with ultrasound. However, most of the RCTs were about the femoral and peroneal nerves. Recently, Arnuntasupakul et al. [12] reported that ultrasound with nerve stimulation guidance for LPBs resulted in a shorter total anesthesia and onset times than US alone. Due to the size and location of the lumbar plexus and sciatic nerves, LPBs and SNBs are advanced regional anesthesia techniques. Different induction pathways for the nerve block may result in different outcomes.

Table 3 Summary of Events of Local Anesthetic Systemic Toxicity (LAST)

Group	Sex	Age(Y)	Weight(kg)	Height(cm)	Signs and Symptoms	Occurrence time	Treatment	Duration time (min)
N	F	35	52.5	155	Lips numbness, Left hand twitch	17	M2	6
N	F	46	55	155	Lips numbness	11	/	5
N	F	65	62.5	163	Agitation, Chest tightness	9	/	3
N	F	19	35.5	149	Tachycardia, Seizures	12/22	M2 P200V	80[a]
U	F	46	54	158	Tongue numbness, Tinnitus	8	M2	9
U	F	53	54	160	Tongue numbness, Left hand and leg twitch	13/17	M2	8
U	F	26	70	161	Tongue numbness	18	/	4
U	F	41	50	156	Unconsciousness, Tachycardia, Hypertension	8	M2 P200	63[a]
U	F	61	60	155	Agitation	9	/	3
U	F	46	60	159	Scream, Unconsciousness	1	M2 P200	100[a]
U	F	32	51	160	Tachycardia	7	M2 D0.5	25
U	M	81	63	152	Right hand twitch, Unconsciousness	4/9	M2	15
U	F	62	58	150	Transient numbness of right hand and leg	20	/	4
U	F	26	46	161	Twitch	12	M2	5
U	F	47	60	145	Hypertension, Tachycardia, Agitation	10	M2	25
U	F	37	48	153	anxiety, Confusion	11	M2	15
M	F	35	64	163	Tinnitus, Whole body numbness	8	M2	10
M	M	21	60	170	Tongue numbness	11	/	6

Treatment: M2 means venous injection of Midazolam 2 mg; P200 means continuous intravenous infusion of Propofol 200 mg with the rate of 3 $mg \cdot kg^{-1} \cdot h^{-1}$; D0.5 means continuous intravenous infusion of Dexmedetomidine with the rate of 0.5 $\mu g \cdot kg^{-1} \cdot h^{-1}$; V means mechanical ventilation. Dosage of local anesthtic: 0.4%Ropivacaine+ 0.4% Lidocaine, 3 mg/kg);
[a]The main reason of long duration time was the use of propofol

Table 4 Associated risk factors for local anesthetic systemic toxicity

Categorical Variables		No. LAST Events(%)	*OR*	95% CI	*P*
Method of Block	N	4(4)			0.037 (N vs U)
	U	12(12)			0.006 (U vs M)
	M	2(2)			0.407 (M vs N)
Needle passes(times)	2–5	11(5.1)	0.58	0.217–1.550	0.272
	6-	7(8.4)	1		
Sex	Male	2(1.3)	1		
	Female	16(11.0)	9.488	2.142–42.093	0.0004
HBV infection	negative	11(4.4)	1		
	positive	7(13.5)	3.352	1.233–9.108	0.013
Renal disease	negative	17(6.1)	1		
	positive	1(4.5)	0.731	0.093–5.766	0.765
Diabetes	negative	18(6.3)			
	positive	0(0)			1.00

Data are expressed as number and %
Abbreviations: *Group U* nerve block with ultrasound guidance, *Group N* nerve block with nerve stimulation-guidance, *group M* nerve block with combined guidance

Furthermore, due to comorbidities, some of the enrolled patients may have already had minor pathological changes in the targeted nerves, which may have affected the onset and restoration times.

The incidence of LAST was 6%,which is much higher than previously reported [1]. LAST can occur as a result of the patient's risk factors and current medications, inadvertent injection of LAs directly into the vascular system, exceeding the maximum LA dose, or immediate LA absorption upon injection into an extremely vascularized area [18]. It has been widely reported that US is safer than NS because US can provide direct visualization of the target nerve, surrounding tissues, and LA spread [9, 20]. However, in our study, approximately two-thirds of the patients who experienced LAST were in group U. There are two main reasons for this finding. First, a fair number of patients in our study were infected with HBV or had a renal diseases and thus may be more susceptible to LAST [21]. Second, the lumbar plexus and sciatic nerves are difficult to visualize due to their depth. To obtain a better view of tissues near the nerve, the block needle and the injected LAs, an ultrasonic probe must be applied with some pressure near the injection site. This pressure slows the blood flow in the deep, small vessels, and it is difficult to examine the deep, small vessels using Doppler ultrasonography, especially with slow flow [22]. The continuous pressure caused by the ultrasonic probe makes deep, small vessels "invisible" and thus increased the difficulty of avoiding injecting LAs into extremely vascularized areas, resulting in LAST. The nerve stimulator has advantages over US in terms of determining the relative positions of the needle tip and nerves. When the needle tip is near an extremely vascularized area, the electric current decreases, resulting in failure to induce muscle twitching. In group M, after ultrasound guidance, the rate of failure to induce twitching in the quadriceps and gastrocnemius distribution was 10 and 12%, respectively. Under these circumstances, the distance between the tip and the targeted nerve needed to be adjusted. Therefore, the likelihood of injecting LAs into extremely vascularized areas was less than that with US alone.

The patient's weight, comorbidities, use of other medications, genetics, allergies, and other physiological limitations also affecting the incidence of LAST [23]. Factors affected systemic LA absorption, the peak plasma LA concentration and the time to reach that peak are all related to LAST. Bupivacaine and ropivacaine are degraded in the liver by α1-acid glycoprotein (AAG) [21]. Patients with liver diseases would have a decreased rate of LAs clearance due to a reduced AAG concentration, which may increase the incidence of LAST. However, even in patients with advanced liver dysfunction, the synthesis of AAG is still maintained [21, 24]. In patients with hepatic dysfunction, single-dose blocks can usually be performed safely with a normal dose of LAs [25]. This finding indicates that the decreased clearance of LAs caused by isolated hepatic dysfunction is not the main reason for LAST in this study. However, as shown in Tab 4, patients infected with HBV had a higher risk of LAST in this study. Patients who are infected with HBV may develop chronic liver disease. Patients with chronic liver disease usually have vascular dysfunction, especially angiogenesis, microvascular derangements and microcirculatory dysfunction [26, 27]. Cirrhosis causes numerous microscopic vessel aberrations, and these vessels may become entangled with each other, resulting in sharp bends, anomalous branching patterns, abnormal branching angles and tortuosity [28]. McAvoy et al. [29] demonstrated that patients with cirrhosis had selective regional increases in blood flow in the splanchnic and hepatic circulations but diminished flow in the peripheral limbs. Neovascularization and slower blood flow make it easier to inject LAs into extremely vascularized areas, especially for the use of ultrasound, resulting in an increased incidence of LAST. Vascular endothelial growth factor (VEGF) and bone morphogenetic protein 9 (BMP-9) have been widely reported to promote angiogenesis [30]. Higher BMP-9 levels in human serum are accompanied by advanced stages of liver fibrosis, while BMP-9 overexpression accelerated liver fibrosis and BMP-9 knockdown attenuated the liver fibrosis in a mouse model [31]. The plasma VEGF level was elevated in patients with cirrhosis, especially in those with spider angiomas [27]. Higher serum levels of BMP-9 and VEGF in patients with HBV indicated more advanced stages of liver dysfunction and increased new blood vessel formation. However, further efforts are needed to determine the relationship of VEGF and BMP-9 with HBV infection. VEGF and BMP-9 may be promising prognostic indicators for the incidence of LAST after deep nerve block in patients with HBV.

Herein, women were more likely to experience LAST, which is in consistent with the latest regional anesthesia and pain medicine practice advisory on LAST [1]. Some enrolled patients who experienced LAST were HBV carriers. The increased risk of LAST in females may be related to HBV infection. Under physiological conditions, the estrogen/estrogen receptor α (ER/ER α) axis has a protective effect against HBV-associated liver damage, and postmenopausal hormone replacement therapy results in a lower risk of hepatocellular carcinoma in HBV positive women [32]. In a female cirrhosis rat model the mRNA expression of ER α was lower in that of a sham rats and the ability of 17β-estradiol to alleviate relevant complications was diminished [33]. This finding indicates that female HBV carriers might have a lower level of ER/ER α, which made them more susceptible to LAST. Further efforts are needed to investigate the underlying mechanism.

There are a number of limitations to this study. First, it was not possible to blind the anesthesiologist performing the nerve block, and we could not exclude the potential influence of a performance bias in this study. Second, although we made efforts to maintain blinding among the investigators, patients, and statistician, it may be partial blinding due to the muscle contractions elicited by nerve stimulation, counting the number of needle redirections and so on. We attempted to minimize this bias by only involving staff anesthesiologists experienced in peripheral nerve blockades using both guidance modalities. Third, there is some limitation related to the techniques and equipment used in this single-center study, so the results cannot be generalized to other techniques or peripheral nerve block locations. The degree of advantages and disadvantages provided by ultrasound guided deep nerve block, especially in HBV carriers, is likely to vary by the nerve block site as well. We only demonstrated some interesting phenomenon and did not determine the underlying mechanisms in the present single-center study. A multicenter study and more detailed experiments are needed to verify our results and reveal the mechanisms.

Conclusions

Our results suggest that ultrasound guidance, HBV infection and the female sex are risk factors of LAST in LPBs and SNBs. For patients infected with HBV or female patients undergoing LPBs and SNBs, combined ultrasound and nerve stimulation guidance should be used to improve the safety. The probable mechanisms are as follows:1) angiogenesis and slower blood flow in deeply located small vessels; and 2) the use of nerve stimulation to avoid injecting LAs into extremely vascularized areas.

Abbreviations

BMP-9: Bone Morphogenetic Protein 9; LAs: Local Anesthetics; LAST: Local Anesthetics Systemic Toxicity; LPBs: Lumbar Plexus Blocks; NS: Nerve Stimulator guidance; SNBs: Sciatic Nerve Blocks; US: Ultrasound guidance; VEGF: Vascular Endothelial Growth Factor

Acknowledgments

To our Families and colleagues.

Authors' contributions

ZXH helped design and conduct the study; data collection and manuscript writing. LYJ helped with data analysis and interpretation; and drafting, revision, and final approval of the article. HWQ helped conduct the study and collect data. YCY helped data analysis and revision. GJT helped with study design and data analysis. LKZ helped with study design and revision. YB helped design the study, write this manuscript and revision. All authors have agreed both to be personally accountable for their own contributions and to ensure that questions related to the accuracy or integrity of any part of the work. All authors have read and approved the final manuscript.

References

1. Neal JMB, Michael J, Fettiplace MR, et al. The third American Society of Regional Anesthesia and Pain Medicine practice advisory on local anesthetic systemic toxicity. Reg Anesth Pain Med. 2018;43(2):113–23.
2. Auroy Y, Benhamou D, Bargues L, Ecoffey C, Falissard B, Mercier FJ, Bouaziz H, Samii K. major complications of regional anesthesia in France: the SOS regional anesthesia hotline service. Anesthesiology. 2002;97(5):1274–80.
3. Salinas FV, Hanson NA. Evidence-based medicine for ultrasound-guided regional anesthesia. Anesthesiol Clin. 2014;32(4):771–87.
4. Gelfand HJ, Ouanes JP, Lesley MR, Ko PS, Murphy JD, Sumida SM, Isaac GR, Kumar K, Wu CL. Analgesic efficacy of ultrasound-guided regional anesthesia: a meta-analysis. J Clin Anesth. 2011;23(2):90–6.
5. Liu SS, ZayasVM GMA, Beathe JC, Maalouf DB, Paroli L, Liguori GA, Ortiz J, Buschiazzo V, Ngeow J, Shetty T, Ya Deau JT. A prospective, randomized, controlled trial comparing ultrasound versus nerve stimulator guidance for interscalene block for ambulatory shoulder surgery for postoperative neurological symptoms. Anesth Analg. 2009;109(1):265–71.
6. Williams SR, Chouinard P, Arcand G, Harris P, Ruel M, Boudreault D, Girard F. Ultrasound guidance speeds execution and improves the quality of supraclavicular block. Anesth Analg. 2003;97(5):1518–23.
7. Sauter AR, Dodgson MS, Stubhaug A, Halstensen AM, Klaastad O. Electrical nerve stimulation or ultrasound guidance for lateral sagittal infraclavicular blocks: a randomized, controlled, observer-blinded, comparative study. Anesth Analg. 2008;106(6):1910–5.
8. Chan VW, Perlas A, CJ MC, Brull R, Xu D, Abbas S. Ultrasound guidance improves success rate of axillary brachial plexus block. Can J Anaesth. 2007;54(3):176–82.
9. Barrington MJ, Kluger R. Ultrasound guidance reduces the risk of local anesthetic systemic toxicity following peripheral nerve blockade. Reg Anesth Pain Med. 2013;38(4):289–99.
10. Amin WA, Seada MO, Elkersh MM, Mathai A, Medekova S, Husain T. Comparative study between ultrasound and nerve stimulator guided sciatic nerve block through the anterior approach. Middle East J Anaesthesiol. 2015;23(2):185–91.
11. Danelli G, Fanelli A, Ghisi D, Moschini E, Rossi M, Ortu A, Baciarello M, Fanelli G. Ultrasound vs nerve stimulation multiple injection technique for posterior popliteal sciatic nerve block. Anaesthesia. 2009;64(6):638–42.
12. Arnuntasupakul V, Chalachewa T, Leurcharusmee P, Tiyaprasertkul W, et al. Ultrasound with neurostimulation compared with ultrasound guidance alone for lumbar plexus block: a randomised single blinded equivalence

trial. Eur J Anaesthesiol. 2018;35(3):224–30.
13. Mannion S. Psoas compartment block. Cont Educ Anaesth Crit Care Pain. 2007;7:162–6.
14. Chayen D, Nathan H, Chayen M. The psoas compartment block. Anesthesiology. 1976;45(1):95–9.
15. Horlocker TT. Regional anesthesia and analgesia in the patient receiving thromboprophylaxis. Reg Anesth. 1996;21(6):503–7.
16. Sauter AR, Ullensvang K, Bendtsen TF, Børglum J. The shamrock method a new and promising technique for ultrasound guided lumbar plexus blocks. Br J Anaesth. 2013;111.
17. Yamamoto H, Sakura S, Wada M, Shido A. A prospective, randomized comparison between single- and multiple-injection techniques for ultrasound-guided subgluteal sciatic nerve block. Anesth Analg. 2014; 119(6):1442–8.
18. Fencl JL. Local anesthetic systemic toxicity: perioperative implications. AORN J. 2015;101(6):697–700.
19. Liu SS. Evidence basis for ultrasound-guided block characteristics onset, quality, and duration. Reg Anesth Pain Med. 2016;41(2):205–20.
20. Orebaugh S, Kentor ML, Williams BA. Adverse outcomes associated with nerve stimulator-guided and ultrasound-guided peripheral nerve blocks by supervised trainees: update of a single-site database. Reg Anesth Pain Med. 2012;37(6):577–82.
21. Christie LE, Picard J, Weinberg GL. Local anaesthetic systemic toxicity. BJA Education. 2015;15(3):136–42.
22. Degirmenci NA, Ozakyol AH, Atlanoglu S, Akcan E, Susuz S. Increased incidence of abnormal reflux flow in lower extremity veins of cirrhotic patients by Doppler ultrasonography. Saudi Med J. 2013;34(3):276–81.
23. Wadlund DL. Local anesthetic systemic toxicity. AORN J. 2017;106(5):367–77.
24. El-Boghdadly K, Chin KJ. Local anesthetic systemic toxicity: continuing professional development. Can J Anaesth. 2016;63(3):330–49.
25. Rosenberg PH, Veering BT, Urmey WF. Maximum recommended doses of local anesthetics: a multifactorial concept. Reg Anesth Pain Med. 2004;29(6):564–75 discussion 524.
26. Davies T, Wythe S, O'Beirne J, Martin D, Gilbert-Kawai E. Review article: the role of the microcirculation in liver cirrhosis. Aliment Pharmacol Ther. 2017;46(9):825–35.
27. Li CP, Lee FY, Hwang SJ, Lu RH, Lee WP, Chao Y, Wang SS, Chang FY, Whang-Peng J, Lee SD. Spider angiomas in patients with liver cirrhosis: role of vascular endothelial growth factor and basic fibroblast growth factor. World J Gastroenterol. 2003;9(12):2832–5.
28. Peeters G, Debbaut C, Friebel A, Cornillie P, De Vos WH, Favere K, Vander Elst I, Vandecasteele T, Johann T, Van Hoorebeke L, Monbaliu D, Drasdo D, Hoehme S, Laleman W, Segers P. Quantitative analysis of hepatic macro- and microvascular alterations during cirrhogenesis in the rat. J Anat. 2018;232(3):485–96.
29. NC MA, Semple S, Richards JM, Robson AJ, Patel D, Jardine AG, Leyland K, Cooper AS, Newby DE, Hayes PC. Differential visceral blood flow in the hyperdynamic circulation of patients with liver cirrhosis. Aliment Pharmacol Ther. 2016;43(9):947–54.
30. Jin Y, Kaluza D, Jakobsson L. VEGF, notch and TGFbeta/BMPs in regulation of sprouting angiogenesis and vascular patterning. Biochem Soc Trans. 2014;42(6):1576–83.
31. Li P, Li Y, Zhu L, et al. Targeting secreted cytokine BMP9 gates the attenuation of hepatic fibrosis. Biochim Biophys Acta. 2018;1864(3):709–20.
32. Wang SH, Chen PJ, Yeh SH. Gender disparity in chronic hepatitis B: mechanisms of sex hormones. J Gastroenterol Hepatol. 2015;30(8):1237–45.
33. FY HHLL, Hsu SJ, Wang SS, Hsin IF, Huang HC, Lee JY, Lin HC, Lee SD. The ability of 17 β-estradiol to attenuate intrahepatic vasoconstriction to endothelin-1 in female rats is lost in cirrhosis. Ann Hepatol. 2015;14(3):404–13.

22

A comparison of effects of scalp nerve block and local anesthetic infiltration on inflammatory response, hemodynamic response, and postoperative pain in patients undergoing craniotomy for cerebral aneurysms

Xi Yang†, Jing Ma†, Ke Li, Lei Chen, Rui Dong, Yayuan Lu, Zongze Zhang and Mian Peng*

Abstract

Background: The purpose of this study was to compare the effects of scalp nerve block (SNB) and local anesthetic infiltration (LA) with 0.75% ropivacaine on postoperative inflammatory response, intraoperative hemodynamic response, and postoperative pain control in patients undergoing craniotomy.

Methods: Fifty-seven patients were admitted for elective craniotomy for surgical clipping of a cerebral aneurysm. They were randomly divided into three groups: Group S (SNB with 15 mL of 0.75% ropivacaine), group I (LA with 15 mL of 0.75% ropivacaine) and group C (that only received routine intravenous analgesia). Pro-inflammatory cytokine levels in plasma for 72 h postoperatively, hemodynamic response to skin incision, and postoperative pain intensity were measured.

Results: The SNB with 0.75% ropivacaine not only decreased IL-6 levels in plasma 6 h after craniotomy but also decreased plasma CRP levels and increased plasma IL-10 levels 12 and 24 h after surgery compared to LA and routine analgesia. There were significant increases in mean arterial pressure 2 and 5 mins after the incision and during dura opening in Groups I and C compared with Group S. Group S had lower postoperative pain intensity, longer duration before the first dose of oxycodone, less consumption of oxycodone and lower incidence of PONV through 48 h postoperatively than Groups I and C.

Conclusion: Preoperative SNB attenuated inflammatory response to craniotomy for cerebral aneurysms, blunted the hemodynamic response to scalp incision, and controlled postoperative pain better than LA or routine analgesia.

Keywords: Scalp nerve block, Local anesthetic infiltration, Craniotomy, Postcraniotomy pain, Inflammatory response

* Correspondence: sophie_pm@msn.com
†Xi Yang and Jing Ma contributed equally to this work.
Department of Anesthesiology, Zhongnan Hospital of Wuhan University, 169 Donghu Road, Wuhan, Hubei, China

Background

Moderate to severe postoperative pain after craniotomy has an incidence as high as 80% [1]. Uncontrolled postoperative pain may contribute to increased intracranial pressure (ICP) and hypertension, which may be detrimental, especially for patients with cerebral aneurysms [2]. Therefore, postoperative pain control should be a priority for neurosurgical patients.

An increasing number of studies have suggested that multimodal pain treatment, which combines systemic analgesics and local anesthetics, optimizes pain relief and limits adverse effects of opioids [3, 4]. For example, scalp nerve block and local anesthetic infiltration of the scalp have been proposed to blunt hemodynamic response to craniotomy, decrease opioid consumption, and reduce postoperative pain perception [5–7]. Additionally, both scalp blocks and local anesthetic infiltration were recommended for enhanced recovery after surgery (ERAS) for oncological craniotomies, although the current evidence is not sufficient to create a standardized ERAS protocol for oncological craniotomy [8]. However, whether scalp nerve block or local anesthetic infiltration is more effective for analgesia has not been evaluated in craniotomy for cerebral aneurysms.

Surgery can initiate the inflammatory stress response. Surgical stress induces the migration of inflammatory cells that release cytokines, primarily interleukin (IL)-6, causing a local inflammatory response at the injured site. Then, when cytokines subsequently release into human plasma, systemic inflammation may occur that leads to an increase in C-reactive protein (CRP) and T- and B-cell activation in bone marrow and blood [9]. Later, compensatory anti-inflammatory cytokines, such as IL-10, are produced that cause a reduction in pro-inflammatory cytokine synthesis [10, 11]. Accordingly, acute-phase proteins, such as CRP, and cytokines, such as IL-6 and IL-10, are thought to be early measures of inflammatory response induced by surgical trauma. Local anesthetics via a nerve block have been demonstrated to attenuate the local inflammatory response [12]. For instance, previous animal experiments have demonstrated that C-fiber blockade may inhibit peripheral inflammation in the corresponding innervated zone [12, 13]. Furthermore, in postoperative patients, peripheral nerve blocks have been shown to attenuate postoperative inflammatory response in knee arthroplasty [14, 15]. The scalp is densely innervated with C-fibers (unmyelinated) and A-delta fibers (thinly myelinated) [16].

However, as far as we know, no study has attempted to investigate the impact of scalp nerve block on inflammatory response in the craniotomies.

Therefore, the goal of this prospective, randomized, controlled study was to compare the impact of scalp nerve block and local anesthetic infiltration with 0.75% ropivacaine on postoperative inflammatory response, intraoperative hemodynamic response, pain scores, and oxycodone consumption in the first 48 h postoperatively in patients undergoing craniotomy for cerebral aneurysms.

Methods

Patients

After written informed consent was obtained, 57 adult patients (ASA I or II, aged 18 to 65 years) who were scheduled for an elective craniotomy for surgical clipping of cerebral aneurysm located in the anterior cerebral circulation were included.

We did not enroll patients if they (1) had difficult surgical anatomy or multiple or giant aneurysms, (2) had a previous craniotomy incision, (3) had a history of allergy to opioids or local anesthetics, (4) had a history of drug dependence and alcohol abuse, or (5) could not understand a visual analog scale (VAS) or communicate [scheduled to be sedated postoperatively or a GCS (Glasgow coma score) < 14]. The first author (X.Y.) enrolled the patients in the study.

Anesthesia, surgery and postoperative pain relief

The patients included in the current study were anesthetized by the same anesthesiologist and operated on by the same surgeon. Patients received 0.03 mg/kg IV midazolam as a preanesthetic medication, and 0.25 mg prophylaxis of postoperative nausea and vomiting (PONV) was achieved with palonosetron for all patients.

Anesthesia and monitoring were standardized for all patients. Electrocardiography, pulse oximetry, noninvasive blood pressure, end-tidal CO_2 ($ETCO_2$), nasopharyngeal temperature, and bispectral index (BIS) were continuously monitored during anesthesia and were recorded at fixed intervals of 5 min. Before anesthesia induction, four electrodes for measuring EEG signals were applied to the patient's forehead, as recommended by the manufacturer (BIS Sensor, Covidien B.V. Zaltbommel, Netherlands), and were used to measure BIS values, signal quality index (SQI) and electromyography (EMG). BIS was displayed using an Aspect EEG monitor (A-2000, version 3.2; Aspect Medical Systems, Newton, M.A.). (We wiped clean the skin on the forehead with an alcohol-soaked skin wipe to lower the skin/electrode impedance. When SQI was greater than 50% the BIS values were considered valid. When SQI was less than 50% and the duration exceeded 20% of the total study time, all data for this patient was excluded.) General anesthesia was induced with 1.5–2.0 mg/kg propofol and 0.5–0.8 μg/kg sufentanil, and 0.2 mg/kg cis-atracurium was administered to facilitate orotracheal intubation. After intubation, we placed an arterial catheter to monitor mean arterial pressure (MAP) and collect a blood sample, and an intravenous catheter was placed in the right jugular vein. After intubation, all patients were ventilated mechanically with a tidal volume of 8 ml/kg, and the respiratory rate was adjusted accordingly to maintain 35–40 mmHg of paCO2 (partial pressure of carbon dioxide in the artery). Then, 4–9 mg/kg/h propofol was infused continuously to maintain anesthesia. The infusion rate of propofol was adjusted to keep the BIS within 40–60. Remifentanil was adjusted according to the degree of surgical manipulation (0.1–0.5 μg/kg/min). If intraoperative MAP and heart rate (HR) increased by more than 20% from baseline, supplemental doses of 0.5 μg/kg remifentanil were administered, and the infusion rate of remifentanil was increased by 0.05 μg/kg/min. If the increased MAP and HR did not respond to higher remifentanil infusion rate, nicardipine or esmolol was administered, as appropriate. Considering intraoperative neurophysiological monitoring, we did not administer additional neuromuscular blocker during the surgery. Normothermia was maintained throughout the surgery. Volume was replaced by 0.9% sodium chloride and 130/0.4 hydroxyethyl starch. Patients were extubated after the operation in the post-anesthetic care unit (PACU) when awake and in a neurologically stable condition before being transferred to the neurosurgical intensive care unit (NICU).

All patients were administered oxycodone (0.1 mg/kg) 30 mins before the end of surgery. Oxycodone was also used as rescue analgesia in the first 48 h postoperatively. Pain was evaluated with visual analogue scale (VAS) scores from 0 to 10 (0 = no pain, 10 = worst pain). If a patient reported a VAS more than 3, an intravenous injection of 2 mg of oxycodone was given by a nurse as the rescue analgesia. This dose was administered at 15-min intervals until VAS was less than 3. Oxycodone consumption in the first 48 postoperative hrs and the time to first rescue requirement were recorded.

Randomization

A randomization list was generated, and patients were assigned consecutively to one of three groups by the third author (R.D.), who was not involved in patient care. Scalp nerve block was performed in Group S, local anesthetic infiltration was performed in Group I, and patients in Group C only received sufentanil, remifentanil and oxycodone as analgesics during the intraoperative period.

The patients and the second author (J.M.) who followed the hemodynamic response to skin incision, drew the blood samples, and recorded postoperative pain scores and rescue analgesic consumption were blinded in every case.

Scalp nerve block and local anesthetic infiltration

In Group S, the scalp blocks were performed bilaterally with 15 mL of 0.75% ropivacaine 10 mins before the incision by the anesthesiologist using the method described by Pinosky et al. [17]. The supraorbital and supratrochlear nerves emerge from the orbit, and a 25-gauge needle was introduced above the eyebrow perpendicular to the skin. These nerves were blocked bilaterally with 4 mL of 0.75% ropivacaine. The zygomatico-temporal nerve emerges lateral to the orbit, equal to the position of pterion, and this nerve was blocked bilaterally with 2 mL of 0.75% ropivacaine. The auriculotemporal nerve was blocked bilaterally 1.5 cm anterior to the ear at the level of the tragus, the needle was introduced perpendicularly to the skin and infiltration was performed deep into the fascia and superficially as the needle was withdrawn. Care must be taken to avoid destroying the superficial temporal artery. These nerves were blocked bilaterally with 2 mL of 0.75% ropivacaine. The greater, lesser, and third occipital nerves were blocked bilaterally with 7 mL 0.75% ropivacaine injected using a 22-gauge needle along the superior nuchal line, approximately halfway between the occipital protuberance and the mastoid process.

In Group I, the surgical incision sites were infiltrated with 15 mL of 0.75% ropivacaine 10 mins before the incision by the neurosurgeon. Neither scalp blocks nor local infiltration was performed in Group C.

Outcome measurements

Patient characteristics, type of aneurysm, duration of anesthesia and surgery, total dose of propofol and remifentanil, fluid balance, and number of patients who used nicardipine or esmolol were documented.

Plasma levels of CRP, IL-6, and IL-10 were measured in pre-, intra- and. postoperative periods, and EDTA arterial blood samples were collected to measure the concentrations of CRP, IL-6, and IL-10 in plasma at the following time points: (Baseline) before the induction of anesthesia, (6H) 6 h after incision, and (12H) 12, (24H) 24, (48H) 48, and (72H) 72 h postoperatively. After centrifugation, plasma samples were stored at − 80 °C until analysis. The serum levels of CRP, IL-6, and IL-10 were measured using enzyme-linked immunosorbent assay (Elabscience Biotechnology Co. Ltd., Wuhan, China) following the manufacturer's instructions. The detection levels of cytokines and inflammatory mediators in the assays were 0.4 ng/mL for CRP, 4 pg/mL for IL-6, and 1 pg/mL for IL-10.

MAP and HR were recorded just before anesthesia induction (T1); 5 mins after induction (T2); 5 mins after skin incision (T3); 2 mins (T4) and 5 mins (T5) after the incision; during dura opening (T6); and at the end of surgery (T7).

Postoperative VAS, cumulative oxycodone consumption and postoperative pain control-related side effects such as postoperative nausea and vomiting (PONV), infection and pruritus were recorded 2, 4, 8, 12, 24, and 48 h after recovery of consciousness. Additionally, the time intervals from patient recovery to the first use of oxycodone and consumption of oxycodone 48 h postoperatively were recorded.

The primary endpoint of the current study was the effect of scalp nerve block and local infiltration with 0.75% ropivacaine on postoperative inflammatory response in patients undergoing craniotomy for cerebral aneurysms. The secondary endpoints were the effects of scalp nerve block and local infiltration on the hemodynamic response to skin incision, postoperative pain intensity, cumulative oxycodone consumption and pain control-related side effects 48 h postoperatively.

Statistical analysis

The data are expressed as the mean ± standard deviation (SD), median and interquartile range (IQR, 25–75% percentile) or number (%). The Kolmogorov–Smirnov test was used to assess the normality and homogeneity of all the variables.

Continuous variables were presented as the mean ± SD and analyzed using one-way ANOVA with post hoc correction for multiple comparisons (Bonferroni correction) to determine differences among groups. Categorical variables were described as numbers (%) and were compared using chi-square tests. Biological data (CRP, IL-6, and IL-10 levels) and hemodynamic data (HR, MAP) were compared among groups and over time using repeated-measures ANOVA. Nonnormally distributed continuous variables, such as pain scores, were presented as median and interquartile range (IQR, 25–75 percentile) and were analyzed with nonparametric tests (Kruskal–Wallis test and Mann-Whitney U-test with Bonferroni correction).

On the basis of a previous study [7], we assumed that a difference of 20% in MAP was clinically relevant, and setting α equal to 0.05 and β equal to 0.2, we calculated a necessary sample size of 15 patients per group. Values of $P < 0.05$ were considered significant. SPSS statistical software, version 21.0 (SPSS, Inc., Chicago, Illinois, USA), was used for data analysis.

Results

Patient demographics and perioperative characteristics

Fifty-seven patients agreed and were randomized into the study, and 6 patients were excluded from the study after randomization due to unexpected sedation after surgery and delayed extubation ($n = 5$, 1 in Group C, 2 in Group I and 2 in Group S) or reoperation ($n = 1$ in group I). Thus, the remaining 51 patients were analyzed (18 in Group S, 16 in Group I and 17 in Group C). The consort diagram showed the flow of participants through each stage of a randomized trial (Fig. 1).

The three groups were similar in age, gender, BMI, ASA, type of aneurysm, duration of operation, duration of anesthesia, cumulative dose of propofol, total loss of blood, urine volume and infusion volume. There were significant differences among the study groups ($F = 205.377$; $P < 0.001$, Table 1) for the cumulative dose of remifentanil. Patients in Group C received a higher cumulative dose of remifentanil (4.59 ± 0.64 mg) compared to Group I (3.67 ± 0.38 mg) and Group S (1.40 ± 0.38 mg) ($P < 0.001$, $P < 0.001$, respectively). Patients in Group I consumed more remifentanil during the operation than patients in Group S ($P < 0.001$).

Additionally, 8 patients (47.1%) in Group C, 3 patients (18.8%) in Group I, and 1 patient (5.6%) in Group S used nicardipine during the operation. Nicardipine administration was different among the three groups ($P = 0.017$ according to Fisher's exact test, Table 1), and nicardipine was less frequently required in Group S than in group C ($P = 0.007$, Table 1).

Plasma concentrations of CRP, IL-6, and IL-10

Plasma concentrations of CRP, IL-6, and IL-10 at all time points are displayed in Fig. 2. Plasma CRP levels significantly changed with time in the three groups (main effect of time: $F(3.874, 185.944) = 108.039$, $P < 0.001$). In all groups, CRP levels increased 24 h after surgery, reaching maximum values at 24 h, and subsequently decreased gradually until 72 h after the operation (Fig. 2a). Additionally, there was no significant interaction between analgesia mode and time in plasma levels of CRP (group-time interaction: $F(7.748, 185.944) = 1.43$, $P = 0.069$). Although plasma CRP was not significantly different among the three groups, there was a tendency for lower CRP in Group S compared to Groups C and I 12 and 24 h postoperatively (Fig. 2a).

The same trend applied to IL-6 levels. There was a significant difference over time among the three groups in plasma IL-6 values (main effect of time: $F(2.238, 107.447) = 303.761$, $P < 0.001$). IL-6 values increased 24 h after surgery, reaching peak at 24 h and decreasing gradually until 72 h after the operation (Fig. 2b). Moreover, there was a significant interaction between analgesia mode and time on plasma levels of IL-6 (group-time interaction: $F(4.477, 107.447) = 2.47$, $P = 0.043$), and patients in Group S had lower IL-6 6 h postoperatively compared with those in Groups C and I ($P = 0.001$, and $P = 0.009$, respectively) (Fig. 2b).

Plasma IL-10 levels significantly changed with time in all three groups (main effect of time: $F(3.189, 153.067) = 198.014$, $P < 0.001$). In all three groups, IL-10 levels increased 48 h after surgery, reaching maximum values at 12 h, and subsequently decreased gradually until 72 h after the operation (Fig. 2c). There was a significant interaction between analgesia mode and time on plasma levels of IL-10 (group-time interaction: $F(6.378, 153.067) = 5.107$, $P < 0.01$). Furthermore, patients in Group S had higher IL-10 levels 12 and 24 h postoperatively compared with those in Groups C and I (12 h: $P = 0.012$, and $P < 0.001$, 24 h: $P = 0.011$, and $P < 0.001$, respectively) (Fig. 2c).

Hemodynamic parameters (HRs and MAPs)

HRs were significantly lower in Groups I and S compared to Group C at T3, T4, T5 and T6 (group-time interaction: $F(3.46, 166.075) = 86.081$, $P < 0.001$). Post hoc analysis

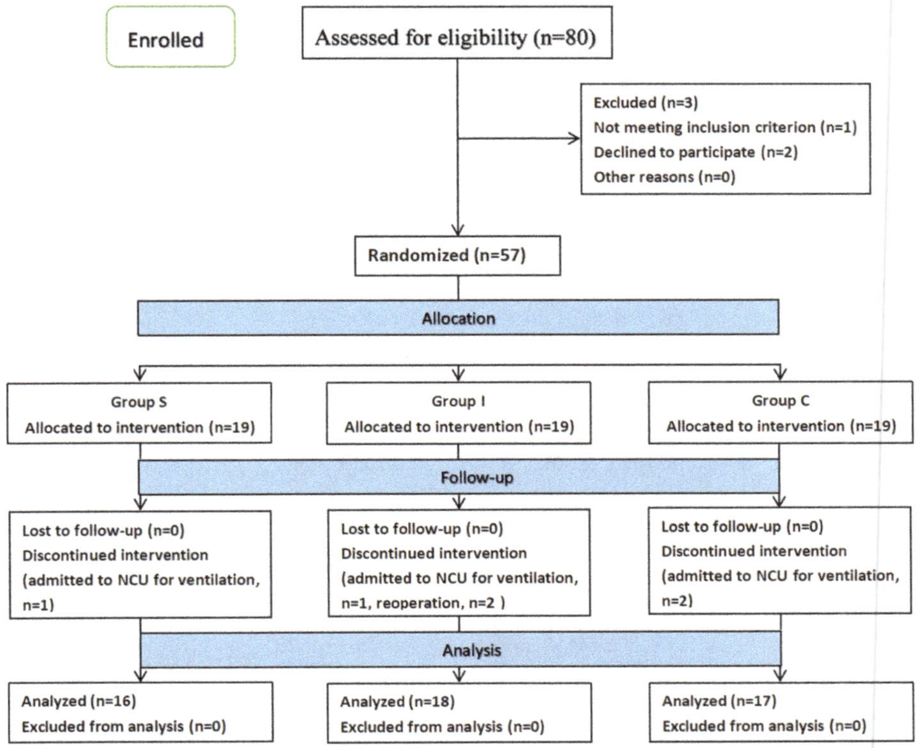

Fig. 1 CONSORT flow diagram

showed significant differences during skin incision (T3) ($P = 0.03$, $P = 0.035$, respectively) and the second (T4) ($P < 0.001$, $P < 0.001$, respectively) and fifth minutes (T5) after incision ($P < 0.001$, $P < 0.001$, respectively) and during dura opening (T6) ($P = 0.032$, $P < 0.001$, respectively). There were no significant differences in HRs between Group S and Group I at any time point ($P > 0.05$) (Fig. 3a)
.

There were significant differences in MAP among the three groups at T3, T4, T5 and T6 (group-time interaction: F(6.995, 167.883) = 24.192, $P < 0.001$). Post hoc analysis showed that MAPs were significantly lower in Group I and Group S compared to Group C during skin incision (T3) (Group S vs. Group C: $P < 0.001$, Group I vs. Group C: $P < 0.001$). Additionally, MAPs in Group S were significantly lower than those in Group I and Group C at the second (T4) and fifth minutes (T5) after the incision and during dura opening (T6) (T4, T5 and T6: Group S vs. Group I, $P < 0.001$; Group S vs. Group C, $P < 0.001$). However, there were no significant differences in MAPs between Groups I and C at T4, T5 and T6 ($P > 0.05$) (Fig. 3b).

Postoperative pain scores and oxycodone consumption

The VAS scores were significantly lower in Group S than in Group C and Group I 2, 4, 8, 12, 24 and 48 h postoperatively ($P < 0.001$, respectively). However, Group I only had lower VAS scores compared to Group C 2 h after surgery ($P = 0.026$) (Fig. 4).

The time intervals from patient recovery to the first use of oxycodone in Groups I and S were significantly longer than those in Group C [5.75(3.58–9.28) and 9.85 (7.93–14.83) vs. 1.5(0.8–3.65) hrs, $P = 0.009$, and $P < 0.001$, respectively]. In addition, the first use of oxycodone in Group S was significantly longer than that in Group I ($P = 0.018$) (Fig. 5a).

Oxycodone consumption after 48 h was significantly higher in Groups C and I than in Group S (27 ± 9.6 and 22.06 ± 12.24 vs. 5.01 ± 4.3 mg, $P < 0.001$, $P < 0.001$, respectively). There was no significant difference in oxycodone consumption between Groups I and C ($P = 0.386$) (Fig. 5b).

Pain control-related adverse events during the study period

Adverse events 48 h after surgery, such as respiration depression, cutaneous pruritus, subcutaneous hematomas, scalp infection, and local anesthetic toxicity were not observed. However, the incidence of PONV was significantly different among the three groups ($P = 0.017$, Table 2.). Five patients (29.4%) in Group C, 4 patients (25%) in Group I and 2 patients (11.1%) in Group S suffered from PONV, and PONV occurred less frequently in Group S

Table 1 Patient Demographics and Perioperative Characteristics

Characteristic	Group C (*n* = 17)	Group I (*n* = 16)	Group S (*n* = 18)	*P* values
Age (years)	54.41 ± 6.62	55.19 ± 5.94	55.94 ± 5.14	NS
Gender (M/F)	4/13	4/12	6/12	NS
BMI (kg/m^2)	22.48 ± 1.30	22.54 ± 0.80	22.51 ± 0.90	NS
ASA (I/II)	7/10	8/8	8/10	NS
Type of aneurysm (number%)				NS
Middle cerebral artery	11 (64.6%)	12 (75%)	13 (72.2%)	
Anterior communicating artery	2 (11.8%)	0	1 (5.6%)	
Posterior communicating artery	2 (11.8%)	2 (12.5%)	3 (16.6%)	
Anterior cerebral artery	2 (11.8%)	2 (12.5%)	1 (5.6%)	
Duration of operation (min)	169.41 ± 44.75	161.88 ± 36.69	155.56 ± 40.94	NS
Duration of anesthesia (min)	252.94 ± 42.65	248.44 ± 36.96	240.28 ± 41.53	NS
Total dose of propofol (mg)	1854.65 ± 375.03	1820.88 ± 233.17	1716.33 ± 206.67	NS
Total dose of remifentanil (mg)	4.59 ± 0.64	3.67 ± 0.38	1.40 ± 0.38	0.000*
Total loss of blood (ml)	370.59 ± 161.11	393.75 ± 166.21	305.56 ± 93.76	NS
Urine volume (ml)	1135.29 ± 337.16	1218.75 ± 335.10	1055.56 ± 261.72	NS
Infusion volume (ml)				
Crystalloids (ml)	1361.76 ± 644.58	1468.75 ± 618.30	1147.22 ± 269.24	NS
Colloids (ml)	1161.76 ± 264.30	1109.38 ± 240.98	1111.11 ± 213.90	NS
Number of use of nicardipine(%)	8 (47.1%)	3 (18.8%)	1 (5.6%)	0.017#
Number of use of esmolol(%)	0	0	0	NA

Values are expressed as mean ± SD or number of patients(%)
The differences among groups were not significant except for the consumption of remifentanil and the use of nicardipine
Group C Control group, *Group I* Local anesthesic infiltrationgroup, *Group S* Scalp nerve block group
Abbreviations: *ASA* American society of anaesthesiologists, *NA* Not applicable, *NS* Not significant
#$P < 0.05$ for Group I and Group S compared with group C. *$P < 0.05$ among three groups

than Group C ($P = 0.012$, Table 2). There were no significantly differences in the incidence of fever or dizziness among groups ($P = 0.721$, $P = 0.462$, respectively, Table 2).

Discussion

This prospective, randomized, controlled study demonstrated that scalp nerve block with 0.75% ropivacaine had a modest preventive effect on postoperative inflammation demonstrated by lower IL-6 concentrations in plasma 6 h after craniotomy for cerebral aneurysms and reduced CRP levels and increased IL-10 levels 12 and 24 h postoperatively. Scalp nerve block blunted the hemodynamic response to skin incision better than local anesthetic infiltration or routine anesthesia. Additionally, both the scalp nerve block and local anesthetic infiltration decreased remifentanil consumption during the operation compared to the control group, and the scalp nerve block group had lower postoperative pain intensity, longer duration before the first dose of oxycodone, less consumption of oxycodone and lower incidence of PONV 48 h postoperatively than the local anesthetic infiltration group and the control group.

Substances released by sensory nerve endings produce inflammation in the target tissue, which is a progress of neurogenic inflammation response [18]. The key point of neurogenic inflammation is the activation of the primary afferent, which cause dorsal root reflexes in the spinal cord [19]. Blocking the nerve through local anesthetics can reduce the release of substances, such as substance P and calcitonin gene–related peptide, and block neural transmission at the site of tissue injury, thereby alleviating the neurogenic inflammatory response [20]. However, the exact mechanisms are still largely unclear.

Therefore, it is possible that in the current study, the reduced concentrations of pro-inflammatory cytokines CRP and IL-6, as well as the increased concentration of anti-inflammatory cytokine IL-10 in plasma, compared to local anesthetic infiltration and routine analgesia, were related to the local anti-inflammatory effects of scalp nerve block. It is possible that scalp nerve block has a greater deafferentation effect than local anesthetic infiltration that prevents the development of peripheral and systemic inflammation. There is also evidence suggesting that inflammation and pain are related [21]. In the current study, patients in the scalp nerve

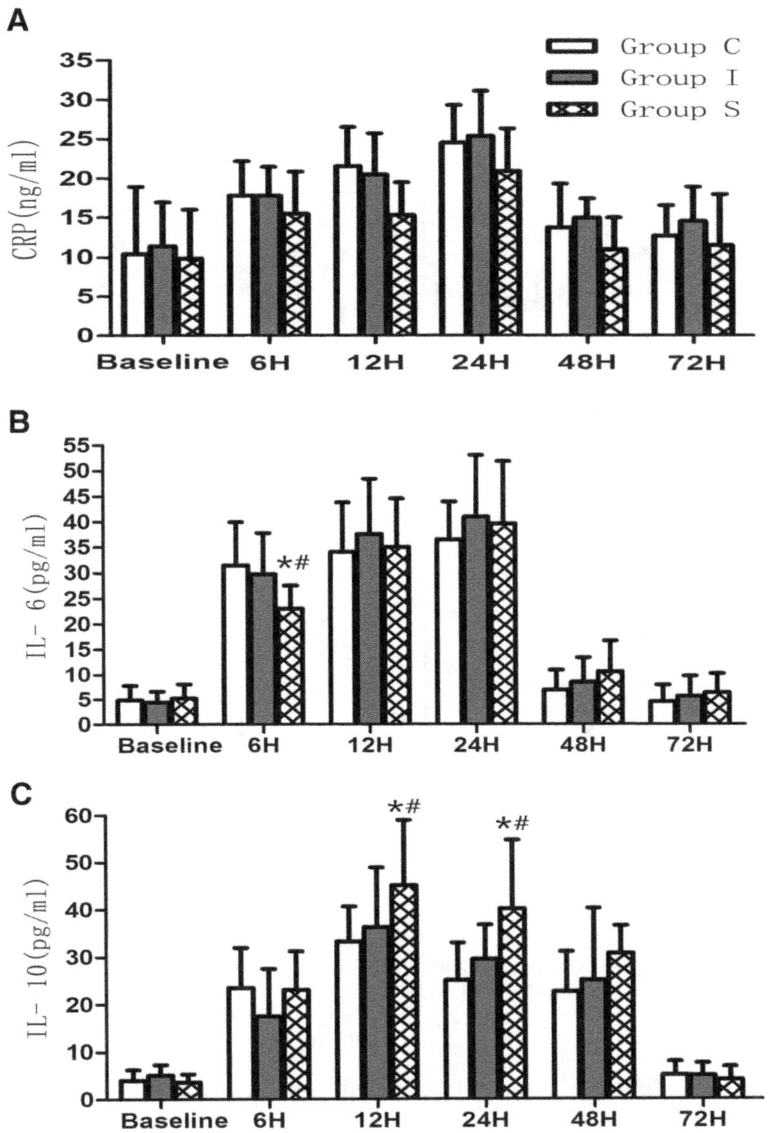

Fig. 2 Concentrations of **a** C-reactive protein (CRP), **b** interleukin-6 (IL-6), and **c** interleukin-10 (IL-10) preoperatively (Pre-op) and 6, 12, 24, 48 and 72 h postoperatively in the three groups studied. Group C: control group, Group I: local anesthetic infiltration group, Group S: scalp nerve block group. $^{*}P < 0.05$, compared to Group C, $^{\#}P < 0.001$, compared to Group I

block group had lower postoperative pain intensity and longer duration before the first dose of oxycodone than patients in the local anesthetic infiltration and routine analgesia groups, supporting our findings that scalp nerve block inhibited craniotomy-induced inflammation.

The effects of neuraxial blockade with local anesthetics on postoperative inflammatory response are still controversial. For example, a previous study suggested that a combined continuous lumbar plexus and sciatic nerve blocks with 0.2% ropivacaine contributed to the attenuation of postoperative inflammatory response, which was demonstrated by decreased CRP and IL-6 concentrations in plasma 24 and 48 h postoperatively [14]. Another clinical study using more extensive nerve blocks, such as epidural analgesia, have also indicated attenuated ex vivo pro-inflammatory cytokine IL-6 and anti-inflammatory cytokine IL-10 production after visceral surgery [22]. However, Moore and coworkers found that the circulating CRP and IL-6 response to pelvic surgery was unaffected by extradural analgesia [23]. This finding is in contrast with the present study where the scalp nerve block inhibited CRP and IL-6. Such discrepancies could originate from the nerve block technique, the type of surgery, and probably the assay used to measure the inflammatory mediator concentration (i.e., ex vivo or in vivo assays).

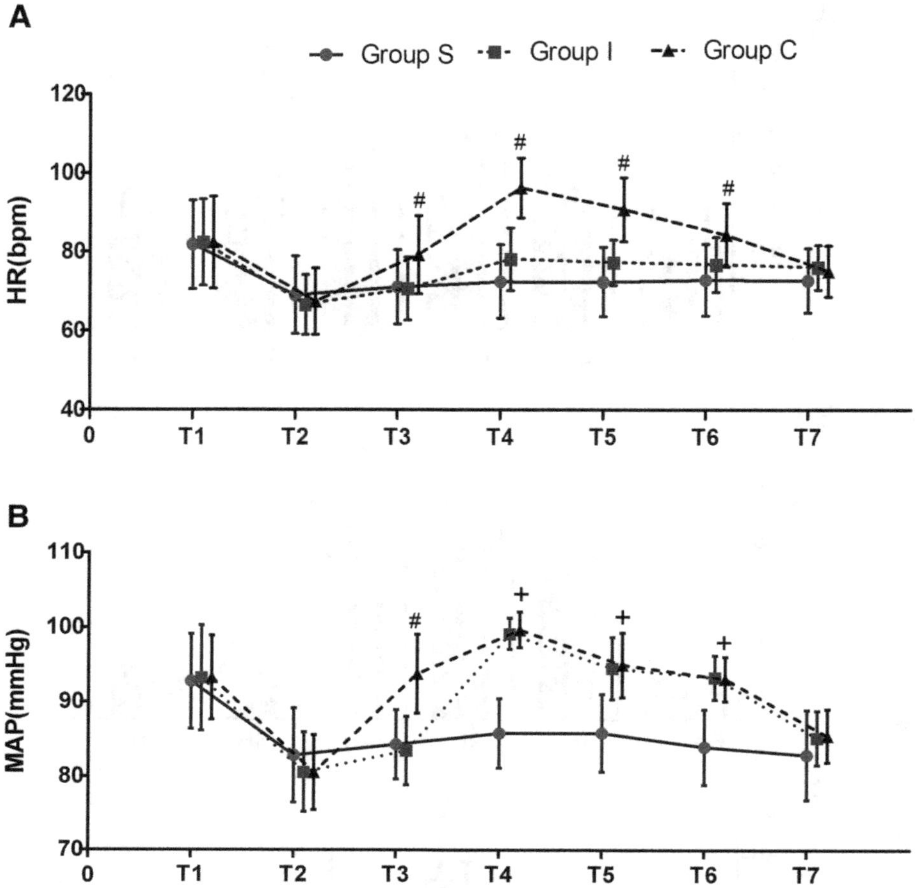

Fig. 3 Comparison of HR and MAP changes during surgery. T1: before anesthesia induction, T2: 5 mins after induction, T3: 5 mins after skin incision, T4: 2 mins after the incision, T5: 5 mins after the incision, T6: during dura opening, and T7: the end of the surgery. Group C: control group, Group I: local anesthetic infiltration group, Group S: scalp nerve block group. $^{\#}P < 0.05$, for Group C compared with Groups I and S, $^{+}P < 0.001$ for Groups I and C compared with Group S

Of note is that, in our study, scalp nerve block only had modest anti- inflammatory effects. Previous studies have indicated the impacts of remifentanil on systemic inflammation. For example, remifentanil has been indicated to reduce plasma IL-6 levels on the seventh day after abdominal surgery [24]. It has also been demonstrated to inhibit exaggerated inflammation after cardiac surgery with cardiopulmonary bypass [25]. In the present study, we found that patients in the scalp nerve block group consumed less remifentanil during the operation than patients in the local anesthetic infiltration group and the routine analgesia group. Therefore, remifentanil requirements may be a confounding factor that hampered the interpretation of the effects of different analgesic modalities on the inflammatory response caused by craniotomy. Furthermore, our study might have been underpowered because of the small study group size, which could also explain the modest anti-inflammatory effects of scalp nerve block. Collectively, our findings suggest a potential anti-inflammatory effect of scalp nerve block with 0.75% ropivacaine, pending further investigations.

Acute increases in MAP and HR could be deleterious for neurosurgical patients with cerebral aneurysm, given that acute arterial hypertension and tachycardia may result in ruptured cerebral aneurysms. In the current study, we found that scalp nerve block blunted hemodynamic response to skin incision and dura opening better than local anesthetic infiltration or routine anesthesia. These results are in line with the study by Gezel et al. [7], in which scalp nerve block with 0.5% bupivacaine was shown to be better at blunting the hemodynamic response to strong nociceptive stimulus, such as head pinning, than local infiltration or routine analgesia [7]. However, the it has also been reported that local infiltration promotes intraoperative hemodynamic stability in patients undergoing craniotomy [26–28]. Our study is inconsistent with these studies. The discrepancy may be explained by different local anesthetic used

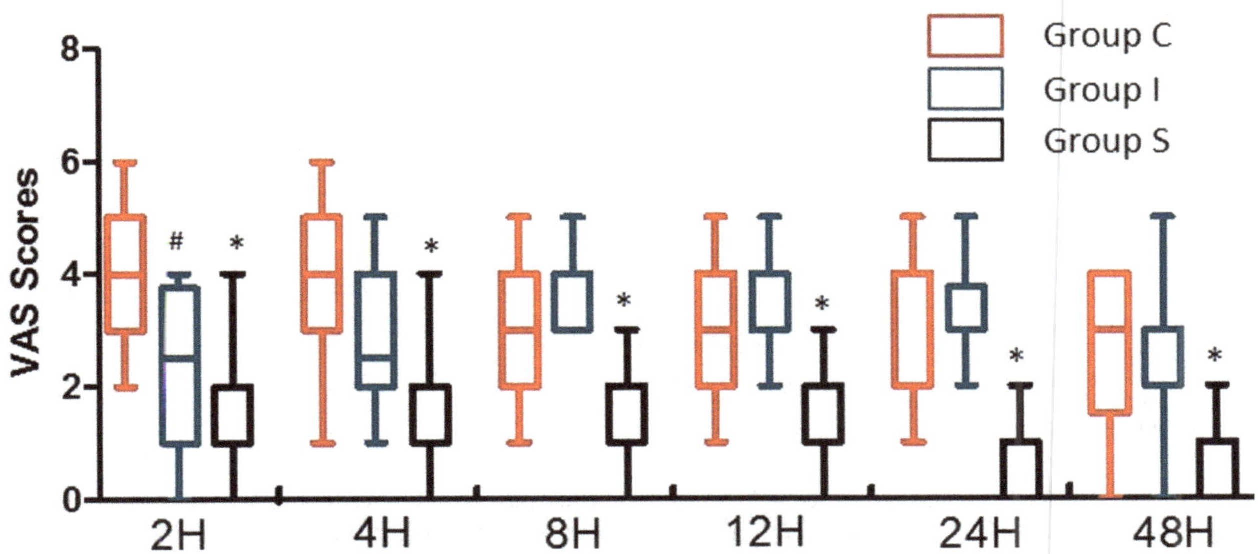

Fig. 4 Comparison of VAS scores postoperatively for all three groups. Group C: control group, Group I: local anesthetic infiltration group, Group S: scalp nerve block group. $^{\#}P < 0.05$, Compared to Group C, $^{*}P < 0.001$ for Group S compared with Groups I and C

(bupivacaine vs. ropivacaine), the time point studies or the nociceptive stimulus.

Both scalp nerve block and local infiltration have been demonstrated to reduce VAS scores and opioid requirements after surgery. For example, a meta-analysis of scalp blocks demonstrated not only a significant reduction in VAS scores 2, 4, 6 and 8 h after the operation, with the most significant mean reduction occurring 1 h after surgery, but also a decrease in opioid requirements over the first 24 h postoperatively. However, few studies have compared the effects of scalp nerve block and local infiltration on postoperative pain control. In the current study, we found that the scalp nerve block group had lower postoperative pain intensity, longer duration of time before the first dose of oxycodone, less consumption of oxycodone and lower incidence of PONV 48 h postoperatively than the local infiltration group and control group. Our study is consistent with the study by Hwang et al. [29], showing that

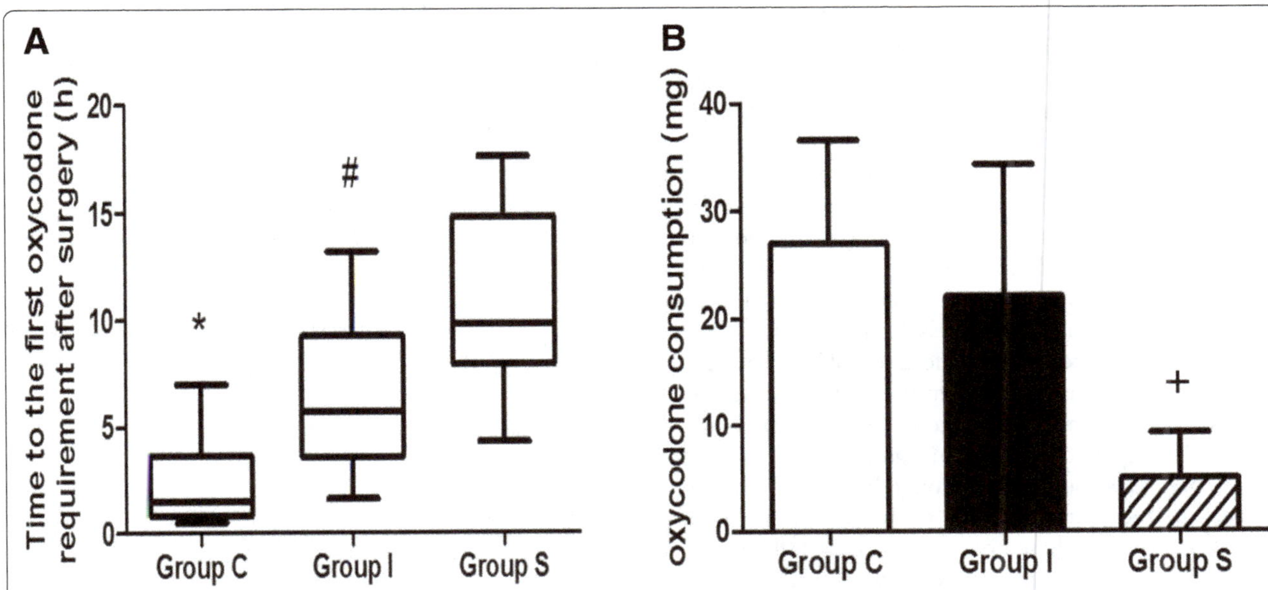

Fig. 5 Comparison of **a** first patient request for rescue analgesia and **b** oxycodone consumption during the first 48 postoperative hrs. Group C: control group Group I: local anesthetic infiltration group, Group S: scalp nerve block group. $^{*}P < 0.01$ for Group C compared with Groups I and S, $^{\#}P < 0.05$ for Group I compared with Group S, $^{+}P < 0.001$ for Group S compared with Groups C and I

Table 2 Pain control related adverse events during the study period (48 h after surgery)

	Group C (n = 17)	Group I (n = 16)	Group S (n = 18)	*P* values
Fever	1 (5.9%)	2 (12.5%)	1 (5.6%)	NS
Nausea and Vomit*	5 (29.4%)	4 (25%)	2 (11.1%)	0.017*
Dizziness	1 (5.9%)	0	1 (5.6%)	NS
Respiration depression	0	0	0	NA
Cutaneous pruritus	0	0	0	NA
Subcutaneous haematomas	0	0	0	NA
Scalp infection	0	0	0	NA
Local anesthetic toxicity	0	0	0	NA

Values are given as number of patients(%)
Group C Control group, *Group I* Local anesthesic infiltration group, *Group S* Scalp nerve block group
Abbreviations: *NA* Not applicable, *NS* Not significant
*P < 0.05 comparison among three groups

scalp blocks with 0.75% levobupivacaine effectively lowered postoperative pain and PCA consumption 72 h after patients underwent frontoparietal craniotomy for aneurysm clipping compared to routine analgesia. In our study, the beneficial effect of the scalp block lasted longer than the expected duration of action. This phenomenon could be explained by preemptive analgesia [30], which commences before surgery and continues in the postoperative period, preventing the establishment of peripheral and central sensitization since we performed the scalp block prior to scalp incision [31].

It is noteworthy that in our study, PONV occurred less frequently in the scalp nerve block group than the local infiltration group and the control group. It is possible that the lower incidence of PONV in the scalp nerve block group was related to less intraoperative remifentanil consumption and postoperative oxycodone use.

The current study has several limitations. First, 0.75% ropivacaine (15 mL, 112.5 mg) was used for the scalp nerve block and local infiltration, but the plasma concentration was not measured, and the maximum recommended dose of ropivacaine is 225 mg with or without epinephrine [32]. Furthermore, in our study, no patient developed side effects related to local anesthetic toxicity. Second, we did not apply isotonic sodium chloride for the scalp nerve block or local infiltration in the control group. Thus, we could not rule out the effects of injection stress. Third, in the present study, we only focused on the effects of different analgesic modalities on systemic inflammatory response but not local inflammatory response at the site of tissue injury. Fourth, because the impact of different analgesic modalities on inflammatory response to craniotomy has been rarely reported, in the current pilot study, the sample size calculation was done based on MAP and not inflammatory markers in response to craniotomy. Accordingly, the present study may not be sufficiently powered to provide strong evidence for the effects of scalp nerve block and local anesthetic infiltration on inflammatory response, hemodynamic response, or postoperative pain control in patients undergoing craniotomy due to the small sample size. A larger study with adequate power is needed to validate our results. Finally, in the current study, we only evaluated the effect of the ropivacaine scalp block on acute pain after craniotomy (48 h postoperatively) but not chronic postcraniotomy headache. These limitations indicate the need for further investigations.

Conclusions

In conclusion, the present study shows that scalp nerve block with 0.75% ropivacaine attenuated inflammatory response to craniotomy for cerebral aneurysms, blunted hemodynamic response to scalp incision, and controlled postoperative pain better than local anesthetic infiltration or routine anesthesia. Scalp nerve block should be considered in conjunction with general anesthesia for aneurysm clipping. Scalp nerve block might exert potential anti-inflammatory neuroanesthetic effects pending further investigations.

Abbreviations

BIS: Bispectral index; CRP: C-reactive protein; EMG: Electromyography; ERAS: Enhanced recovery after surgery; ETCO2: End-tidal CO2; GCS: Glasgow coma score; HR: Heart rate; ICP: Increased intracranial pressure; IL-6: Interleukin-6; IQR: Interquartile range; LA: Local anesthetic infiltration; MAP: Mean arterial pressure; NICU: Neurosurgical intensive care unit; paCO2: Partial pressure of carbon dioxide in the artery; PACU: Post-anesthetic care unit; PONV: Postoperative nausea and vomiting; SNB: Scalp nerve block; SQI: Signal quality index; VAS: Visual analog scale

Acknowledgments

Not applicable.

Authors' contributions

Each author's individual contributions to the manuscript are as follows: XY: This author helped enroll patients in the study and test patient samples. JM: This author helped record experimental data and gather specimens. RD: This author helped group the patients. YYL, LC and KL: These authors helped analyze the data. MP and ZZZ: These authors helped design experiments and write the manuscript. All authors read and approved the final manuscript.

References

1. Flexman AM, Ng JL, Gelb AW. Acute and chronic pain following craniotomy. Curr Opin Anaesthesiol. 2010;23:551–7.
2. Owens WB. Blood pressure control in acute cerebrovascular disease. J Clin Hypertens (Greenwich). 2011;13:205–11.
3. Lee EJ, Lee MY, Shyr MH, Cheng JT, Toung TJ, Mirski MA, Chen TY. Adjuvant bupivacaine scalp block facilitates stabilization of hemodynamics in patients undergoing craniotomy with general anesthesia: a preliminary report. J Clin Anesth. 2006;18:490–4.
4. Guilfoyle MR, Helmy A, Duane D, Hutchinson PJ. Regional scalp block for postcraniotomy analgesia: a systematic review and meta-analysis. Anesth Analg. 2013;116:1093–102.
5. Batoz H, Verdonck O, Pellerin C, Roux G, Maurette P. The analgesic properties of scalp infiltrations with ropivacaine after intracranial tumoral resection. Anesth Analg. 2009;109:240–4.
6. Law-Koune JD, Szekely B, Fermanian C, Peuch C, Liu N, Fischler M. Scalp infiltration with bupivacaine plus epinephrine or plain ropivacaine reduces postoperative pain after supratentorial craniotomy. J Neurosurg Anesthesiol. 2005;17:139–43.
7. Geze S, Yilmaz AA, Tuzuner F. The effect of scalp block and local infiltration on the haemodynamic and stress response to skull-pin placement for craniotomy. Eur J Anaesthesiol. 2009;26:298–303.
8. Hagan KB, Bhavsar S, Raza SM, Arnold B, Arunkumar R, Dang A, Gottumukkala V, Popat K, Pratt G, Rahlfs T, Cata JP. Enhanced recovery after surgery for oncological craniotomies. J Clin Neurosci. 2016;24:10–6.
9. Kishimoto T. The biology of interleukin-6. Blood. 1989;74:1–10.
10. Hildebrand F, Pape HC, Krettek C. The importance of cytokines in the posttraumatic inflammatory reaction. Unfallchirurg. 2005;108:793–4 6-803.
11. Mannick JA, Rodrick ML, Lederer JA. The immunologic response to injury. J Am Coll Surg. 2001;193:237–44.
12. Beloeil H, Ababneh Z, Chung R, Zurakowski D, Mulkern RV, Berde CB. Effects of bupivacaine and tetrodotoxin on carrageenan-induced hind paw inflammation in rats (part 1): hyperalgesia, edema, and systemic cytokines. Anesthesiology. 2006;105:128–38.
13. Gentili ME, Mazoit JX, Samii KK, Fletcher D. The effect of a sciatic nerve block on the development of inflammation in carrageenan injected rats. Anesth Analg. 1999;89:979–84.
14. Bagry H, de la Cuadra Fontaine JC, Asenjo JF, Bracco D, Carli F. Effect of a continuous peripheral nerve block on the inflammatory response in knee arthroplasty. Reg Anesth Pain Med. 2008;33:17–23.
15. Martin F, Martinez V, Mazoit JX, Bouhassira D, Cherif K, Gentili ME, Piriou P, Chauvin M, Fletcher D. Antiinflammatory effect of peripheral nerve blocks after knee surgery: clinical and biologic evaluation. Anesthesiology. 2008; 109:484–90.
16. Bin Saif GA, Ericson ME, Yosipovitch G. The itchy scalp--scratching for an explanation. Exp Dermatol. 2011;20:959–68.
17. Pinosky ML, Fishman RL, Reeves ST, Harvey SC, Patel S, Palesch Y, Dorman BH. The effect of bupivacaine skull block on the hemodynamic response to craniotomy. Anesth Analg. 1996;83:1256–61.
18. Szolcsanyi J. Capsaicin-sensitive sensory nerve terminals with local and systemic efferent functions: facts and scopes of an unorthodox neuroregulatory mechanism. Prog Brain Res. 1996;113:343–59.
19. Willis WD Jr. Dorsal root potentials and dorsal root reflexes: a double-edged sword. Exp Brain Res. 1999;124:395–421.
20. Coderre TJ, Katz J, Vaccarino AL, Melzack R. Contribution of central neuroplasticity to pathological pain: review of clinical and experimental evidence. Pain 1993;52:259–85.
21. Zhang JM, An J. Cytokines, inflammation, and pain. Int Anesthesiol Clin. 2007;45:27–37
22. Beilin B, Bessler H, Mayburd E, Smirnov G, Dekel A, Yardeni I, Shavit Y. Effects of preemptive analgesia on pain and cytokine production in the postoperative period. Anesthesiology. 2003;98:151–5.
23. Moore CM, Desborough JP, Powell H, Burrin JM, Hall GM. Effects of extradural anaesthesia on interleukin-6 and acute phase response to surgery. Br J Anaesth. 1994;72:272–9.
24. De Cosmo G, Sessa F, Fiorini F, Congedo E. Effect of remifentanil and fentanyl on postoperative cognitive function and cytokines level in elderly patients undergoing major abdominal surgery. J Clin Anesth. 2016;35:40–6.
25. von Dossow V, Luetz A, Haas A, Sawitzki B, Wernecke KD, Volk HD, Spies CD. Effects of remifentanil and fentanyl on the cell-mediated immune response in patients undergoing elective coronary artery bypass graft surgery. J Int Med Res. 2008;36:1235–47.
26. Bloomfield EL, Schubert A, Secic M, Barnett G, Shutway F, Ebrahim ZY. The influence of scalp infiltration with bupivacaine on hemodynamics and postoperative pain in adult patients undergoing craniotomy. Anesth Analg. 1998;87:579–82.
27. Mohammadi SS, Shahbazian E, Shoeibi G, Almassi F. Effect of scalp infiltration with bupivacaine on early hemodynamic responses during craniotomy under general anesthesia. Pak J Biol Sci. 2009;12:603–6.
28. Hartley EJ, Bissonnette B, St-Louis P, Rybczynski J, McLeod ME. Scalp infiltration with bupivacaine in pediatric brain surgery. Anesth Analg. 1991; 73:29–32.
29. Hwang JY, Bang JS, Oh CW, Joo JD, Park SJ, Do SH, Yoo YJ, Ryu JH. Effect of scalp blocks with levobupivacaine on recovery profiles after craniotomy for aneurysm clipping: a randomized, double-blind, and controlled study. World Neurosurg. 2015;83:108–13.
30. Kaye AD, Baluch A, Kaye AJ, Gebhard R, Lubarsky D. Pharmacology of cyclooxygenase-2 inhibitors and preemptive analgesia in acute pain management. Curr Opin Anaesthesiol. 2008;21:439–45.
31. Kissin I. Preemptive analgesia. Anesthesiology. 2000;93:1138–43.
32. Rosenberg PH, Veering BT, Urmey WF. Maximum recommended doses of local anesthetics: a multifactorial concept. Reg Anesth Pain Med. 2004;29: 564–75 discussion 24.

23

Cytotoxicity of amide-linked local anesthetics on melanoma cells via inhibition of Ras and RhoA signaling independent of sodium channel blockade

Qinghong Zheng, Xiaohong Peng and Yaqin Zhang*

Abstract

Background: Substantial clinical and preclinical evidence have indicated the association between amide-linked local anesthesia and the long-term outcomes of cancer patients. However, the potential effects of local anesthesia on cancer recurrence are inconclusive and the underlying mechanisms remain poorly understood.

Methods: We systematically examined the effects of three commonly used local anesthetics in melanoma cells and analyzed the underlying mechanisms focusing on small GTPases.

Results: Ropivacaine and lidocaine but not bupivacaine inhibited migration and proliferation, and induced apoptosis in melanoma cells. In addition, ropivacaine and lidocaine but not bupivacaine significantly augmented the in vitro efficacy of vemurafenib (a B-Raf inhibitor for melanoma with BRAF V600E mutation) and dacarbazine (a chemotherapeutic drug). Mechanistically, ropivacaine but not bupivacaine decreased the activities of Ras superfamily members with the dominant inhibitory effects on RhoA and Ras, independent of sodium channel blockade. Rescue studies using constitutively active Ras and Rho activator calpeptin demonstrated that ropivacaine inhibited migration mainly through RhoA whereas growth and survival were mainly inhibited through Ras in melanoma cells. We further detected a global reduction of downstream signaling of Ras and RhoA in ropivacaine-treated melanoma cells.

Conclusion: Our study is the first to demonstrate the anti-melanoma activity of ropivacaine and lidocaine but not bupivacaine, via targeting small GTPases. Our findings provide preclinical evidence on how amide-linked local anesthetics could affect melanoma patients.

Keywords: Local anesthetics, Ras, RhoA, Voltage-gated sodium channel, Melanoma

Background

Melanoma is a highly aggressive skin malignancy with increasing incidence over the past decades [1]. The current treatment include radio-chemotherapy for early stage of melanoma, targeted therapy such as B-raf inhibitor vemurafenib for metastatic melanoma [2], surgery to remove the tumor at all stages of melanoma [3]. Several retrospective studies of patients undergoing cancer surgery indicate that the choice of anesthetic technique might translate into a clinical benefit such as prolonged survival after cancer surgery [4]. In particular, local anesthesia has been shown to reduce tumor metastasis and recurrence in patients undergoing surgery with breast or prostate cancer [5, 6]. Additionally, regional anesthesia in combination with or without general anesthesia would result in improved overall survival in patients with colorectal cancer [7].

In line with clinical observations, preclinical studies suggest that amide-linked local anesthetics have anti-tumor effects. Ropivacaine, lidocaine and bupivacaine are amide-linked local anesthetics and act on neuron cells via blocking voltage-gated sodium-channel (VGSC)

* Correspondence: minizhang0616@163.com
Department of Anesthesia, Wuhan Fourth Hospital; Puai Hospital, Tongji Medical College, Huazhong University of Science and Technology, 473 Hanzheng Street, Qiaokou District, Wuhan 430033, Hubei, China

and subsequent depolarization suppression [8]. They have been shown to exhibit anti-proliferative, anti-metastatic and pro-apoptotic potential on cell culture and xenograft mouse models in a variety of cancers [9–13]. In addition, local anesthetics preferentially target cancer stem cells [14]. Apart from their direct inhibitory effects on tumor cells, ropivacaine and lidocaine also negatively affect tumor microenvironment, such as angiogenesis [15, 16].

In this study, we thoroughly investigated the effect of ropivacaine, lidocaine and bupivacaine alone and their combination with anti-melanoma drugs on melanoma cell migration, proliferation and survival. We show that ropivacaine and lidocaine but not bupivacaine has anti-melanoma activity and acts synergistically with standard of care drugs in melanoma. We further demonstrate that the underlying mechanisms are via targeting RhoA and Ras signaling pathways, and this is in a VGSC blockade-independent manner.

Methods

Cell culture and drug reconstitution

Human melanoma cell lines A375 and A431 (Cell Lines Service, Germany) were cultured in RPMI 1640 medium (Invitrogen, US) supplemented with 2 mM glutamine and 10% heat-inactivated fetal bovine serum (Gibco, US). Ropivacaine and bupivacaine (Sigma, US) were dissolved in water and lidocaine was reconstituted in Hanks Balanced Salt Solution. Veratridine (R&D Systems, US), vemurafenib (LC Laboratories, US), calpeptin (Sigma, US) and dacarbazine (Selleckchem, US) were reconstituted in dimethyl sulfoxide (DMSO). Tetrodotoxin (Sigma, US) was dissolved in citrate buffer.

Proliferation assay

5×10^3 cells were seeded to each well in a 96-well plate. The next day, cells were treated with drugs at various concentrations for 72 h. Proliferation was measured using bromodeoxyuridine / 5-bromo-2′-deoxyuridine (BrdU) Cell Proliferation Assay Kit (Abcam, US) as per manufacturer's protocols.

Measurement of cell apoptosis and migration

Migration assay was performed using the Boyden chamber (Cell Biolabs Inc. US) with transwell inserts of 8 μm pore size as described in our previous study [17]. The migrated cells from five random fields were counted under the microscope (Zeiss, Germany). Apoptosis assay was assessed by flow cytometry of Annexin V staining as described in our previous study [13]. The treatment duration for migration and apoptosis were 8 h and 72 h, respectively.

Western blot analyses

After 24 h drug treatment, total protein was extracted using lysis buffer contained 4% SDS, protease inhibitor cocktail and phosphatase inhibitor (Roche, US). Equal amount of total proteins was resolved using denaturing sodium dodecyl sulfate-polyacrylamide gel electrophoresis and analyzed by Western blot. Antibodies used in WB analyses include anti-p-MYPT1 (Cell Signaling, Cat. No.4563), anti-p-MLC (Cell Signaling, Cat.No.3671), anti-MLC (Cell Signaling, Cat.No.3672), anti-MYPT1 (Cell Signaling, Cat. No.2634), anti-p-Raf (Abcam, Cat. No. ab135559), anti-Raf (Abcam, Cat. No. ab137435), anti-p-ERK (Santa Cruz, Cat. No. sc-16,982), anti-ERK (Santa Cruz, Cat. No. sc-292,838), anti-Ras(Q61L) antibody (NewEast Biosciences, Cat. No. NEBA10195) and anti-β-actin (Santa Cruz, Cat. No. sc-130,656). Immunoblots shown in the accompanying figures are representative of three independent experiments.

Measurement of RhoA, Rac1 and Ras activity

After 24 h drug treatment, cellular RhoA, Rac1 and Ras activities were assessed using total cell lysates and were measured using RhoA G-LISA Activation Assay Kit, Rac1 G-LISA Activation Assay Kit and Ras G-LISA Activation Assay Kit (Cytoskeleton Inc. US).

Plasmid transfection

Cells were transfected with control plasmid (pSecTag2A vector) and pHras (Q61L). Constitutively active Ras (Q61L) was cloned to pSecTag2A from Addgene plasmid # 83186. Plasmid DNA transfection was performed using Lipofectamine 2000 transfection reagent (Invitrogen) as per the manufacture's protocol. Cells were processed for cellular assays at 48 h post-transfection.

Statistical analyses

All data are expressed as mean and standard error measurement (SEM) to indicate data variability. Comparisons of categorical variables by student t test or one way ANOVA were performed using Prism version 8.0 (GraphPad Inc., USA). *P*-value < 0.05 was defined as statistically significant.

Results

Ropivacaine and lidocaine but not bupivacaine demonstrates anti-migratory, anti-proliferative and pro-apoptotic effects to melanoma cells

We first analyzed the effects of three commonly used local anesthetics on melanoma cells migration, growth and survival. Two human cell lines modeling in vitro melanoma with varying cellular origin and genetic profiling were chosen in this study. A375 harbors BRAF V600E mutation and is p53 positive whereas A431 contains wildtype BRAF [18]. Ropivacaine, lidocaine and bupivacaine at concentration range from 0.2 to 2 mM were tested. As shown in Fig. 1a and b, and supplementary Figs. 1 and 2, ropivacaine and lidocaine significantly inhibited both A375 and A431 cell migration in a concentration-dependent manner. In addition, ropivacaine and lidocaine decreased proliferation as shown by BrdU level and induced apoptosis as shown by Annexin V percentage in melanoma cells (Fig. 1c and d, and supplementary Figs. 3 and 4). Notably, ropivacaine is more potent than lidocaine in melanoma cells. We also observed that the starting concentration (0.25 mM) required to inhibit migration is the lowest compared to the concentration (0.5 mM) needed to inhibit proliferation and induce apoptosis, suggesting that ropivacaine is more effective in inhibiting migration than growth and survival in melanoma cells. In contrast, bupivacaine up to 2 mM did not affect melanoma cell migration, growth or survival (Fig. 1).

Ropivacaine and lidocaine but not bupivacaine augments the inhibitory effects of vemurafenib and dacarbazine in melanoma cells

We next determined the combinatory effects of local anesthetics with drugs commonly used for melanoma treatment. Dacarbazine is a chemotherapeutic drug for metastatic melanoma [19] and vemurafenib is a B-Raf enzyme inhibitor to treat late stage of melanoma with BRAF V600E mutation [20]. The dose we had selected for combination studies is the dose that gives moderate effect as single drug alone. We found that ropivacaine and lidocaine significantly enhanced the in vitro efficacy of dacarbazine in suppressing migration and proliferation,

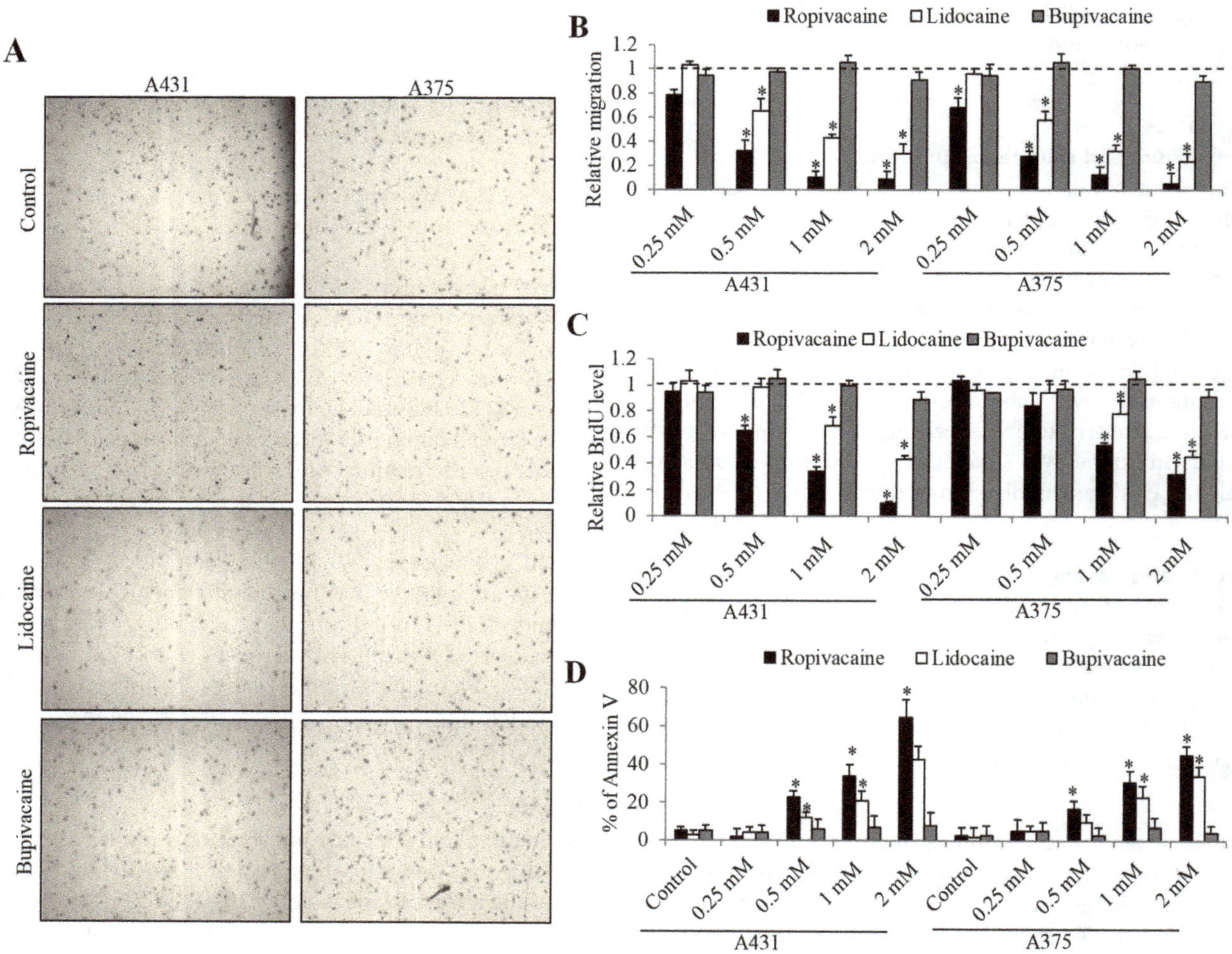

Fig. 1 The inhibitory effects of local anesthetics on melanoma cell migration, growth and survival. (**a**) Representative images of melanoma cell migration in the absence and presence of 1 mM ropivacaine, lidocaine or bupivacaine. (**b**) Quantification of five random fields per sample using NIH ImageJ software shows the anti-migratory effects of ropivacaine and lidocaine but not bupivacaine in A375 and A431 cells. The differential effects of three local anesthetics at concentration range from 0.25 to 2 mM on melanoma cell proliferation (**c**) and survival (**d**). Annexin V-positive cells were considered as apoptotic cells. The data were derived from three independent experiments and presented as mean ± SEM. *$p < 0.05$, compared to control

and inducing apoptosis in melanoma cells (Fig. 2 and supplementary 5 to 8). Similarly, the combination of vemurafenib with ropivacaine or lidocaine is more effective than vemurafenib alone (Fig. 2). The combinatory effects of local anaesthetics with vemurafenib or dacarbazine are likely to be synergistic. For example, the Annexin V% in the combinatory group is more than the sum of Annexin V% in two single drugs. We did not observe further inhibition of the combination of bupivacaine with vemurafenib or dacarbazine in melanoma cells (Fig. 2). These results demonstrate that ropivacaine and lidocaine but not bupivacaine acts synergistically with both targeted therapy or chemo therapy drugs in melanoma cells.

Ropivacaine but not bupivacaine inhibits GTPases activities in melanoma cells in a voltage-gated sodium channel (VGSC)-independent manner

RhoA, Rac1 and Ras are members of Ras super family of small GTPases that are critically involved in tumor cell biological activities such as migration, growth and survival [21]. Our previous study has revealed that ropivacaine inhibited esophageal carcinoma cells via targeting

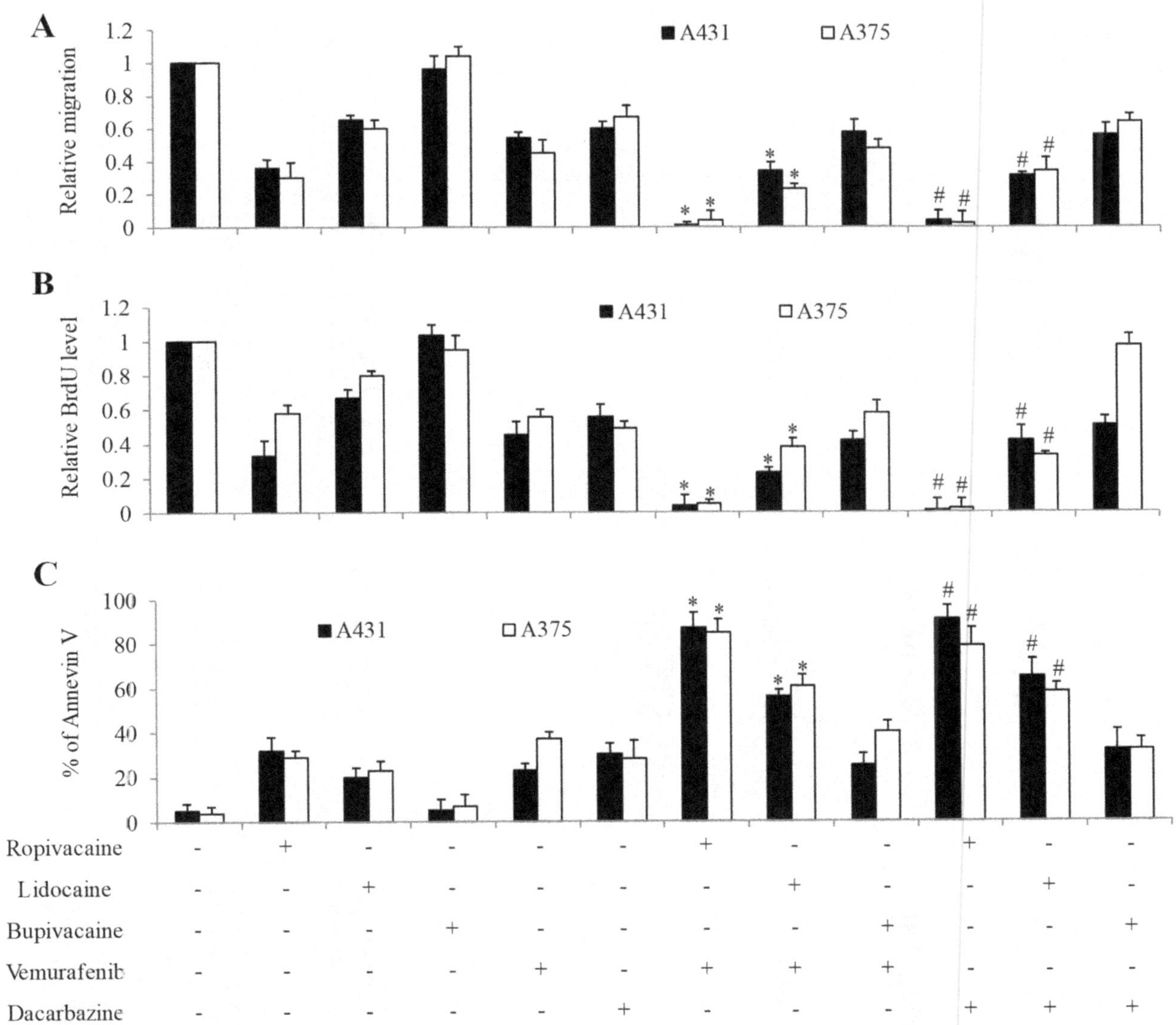

Fig. 2 The combinatory effects of local anesthetics with vemurafenib and dacarbazine on melanoma cell migration, growth and survival. Ropivacaine and lidocaine but not bupivacaine significantly further enhanced the anti-migratory (**a**), anti-proliferative (**b**) and pro-apoptotic (**c**) effects of vemurafenib and dacarbazine. Vemurafenib at 1 μM and dacarbazine at 50 μM were used for the combination studies. Ropivacaine, lidocaine and bupivacaine at 0.5 mM, 1 mM and 1 mM were used for migration, proliferation and apoptosis assays, respectively. The data were derived from three independent experiments and presented as mean ± SEM. *$p < 0.05$, compared to vemurafenib; #$p < 0.05$, compared to dacarbazine

Rac1 [17]. To understand the molecular mechanism of ropivacaine's action in melanoma cells, we investigated the effects of ropivacaine on small GTPases. We found that ropivacaine significantly decreased RhoA, Rac1 as well as Ras activities in melanoma cells (Fig. 3a to c). Similar to ropivacaine, we found that lidocaine also significantly decreased the activities of RhoA, Rac1 and Ras in melanoma cells (Supplementary Fig. S9). In contrast, bupivacaine which did not display inhibitory effects on melanoma cells did not affect RhoA, Rac1 and Ras activities (Fig. 3a to c), suggesting the specific inhibitory effects of ropivacaine on these small GTPases. Additionally, ropivacaine decreased RhoA and Ras activities to a larger extent than Rac1 activity, suggesting that the dominant effects of ropivacaine are inhibition of RhoA and Ras rather than Rac1 in melanoma cells.

We next determined whether the inhibitory effects of ropivacaine on small GTPases were associated with ropivacaine's action on voltage-gated sodium channels (VGSC) [8]. We found that VGSC activator vetratridine at concentrations that abolished amide-linked local anesthesia-induced membrane depolarization [22] did not affect melanoma cell RhoA, Rac1 or Ras activity (Fig. 3d to f). Furthermore, VGSC blocker tetrodotoxin at the concentration that inhibits all VGSCs in excitable membranes [23] did not affect these small GTPases activities (Fig. 3d to f). The addition of tetrodotoxin did not abolish the inhibitory effects of ropivacaine on RhoA and Ras activities (Supplementary Fig. 10). These results suggest that the inhibitory effects of ropivacaine on small GTPases are not associated with sodium channel blockade.

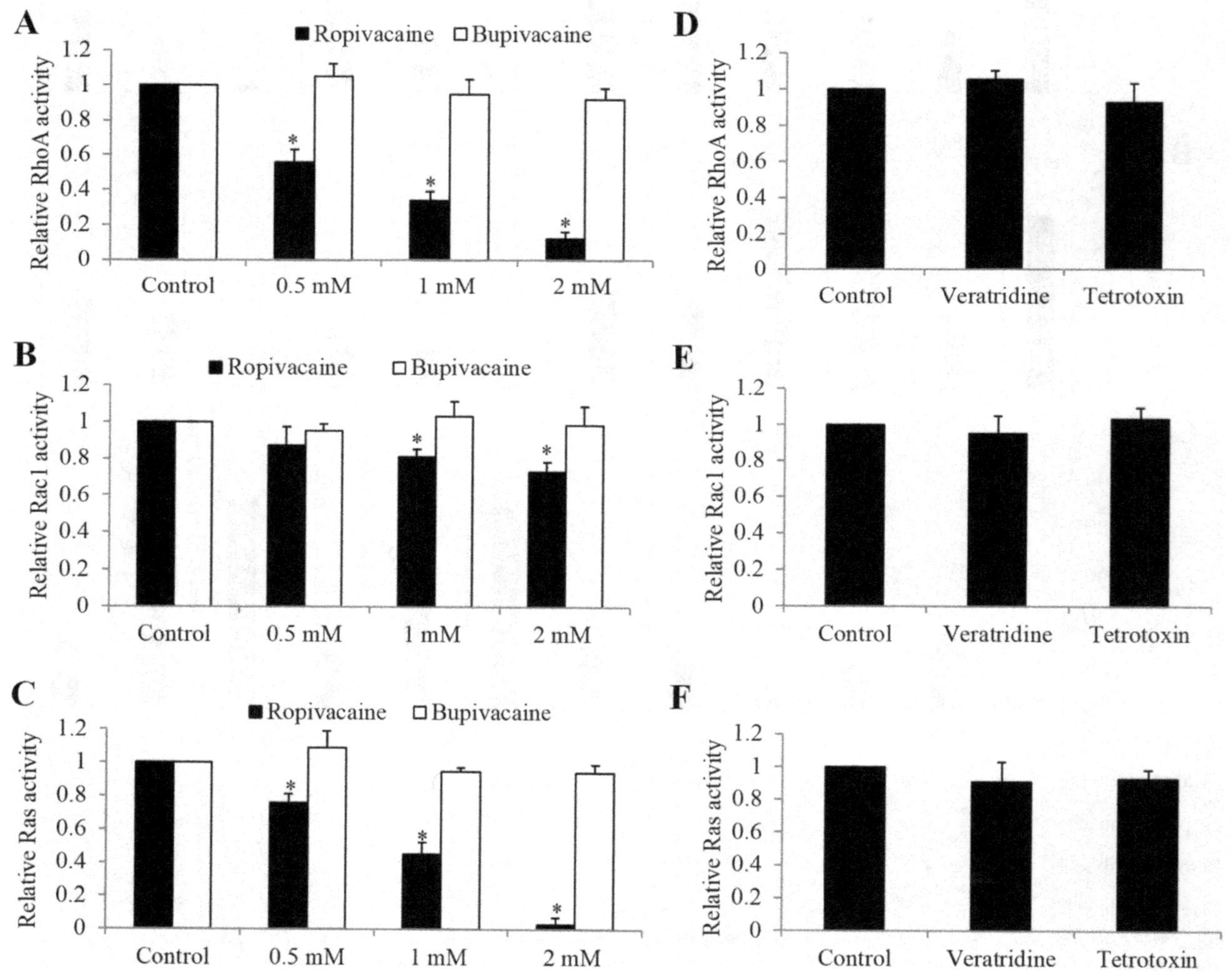

Fig. 3 Ropivacaine but not bupivacaine or sodium channel inhibitor and activator decreased RhoA, Rac1 and Ras activities in melanoma cells. Ropivacaine but not bupivacaine significantly decreased RhoA (**a**), Rac1(**b**) and Ras (**c**) activities in A431 cells. Sodium channel activator veratridine (0.03 mM) and blocker tetrodotoxin (100 nM) did not affect RhoA (**d**), Rac1 (**e**) and Ras (**f**) activity in A431 cells. The data were derived from three independent experiments and presented as mean ± SEM. *$p < 0.05$, compared to control

Ropivacaine acts on melanoma cells via inhibiting Ras and RhoA signalling pathways

To confirm that ropivacaine acts on melanoma cells via targeting small GTPases, we attempted to rescue ropivacaine's inhibitory effects using genetic and pharmacological approaches. We overexpressed constitutively active Ras (Q61L) in A431 melanoma cells and observed the increased mRNA and protein level of Ras (Q61L) as well as increased Ras activity (Fig. 4a and Supplementary Fig. 11). As expected, the decreased Ras activity by ropivacaine was rescued by Ras (Q61L) overexpression. Notably, we further found that overexpression of constitutively active Ras partially but significantly abolished the inhibitory effects of ropivacaine on melanoma cell migration, growth and survival (Fig. 4b to d), demonstrating that Ras inhibition is involved in ropivacaine's ability in inhibiting melanoma cell migration, growth and survival. In addition, Rho activator I calpeptin [24] also partially but significantly reversed the anti-migratory and anti-proliferative but not pro-apoptotic effects of ropivacaine (Fig. 4e to h), indicating that RhoA inhibition is involved in ropivacaine's ability in inhibiting melanoma cell migration and growth but not survival. Consistently, western blot analysis of phosphorylation level of the essential molecules downstream of Ras and RhoA signalling in cells exposed to ropivacaine demonstrated the decreased phosphorylation of Raf and MEK, MYPT1 and MLC (Fig. 4i), demonstrating that ropivacaine inhibits Ras/Raf/ERK and RhoA/MYPT1/MCL signalling pathways in melanoma cells.

Discussion

In this present study, we found that ropivacaine and lidocaine but not bupivacaine resulted in significant inhibitions of cell migration and growth, and

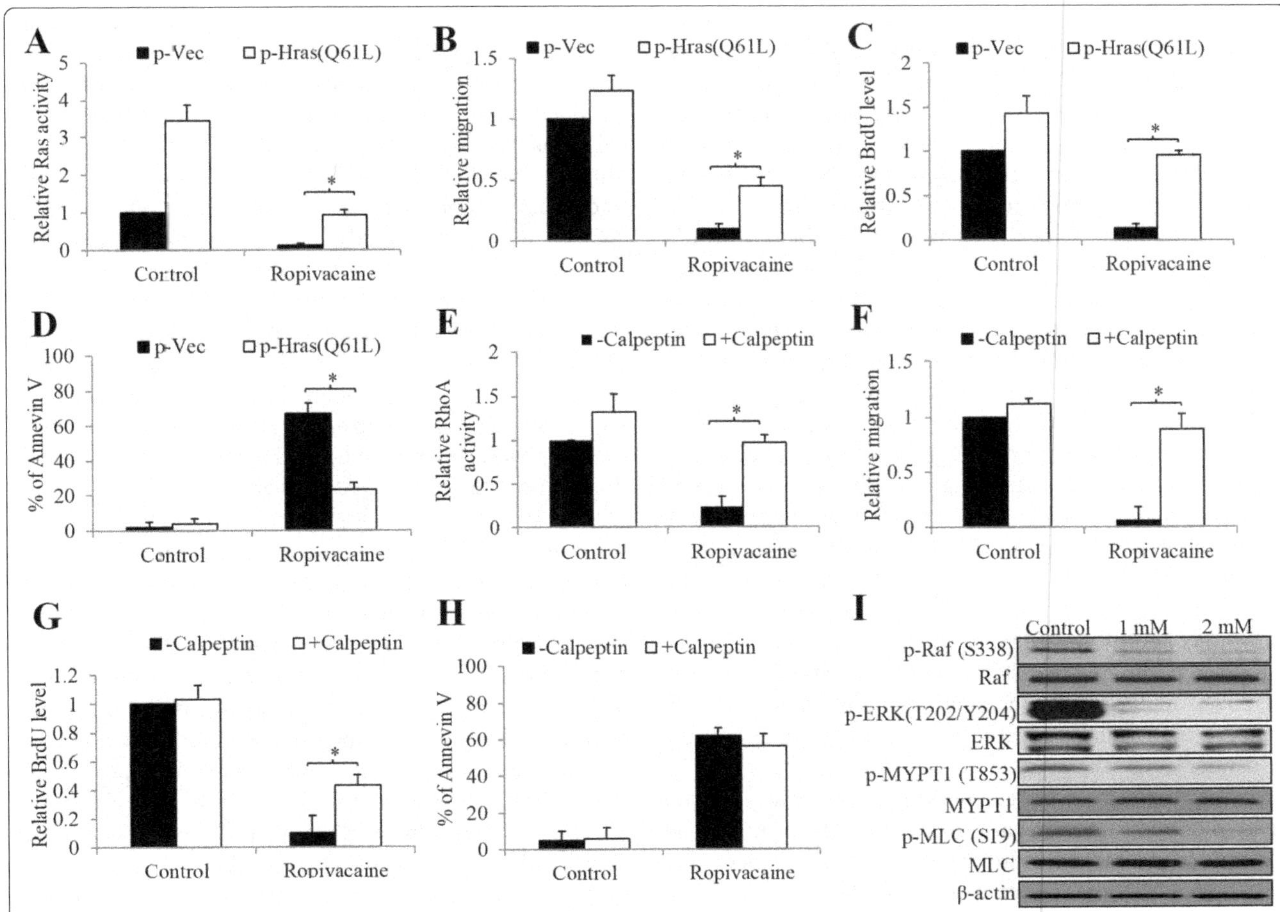

Fig. 4 Ropivacaine's inhibitory effects were abolished by active Ras overexpression or RhoA activator in melanoma cells. Overexpression of constitutively active Ras significantly reversed the effects of ropivacaine (2 mM) in decreasing Ras activity (**a**), inhibiting migration (**b**), decreasing BrdU level (**c**) and inducing apoptosis (**d**) in A431 cells. RhoA activator calpeptin significantly reversed the effects of ropivacaine (2 mM) in decreasing RhoA activity (**e**), inhibiting migration (**f**) and decreasing BrdU level (**g**) in A431 cells. (**h**) Calpeptin did not reverse ropivacaine's effect in inducing apoptosis in A431 cells. (**i**) Western blot of A431 cells treated with ropivacaine for 24 h. Representative western blot photos were shown. $^{*}p < 0.05$, compared to p-Vec or -Calpeptin

induction of cell apoptosis in melanoma. This is consistent with the previous study showing the cytotoxic effects of local anesthesia through lidocaine and ropivacaine on a human melanoma cell line [25]. Our study further extends the previous study by showing that 1) bupivacaine is not toxic to melanoma cells; 2) local anesthetics have differential effects on the varying biological activities of melanoma cells; and 3) the molecular mechanisms are via targeting small GTPases.

After treatment of ropivacaine and lidocaine but not bupivacaine at concentration range from 0.25 to 2 mM, we observed a significant reduction on the migrated cell number and BrdU level, and an increase in the percentage of Annexin V in two cell lines which represent human melanoma model with different cellular origin and oncogenic mutations (Fig. 1). The mean peak plasma concentrations of local anesthetics following transversus abdominis plane block is between 1 and 3 μM [26]. Similarly, Li et al's work referred 0.02 to 0.1 mM as clinical relevance doses of local anesthetics [27]. The rational of testing concentration of local anesthetics that far exceeds the plasma concentration is because local anesthetics have wide range of uses in clinical practice and their plasma concentrations can vary widely. In addition, the surrounding tissues of tumor could be infiltrated with local anesthetic at the concentration range of clinical preparations. For example, the local infiltration concentration of ropivacaine can reach ~ 8 mM [27]. It is interesting to note that ropivacaine and lidocaine are more effective in inhibiting migration and growth than inducing apoptosis, suggesting that their anti-migratory and anti-proliferative effects are more pronounce in melanoma cells. This is supported by our previous study that ropivacaine potently inhibits esophageal cancer cell migration without affecting survival [17]. In addition, both ropivacaine and lidocaine significantly enhanced the in vitro efficacy of vemurafenib and dacarbazine in melanoma cells (Fig. 2). This is consistent with the previous work [13, 17], demonstrating the enhanced efficacy between amide-linked local anaesthetic and anti-cancer agents in cancer cells.

Although the anti-cancer activity of bupivacaine has been demonstrated in various cancers, including gastric cancer, prostate cancer and ovarian cancer [9, 28], our work and Li et al's work demonstrate that bupivacaine does not affect melanoma migration, growth and survival [29]. In addition, bupivacaine does not inhibit breast cancer cell function [30]. Bupivacaine has been shown to augment chemotherapeutic agents' efficacy in ovarian cancer and gastric cancer [9]. In gastric cancer model, we also demonstrated that bupivacaine acts synergistically with chemo drugs [17]. However, we did not observe any combinatory effects in melanoma cells when bupivacaine was combined with standard of care drugs for melanoma (Fig. 2). The differential effects observed in different types of cancers suggest that the anti-cancer activity of bupivacaine is cancer type-dependent.

The majority of melanoma cases demonstrate oncogenic activation of the KIT—NRAS—BRAF—MEK—ERK central axis that is a major regulator of cell differentiation and proliferation [31]. We identified that Ras and RhoA were the targets of ropivacaine in melanoma cells. Ropivacaine inhibited Ras and RhoA activities, and their global downstream signalling (Fig. 3 and 4a to c and i). The lack of changes in Ras and RhoA activities in melanoma cells following bupivacaine treatment (Fig. 3a to c) may also explain their unchanged migration, growth and survival behaviours. Particularly, we further revealed that ropivacaine inhibited migration mainly via suppressing RhoA whereas induced apoptosis mainly via inhibiting Ras in melanoma cells (Fig. 4a to h), and furthermore that this was not dependent on VGSC (Fig. 3d to f). As amide-linked local anesthetics, ropivacaine, lidocaine and bupivacaine act on neuron cells via blocking VGSC [8]. In our study, we found that ropivacaine acts on melanoma cells in a VGSC-independent manner. Other relevant studies including our previous work also demonstrate that the anti-cancer activities of local anesthetics are not through blocking VGSC [17, 32]. This might explain the differential activity of local anesthetics in cancer. We previously showed that ropivacaine targeted small GTPases via inhibiting prenylation in esophageal cancer cells [17]. Given our results that the activities of all tested small GTPases were affected by ropivacaine, we speculate that prenylation inhibition is likely to be involved in ropivacaine's action in melanoma cells.

In conclusion, we have demonstrated a direct inhibitory effect of ropivacaine and lidocaine but not bupivacaine on melanoma cells, which are associated with sodium channel-independent inhibition of Ras and RhoA signaling (Supplementary Fig. 12). These findings indicate the differential effects of local anesthetics in cancer, depending on cancer types. Our findings provide experimental evidence and rationale to select the optimal anaesthetic regimens to further benefit melanoma patient care. However, we would also like to highlight that our work is not without limitations. Given the complexity in in vivo microenvironment and clinical settings, further large-scale prospective clinical trials are warranted to determine the effects of local anesthetics on longer-term reoccurrence or metastasis in patients with melanoma.

Supplementary information

Additional file 1 Figure S1. The inhibitory effects of local anesthetics on melanoma cell migration. **Figure S2.** The inhibitory effects of local anesthetics on melanoma cell migration. **Figure S3.** The inhibitory effects of local anesthetics on melanoma cell survival. **Figure S4**. The inhibitory effects of local anesthetics on melanoma cell survival. **Figure S5.** The combinatory effects of local anesthetics with vemurafenib and dacarbazine on melanoma cell migration. **Figure S6**. The combinatory effects of local anesthetics with vemurafenib and dacarbazine on melanoma cell migration. **Figure S7.** The inhibitory effects of local anesthetics on melanoma cell survival. **Figure S8.** The inhibitory effects of local anesthetics on melanoma cell survival. **Figure S9.** Lidocaine decreased RhoA, Rac1 and Ras activities in melanoma cells. **Figure S10.** Tetrodotoxin does not abolish the inhibitory effect of ropivacaine in decreasing small GTPases activities in melanoma cells. **Figure S11.** Overexpression of Ras(Q61L) in A431 cells. **Figure S12.** The molecular mechanisms of ropivacaine's action on melanoma.

Abbreviations

BrdU: Bromodeoxyuridine / 5-bromo-2'-deoxyuridine; DMSO: Dimethyl sulfoxide; SEM: Standard error measurement; VGSC: Voltage-gated sodium-channel

Acknowledgements

Not applicable.

Authors' contributions

QHZ and YQZ designed the experiments. QHZ and XHP performed each of the tests and collated the data. QHZ and YQZ analysed the results and prepared the manuscript. The author(s) read and approved the final manuscript.

References

1. Siegel RL, Miller KD, Jemal A. Cancer statistics, 2015. CA Cancer J Clin. 2015; 65(1):5–29.
2. Fisher R, Larkin J. Vemurafenib: a new treatment for BRAF-V600 mutated advanced melanoma. Cancer Manag Res. 2012;4:243–52.
3. Valko-Rokytovska M, Bruchata K, Simkova J, Milkovicova M, Kostecka Z. Current trends in the treatment of malignant melanoma. Neoplasma. 2016; 63(3):333–41.
4. Gottschalk A, Sharma S, Ford J, Durieux ME, Tiouririne M. Review article: the role of the perioperative period in recurrence after cancer surgery. Anesth Analg. 2010;110(6):1636–43.
5. Exadaktylos AK, Buggy DJ, Moriarty DC, Mascha E, Sessler DI. Can anesthetic technique for primary breast cancer surgery affect recurrence or metastasis? Anesthesiol. 2006;105(4):660–4.
6. Biki B, Mascha E, Moriarty DC, Fitzpatrick JM, Sessler DI, Buggy DJ. Anesthetic technique for radical prostatectomy surgery affects cancer recurrence: a retrospective analysis. Anesthesiol. 2008;109(2):180–7.
7. Chen WK, Miao CH. The effect of anesthetic technique on survival in human cancers: a meta-analysis of retrospective and prospective studies. PLoS One. 2013;8(2):e56540.
8. Heavner JE. Local anesthetics. Curr Opin Anaesthesiol. 2007;20(4):336–42.
9. Xuan W, Zhao H, Hankin J, Chen L, Yao S, Ma D. Local anesthetic bupivacaine induced ovarian and prostate cancer apoptotic cell death and underlying mechanisms in vitro. Sci Rep. 2016;6:26277.
10. Bundscherer A, Malsy M, Gebhardt K, Metterlein T, Plank C, Wiese CH, Gruber M, Graf BM. Effects of ropivacaine, bupivacaine and sufentanil in colon and pancreatic cancer cells in vitro. Pharmacol Res. 2015;95-96:126–31.
11. Wang HW, Wang LY, Jiang L, Tian SM, Zhong TD, Fang XM. Amide-linked local anesthetics induce apoptosis in human non-small cell lung cancer. J Thorac Dis. 2016;8(10):2748–57.
12. Xing W, Chen DT, Pan JH, Chen YH, Yan Y, Li Q, Xue RF, Yuan YF, Zeng WA. Lidocaine induces apoptosis and suppresses tumor growth in human hepatocellular carcinoma cells in vitro and in a Xenograft model in vivo. Anesthesiol. 2017;126(5):868–81.
13. Zheng Q, Peng X, Yu H. Local anesthetic drug inhibits growth and survival in chronic myeloid leukemia through suppressing PI3K/Akt/mTOR. Am J Med Sci. 2018;355(3):266–73.
14. Ni J, Xie T, Xiao M, Xiang W, Wang L. Amide-linked local anesthetics preferentially target leukemia stem cell through inhibition of Wnt/beta-catenin. Biochem Biophys Res Commun. 2018;503(2):956–62.
15. Gao J, Hu H, Wang X. Clinically relevant concentrations of lidocaine inhibit tumor angiogenesis through suppressing VEGF/VEGFR2 signaling. Cancer Chemother Pharmacol. 2019;83(6):1007–15.
16. Yang J, Li G, Bao K, Liu W, Zhang Y, Ting W. Ropivacaine inhibits tumor angiogenesis via sodium-channel-independent mitochondrial dysfunction and oxidative stress. J Bioenerg Biomembr. 2019;51(3):231–8.
17. Zhang Y, Peng X, Zheng Q. Ropivacaine inhibits the migration of esophageal cancer cells via sodium-channel-independent but prenylation-dependent inhibition of Rac1/JNK/paxillin/FAK. Biochem Biophys Res Commun. 2018;501(4):1074–9.
18. Giard DJ, Aaronson SA, Todaro GJ, Arnstein P, Kersey JH, Dosik H, Parks WP. In vitro cultivation of human tumors: establishment of cell lines derived from a series of solid tumors. J Natl Cancer Inst. 1973;51(5):1417–23.
19. Serrone L, Zeuli M, Sega FM, Cognetti F. Dacarbazine-based chemotherapy for metastatic melanoma: thirty-year experience overview. J Exp Clin Cancer Res. 2000;19(1):21–34.
20. Bollag G, Tsai J, Zhang J, Zhang C, Ibrahim P, Nolop K, Hirth P. Vemurafenib: the first drug approved for BRAF-mutant cancer. Nat Rev Drug Discov. 2012; 11(11):873–86.
21. Wennerberg K, Rossman KL, Der CJ. The Ras superfamily at a glance. J Cell Sci. 2005;118(Pt 5):843–6.
22. Barshack I, Levite M, Lang A, Fudim E, Picard O, Ben Horin S, Chowers Y. Functional voltage-gated sodium channels are expressed in human intestinal epithelial cells. Digestion. 2008;77(2):108–17.
23. Catterall WA. Neurotoxins that act on voltage-sensitive sodium channels in excitable membranes. Annu Rev Pharmacol Toxicol. 1980;20:15–43.
24. Schoenwaelder SM, Burridge K. Evidence for a calpeptin-sensitive protein-tyrosine phosphatase upstream of the small GTPase rho. A novel role for the calpain inhibitor calpeptin in the inhibition of protein-tyrosine phosphatases. J Biol Chem. 1999;274(20):14359–67.
25. Kang DK, Zhao LY, Wang HL. cytotoxic effects of local anesthesia through lidocaine/ropivacaine on human melanoma cell lines. Rev Bras Anestesiol. 2016;66(6):594–602.
26. Trabelsi B, Charfi R, Bennasr L, Marzouk SB, Eljebari H, Jebabli N, Sassi MB, Trabelsi S, Maghrebi H. Pharmacokinetics of bupivacaine after bilateral ultrasound-guided transversus abdominis plane block following cesarean delivery under spinal anesthesia. Int J Obstet Anesth. 2017;32:17–20.
27. Li R, Xiao C, Liu H, Huang Y, Dilger JP, Lin J. Effects of local anesthetics on breast cancer cell viability and migration. BMC Cancer. 2018;18(1):666.
28. Dan J, Gong X, Li D, Zhu G, Wang L, Li F. Inhibition of gastric cancer by local anesthetic bupivacaine through multiple mechanisms independent of sodium channel blockade. Biomed Pharmacother. 2018;103:823–8.
29. Li T, Chen L, Zhao H, Wu L, Masters J, Han C, Hirota K, Ma D. Both bupivacaine and Levobupivacaine inhibit colon cancer cell growth but not melanoma cells in vitro. J Anesth. 2019;33(1):17–25.
30. Ecimovic P, Murray D, Doran P, Buggy DJ. Propofol and bupivacaine in breast cancer cell function in vitro - role of the NET1 gene. Anticancer Res. 2014;34(3):1321–31.
31. Ji Z, Flaherty KT, Tsao H. Targeting the RAS pathway in melanoma. Trends Mol Med. 2012;18(1):27–35.
32. Piegeler T, Votta-Velis EG, Liu G, Place AT, Schwartz DE, Beck-Schimmer B, Minshall RD, Borgeat A. Antimetastatic potential of amide-linked local anesthetics: inhibition of lung adenocarcinoma cell migration and inflammatory Src signaling independent of sodium channel blockade. Anesthesiol. 2012;117(3):548–59.

24

Ethnic considerations in the upper lip bite test: The reliability and validity of the upper lip bite test in predicting difficult laryngoscopy in Koreans

Jong Chan Kim, Yumin Ki, Jihee Kim and So Woon Ahn*

Abstract

Background: Several methods have been used to predict difficult tracheal intubation. Among recently suggested methods, the upper lip bite test (ULBT) could serve as a good predictor. Soft tissue and skeletal hard tissue profiles are affected by many factors including ethnicity. We aimed to assess the clinical utility of the ULBT in Koreans while considering ethnic differences.

Methods: Three-hundred-forty-four Korean patients undergoing general anesthesia with orotracheal intubation were included. Preoperatively, we recorded the patient's Modified Mallampati (MMT) classification, ULBT ratings, and the Cormack–Lehane grade.

Results: The area under the receiver operating characteristic (ROC) curve (AUC) was lower for the ULBT than the MMT (95% confidence interval: 0.0697–0.191, $p < 0.0001$). The ULBT showed high accuracy (73.83%) and specificity (98.04%). On the other hand, the ULBT showed significantly lower sensitivity (4.49%). Only nine of 344 Korean patients could not bite their upper lip; among them, only three presented a difficult laryngoscopic view.

Conclusions: One factor related to the low sensitivity is the low incidence of a grade III ULBT in Koreans. In Asians, the scarcity of a grade III ULBT is explainable as a result of anteriorly displaced temporomandibular joints and redundant lip soft tissues. Despite its high specificity, the low sensitivity and AUC of the ULBT mean that the test results should be interpreted cautiously in Koreans. Ethnic differences should be considered when evaluating parameters related to soft tissues such as the ULBT.

Background

Predicting difficult laryngoscopic endotracheal intubation (TI) is an important concern for anesthesiologists. Anticipated difficulties offer opportunities to prepare alternative methods and use proper advanced management techniques. The Mallampati classification and other methods have been used to evaluate anatomical structures during the preoperative period for airway assessment.

Khan et al. suggested the upper lip bite test (ULBT) to, evaluates the ability of a patient to cover the mucosa of the upper lip with the lower incisors [1]. This simple bedside test was shown to have a good predictive value, specificity, and accuracy without the need for a light or sitting position [1, 2].

This method was based on cephalometric measurements, which differed in skeletal hard tissue and soft tissue profiles of Asian and Caucasian populations [3–10]. The ULBT evaluates mandibular movement, which reflects not only differences in skeletal hard tissue but also the conjointed movements of the ligaments, connective tissues, and soft tissues. In our experiences and other studies, there are some differences in ULBT in Koreans [11]. We suppose these discrepancies might be derived from cephalometric differences in Asian.

* Correspondence: iatria@hanmail.net
Department of Anesthesiology and Pain Medicine, CHA Bundang Medical Center, CHA University, 59 Yatap-ro, Bundang-gu, Seongnam-si, Gyeonggi-do 13496, South Korea

This study aimed to assess the differences in the ULBT in Koreans while considering ethnic differences. We tried to figure out the influence of the cephalometric differences to ULBT in Koreans.

Methods

After obtaining approval from the Severance Hospital Institutional Review Board (IRB number: 4–2008-0583), the trial was performed at Yonsei University Severance Hospital.

The written informed consent was obtained from all subjects participating in the trial.

Three hundred forty-four Korean adult patients undergoing general anesthesia with orotracheal intubation were included in our registered prospective observational study. (ClinicalTrials.gov identifier: NCT01908218, Principal investigator: So Woon Ahn, Date of registration JUL 2013). This manuscript adheres to the applicable EQUATOR Network guidelines. Patients were excluded if they had facial anomalies, had temporomandibular(TM) joint disorder, were edentulous or required a rapid sequence induction. In the pre-anesthetic care unit, we recorded each patient's age, sex, weight, height, American Society of Anesthesiologists (ASA) classification, Modified Mallampati (MMT) class [12], ULBT ratings [1], inter-incisor distance (With the mouth open maximally, measure the distance between the incisors, IID), thyromental distance (distance from the thyroid notch to the tip of the jaw, TMD), sternomental distance (distance from the chin (mentum) to the top of the notch of the thyroid cartilage, SMD) in sitting and fully head-extended position. The choice of the anesthesia induction technique was left to the attending anesthesiologist. After the loss of a response to a train- of -four or single- twitch ulnar nerve stimulation, laryngoscopy was performed by three skilled anesthesiologists (trained for at least four years, > 1000 endotracheal intubations) using a Macintosh laryngoscope with a size 3 or 4 blades. After obtaining a view of the glottis by direct laryngoscopy, the anesthesiologist assessed the Cormack - Lehane grade [13]. Grades 1 and two were considered as easy laryngoscopies. Grades 3 and 4 were considered difficult laryngoscopies from the inability to visualize the vocal cords. Grading was checked with no external laryngeal pressure. After the first attempted laryngoscopic view with Cormack –Lehane grade 3 or 4, external laryngeal pressure (backward upward rightward pressure maneuver [BURP]) was applied. [12] In the case of a second failed endotracheal intubation, an attempt with another intubation method such as fiber-optic bronchoscopy or video laryngoscopy assisted intubation was attempted and recorded.

Based on an institutional pilot study, the area under the receiver operating characteristic (ROC) curve (AUC)s of the MMT and ULBT were 0.61 and 0.52, respectively. We determined that 344 patients would be required to demonstrate a difference between two predicting tools with a type 1 error (α) of 5% and power (1-β) of 90%(two-sided) using the PASS program (NCSS, Kaysville, UT, USA).

For continuous variables, a Student's t-test was used to assess differences in means between the groups. For categorical data, a chi-square test was used to assess differences in proportions across the categories. The cut-off points of thyromental, sternomental and mouth opening distances were obtained from the analysis on the ROC which was calculated maximize the sensitivity and specificity [14]. Each test, individually and together with various combinations, was evaluated by its calculated sensitivity, specificity, positive predictive value (PPV) and negative predictive value (NPV). A comparison of the predictability for each test was performed using AUCs. The significance of the difference between the two areas was assessed using the method described by Delong [15]. Statistical analysis was done by SPSS, version 22.0 (SPSS, Inc., Chicago, IL, USA) and Medcalc 14.8.1 (MedCalc Software, Ostend, Belgium).

Results

Data were collected from four hundred forty-four elective surgical patients. Seventy-five patients were excluded because they were edentulous or the patients did not undergo TI because of changes in their anesthetic plans. A total of 344 patients' data were analyzed (Fig. 1, Table 1).

During direct laryngoscopy, 89 patients presented with a difficult laryngoscopic view (Cormack–Lehane grade of 3 or 4) without external manipulation (Table 2). Among

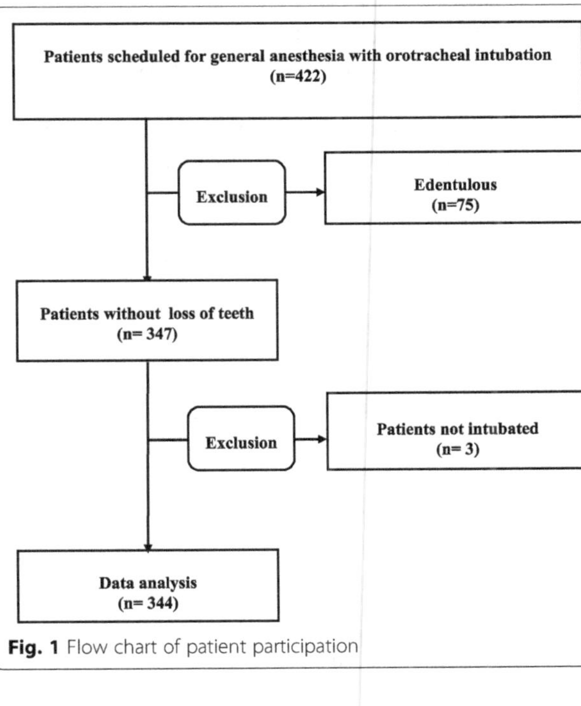

Fig. 1 Flow chart of patient participation

Table 1 Patients' characteristics

All patients $n = 344$	CL grade 1 & 2 = easy laryngoscopy $n = 255$	CL 3 & 4 = difficult laryngoscopy $n = 89$	P -value
Men [n (%)]	104 (68%)	49 (32%)	0.025‡
Women [n (%)]	151 (79.1%)	40 (20.9%)	
Age (yr)	43.17 ± 15.26	51.13 ± 15.19*	< 0.001
Height (cm)	162.86 ± 9.91	163.45 ± 8.99	0.786
Weight (Kg)	62.80 ± 11.60	62.70 ± 9.42	0.764
Body mass index (kg/m^2)	23.60 ± 3.32	23.45 ± 2.75	0.784†
ASA			
1	152(59.6%)	31(34.8%)	
2	97(38.0%)	56(62.9%)	
3	6(2.4%)	2(2.2%)	
Inter-Incisor distance (mm)	45.45 ± 7.20	41.15 ± 6.07*	<.0001†
Thyromental distance (mm)	84.18 ± 15.30	78.98 ± 11.26*	0.0002†
Sternomental distance (mm)	182.33 ± 22.38	173.83 ± 19.38*	0.003†

Values are number (proportion) or mean ± standard deviation; ‡, The Chi-square test; §, The Fisher exact test; †, The Mann–Whitney U test.CL grade: Cormack-Lehane grade

these patients, 86 could be intubated by applying external laryngeal pressure, and two required alternative techniques. One patient was intubated using video laryngoscopy (Glidescope®, Saturn Biomedical Systems, Burnaby, BC, Canada) and another patient was intubated with the use of fiber-optic devices. Moreover, one patient was intubated successfully after multiple laryngoscopic trials while waiting for the preparation of alternative devices.

An MMT class > II, IID ≤ 4.5 cm, TMD ≤ 8.3 cm, and SMD ≤ 17.9 cm were defined as cut-off points for difficult intubation (Table 3).

Table 4 shows the true positive, false positive, true negative, false negative, accuracy, sensitivity, specificity, PPV, and NPV; moreover, AUCs obtained from the ROC analysis are shown for the MMT and ULBT (Appendix).

The AUC, the primary endpoint of this trial, was lower for the ULBT than the MMT (the difference between the areas: 0.13, 95% confidence interval: 0.0697–0.191, $p < 0.0001$, Table 3, Fig. 2).

In our study, the accuracy of the ULBT (73.83%) was higher than that of the MMT (62.80%), and the specificity of the ULBT (98.04%) was higher than that of the MMT (61.18%). Particularly, the ULBT showed significantly lower sensitivity (4.49%) compared with that of the MMT in our trial (67.42%). The prevalence of a difficult laryngoscopy (DL) was 25.87% (89 of 344), and the percentage of patients with an MMT class > II was 67.4% (60 of 344), while only nine patients (2.6%) showed a grade III ULBT (Table 2).

Discussion

Our study demonstrates the ULBT shows particularly high specificity, low false-positive rates and high accuracy in Koreans. The differences were due to lower incidence of high-grade ULBT in Korean than in other ethnities [2, 16, 17]. According to a review of several works of literature, such character might be explainable with the soft tissue redundancy and skeletal variance in Far East Asians.

Several methods such as the MMT classification, IID, TMD, and SMD have focused on one or more patient-related factors that may identify those at risk for a

Table 2 Relationship between pre-anaesthetic assessment classifications and Cormack and Lehane grade

	Cormack and Lehane grade		
Pre-anaesthetic test	1 & 2(%) (n = 255)	3 & 4(%) (n = 89)	p
Modified Mallampati			
Class 1 & 2	156(61.2)	29(32.6)	<.001
Class 3 & 4	99(38.8)	60(67.4)	
Upper lip bite			
Class 1 & 2	250(98.0)	85(95.5)	0.245
Class 3	5(2.0)	4(4.5)	

Values are number (proportion); * The Chi-square test

Table 3 Receiver operating characteristic (ROC) analysis for difficult intubation

Variables	AUC Value (95% CI)
IID ≤ 4.5 cm	0.664 (0.611–0.713)
TMD ≤ 8.3 cm	0.622 (0.568–0.673)
SMD ≤ 17.9 cm	0.629 (0.576–0.680)
MMT	0.643 (0.590–0.694)
ULBT	0.513 (0.458–0.567)

Values are number (confidence interval). *IID* inter-incisor distance, *TMD* thyromental distance, *SMD* Sternomental distance (SMD), *MMT* Modified Mallampati test, *ULBT* upper lip bite test, *AUC* areas under the ROC curves, *CI* confidence interval

Table 4 Predictive values for the Upper lip bite test (ULBT) and the modified Mallampati test (MMT) to predict the occurrence of a grade 3 or 4 according to the Cormack-Lehane grade

Outcome of calculations	ULBT ($n = 344$)	MMT ($n = 344$)
True-Positive	4	60
False-Positive	5	99
True-Negative	250 (74.63%)	156 (84.32%)
False-Negative	85 (25.37%)	29 (15.68%)
Accuracy (%)	73.83	62.80
Sensitivity (%)	4.49	67.42
Specificity (%)	98.04	61.18
Positive prediction value (%)	44.44	37.74
Negative Prediction value (%)	74.63	84.32
AUC of ROC-curve	0.513	0.643

Values are number (proportion)

difficult TI before the induction of anesthesia [16, 18–20]. Concerning applicability, the ULBT does not require an additional light, restriction of phonation, or for the patient to be in the sitting position. The ULBT has been used as a simple bedside test for a DL with good predictive accuracy. It could serve as a good predictor for difficult laryngoscopic intubation because the range and freedom of mandibular movement and the architecture of the teeth have pivotal roles in facilitating laryngoscopic intubation [1]. The ULBT showed higher accuracy (75.9–91%) in previous studies than the MMT (63.7–67.7%) [1, 2, 21, 22] and good predictability with a high AUC value (0.604–0.85) [1, 2, 22]. The percentage of correctly predicted easy laryngoscopies among all laryngoscopies (the specificity) of the ULBT was very high (82.35–92.5%) [1, 2, 23, 24].

The nature of the soft tissue profile is affected by many factors other than the skeletal hard tissue profile, including ethnicity. The ULBT evaluates the range and

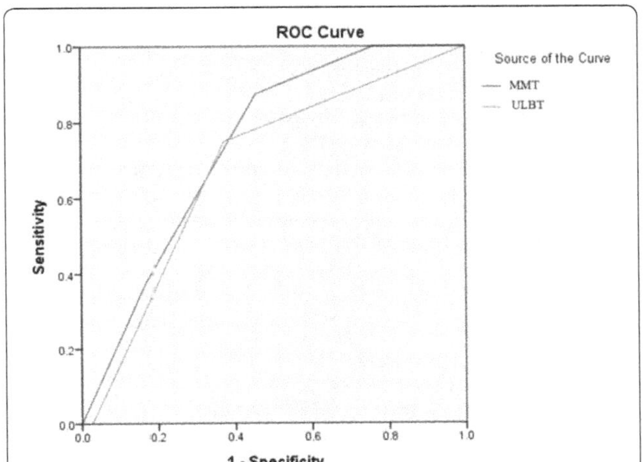

Fig. 2 ROC curves of MMT and ULBT

freedom of mandibular movement and the architecture of the teeth. Mandibular movement is the conjoined movements of skeletal hard tissue, ligament, and soft tissue [25]. Furthermore, the ULBT classification is based on the upper lip mucosa, which is soft tissue [1].

From our observational results comparing the ULBT with the MMT, which has been used widely, the AUC of the MMT in Koreans was 0.627, which is indicative of unreliable predictability similar to those found in recent meta-analyses [5, 26]. However, the AUC of the ULBT was 0.519, which implies predictability that is much lower than those in other studies of different ethnicities (0.604–0.826) [1, 2, 27]. The NPV of the MMT is higher than that of the ULBT. A high AUC value and high NPV mean that the MMT is highly reliable and likely to detect an easy laryngoscopic view. The ULBT has a lower PPV than the MMT. Therefore, many positive results from this procedure are false positives. However, the PPV and NPV are not intrinsic and also depend on the prevalence, which was very low for positive results. In this trial, the prevalence of high-grade ULBT values was 2.6% (9 of 344). This result is also similar to that of another study on Koreans (16 of 305) [11]. We speculated that differences in the soft tissue and bony structure in line with ethnic differences might explain the differences between the ULBT and MMT results. Our results also indicated that the ULBT has higher accuracy and specificity than the MMT. However, sensitivity was much lower (4.49%) compared with that of the MMT in our trial (67%) and consistent with ULBT data from previous trials (28.2–76.5%) [1, 2, 21, 22, 28]. This means that many patients with a DL will not be identified by the ULBT (a large number of patients will have false-negative tests).

$$\text{Sensitivity} = \frac{\text{Number of true positives}}{\text{Number of true positives} + \text{Number of false negatives}}$$

We deduced that one of the factors causing the low sensitivity was the low incidence of a grade III ULBT in Korean subjects. In our study, only nine patients of 344 could not bite their upper lip, and only three of them presented a difficult laryngoscopic view. In Korea, a grade III ULBT is rarely observed [11]. There can be several reasons for this, with ethnic cephalometric differences possibly being one reason. Several studies were published comparing soft tissues between different ethnic groups in orthodontics and the field of maxillofacial surgery [3, 4, 6, 7, 10, 29–32].

In a comparison of Southern Chinese and British Caucasian cephalometric standards, Chinese upper lips were longer with a more acute angulation than those of Caucasians [7]. Moreover, Korean subjects had a lower angle of nasal inclination, and a higher degree of lip protrusion compared with European-American adults and the upper and lower lips were positioned more anteriorly

[3]. Chang and colleagues conducted a morphometric analysis comparing Asian and European-American subjects [32]. Far East Asian (Chinese, Japanese, Korean, and Taiwanese) men seemed to have a significantly shorter cranium and smaller anterior cranial base angles. Compared with Caucasians, Asians with clinically acceptable occlusions tended to have a shorter midface, prominent mandibles, and an anteriorly displaced TMJ in the posterior cranial base [32]. It was also noted that these features resulted from the relative retrusion of the nasomaxillary complex and the relatively forward position of the mandible.

Therefore, in Asians, the scarcity of a grade III ULBT is explainable as a result of an anteriorly displaced TMJ and redundant soft lip tissues. It is clear that the ULBT shows a much lower false-positive rate, lower sensitivity, and higher PPV than other predictive methods.

Limitations

One of the limitations of a test to predict a DL is the discrepancy between a DL and difficult intubation. Patients who presented with a DL (Cormack–Lehane grade 3 or 4) could easily be classified as a grade II or better with the application of external pressure to the larynx (the BURP maneuver) to move the epiglottis. These patients would have been described as having an easy TI. Therefore, it is difficult to predict a difficult TI (DTI) only by mandibular movement, and a DL does not predict a DTI.

Moreover, in this trial, the prevalence of a DL was 25.87% (89 of 344), and the DTI/DL ratio was 3.4% (3/89). These are similar to the results shown in previous studies (4.3–77.8%) [20, 33, 34]. And, even though we used nerve stimulation for checking the achievement of muscle relaxation, the methodological limitation might exist cause we didn't protocolize the technique of anesthetic induction, so it is possible that direct laryngoscopy and endotracheal intubation has not been performed under the same conditions in all patients. We didn't collect the data of surgery that patients underwent. It could be comparable, but we just wanted to evaluate the predictability of ULBT and had excluded patients who had considerable abnormalities to airway prediction and evaluation.

Conclusions

In Koreans, the ULBT shows very high specificity. The ULBT presented low false-positive rates and high accuracy. Cephalometric ethnical differences may present in Far East Asians are one reason. Therefore, especially in Asians, soft tissue redundancy and skeletal variance should be considered based on ethnic differences when evaluating parameters related to soft tissue such as the ULBT.

Abbreviations

ASA: American Society of Anesthesiologists; AUC: The area under the receiver operating characteristic curve; BURP: Backward upward rightward pressure maneuver; DL: Difficult laryngoscopy; DTI: Difficult tracheal intubation; IID: Inter-incisor distance; MMT: Modified Mallampati test; NPV: Negative predictive value; PPV: Positive predictive value; ROC: Receiver operating characteristic; SMD: Sternomental distance; TI: Tracheal Intubation; TMD: Thyromental distance; ULBT: The upper lip bite test

Acknowledgments

None.

Authors' contributions

Dr. JCK: Contributed to performing all statistical analysis and interpretation of data, writing the manuscript. Dr. YK: Performing all statistical analysis, obtaining study participants. Dr. JK: Obtaining study participants and acquisition of data. Dr. SWA: Contributed to the design of the work, drafting the manuscript, revising it critically for important intellectual content. All authors have read and approved the final version of this manuscript.

References

1. Khan ZH, Kashfi A, Ebrahimkhani E. A comparison of the upper lip bite test (a simple new technique) with modified Mallampati classification in predicting difficulty in endotracheal intubation: a prospective blinded study. Anesth Analg. 2003;96(2):595–9.
2. Eberhart LH, Arndt C, Cierpka T, Schwanekamp J, Wulf H, Putzke C. The reliability and validity of the upper lip bite test compared with the Mallampati classification to predict difficult laryngoscopy: an external prospective evaluation. Anesth Analg. 2005;101(1):284–9.
3. Hwang HS, Kim WS, McNamara JA Jr. Ethnic differences in the soft tissue profile of Korean and European-American adults with normal occlusions and well-balanced faces. Angle Orthod. 2002;72(1):72–80.
4. Ioi H, Nakata S, Nakasima A, Counts AL. Comparison of cephalometric norms between Japanese and Caucasian adults in antero-posterior and vertical dimension. Eur J Orthod. 2007;29(5):493–9.
5. Lee A, Fan LT, Gin T, Karmakar MK, Ngan Kee WD. A systematic review (meta-analysis) of the accuracy of the Mallampati tests to predict the difficult airway. Anesth Analg. 2006;102(6):1867–78.
6. Miyajima K, McNamara JA Jr, Kimura T, Murata S, Iizuka T. Craniofacial structure of Japanese and European-American adults with normal occlusions and well-balanced faces. Am J Orthod Dentofac Orthop. 1996;110(4):431–8.
7. Cooke MS, Wei SH. A comparative study of southern Chinese and British Caucasian cephalometric standards. Angle Orthod. 1989;59(2):131–8.
8. Park IC, Bowman D, Klapper L. A cephalometric study of Korean adults. Am J Orthod Dentofac Orthop. 1989;96(1):54–9.
9. Wu J, Hagg U, Rabie AB. Chinese norms of McNamara's cephalometric analysis. Angle Orthod. 2007;77(1):12–20.
10. Alcalde RE, Jinno T, Pogrel MA, Matsumura T. Cephalometric norms in Japanese adults. J Oral Maxillofac Surg. 1998;56(2):129–34.
11. Seo SH, Lee JG, Yu SB, Kim DS, Ryu SJ, Kim KH. Predictors of difficult intubation defined by the intubation difficulty scale (IDS): predictive value of 7 airway assessment factors. Korean J Anesthesiol. 2012;63(6):491–7.
12. Samsoon GL, Young JR. Difficult tracheal intubation: a retrospective study. Anaesthesia. 1987;42(5):487–90.
13. Cormack RS, Lehane J. Difficult tracheal intubation in obstetrics. Anaesthesia. 1984;39(11):1105–11.
14. Perkins NJ, Schisterman EF. The inconsistency of "optimal" cutpoints obtained using two criteria based on the receiver operating characteristic curve. Am J Epidemiol. 2006;163(7):670–5.
15. DeLong ER, DeLong DM, Clarke-Pearson DL. Comparing the areas under two or more correlated receiver operating characteristic curves: a nonparametric approach. Biometrics. 1988;44(3):837–45.
16. Mahmoodpoor A, Soleimanpour H, Golzari SE, Nejabatian A, Pourlak T, Amani M, Hajmohammadi S, Hosseinzadeh H, Esfanjani RM. Determination of the diagnostic value of the modified Mallampati score, upper lip bite test and facial angle in predicting difficult intubation: a prospective descriptive study. J Clin Anesth. 2017;37:99–102.
17. Myneni N, O'Leary AM, Sandison M, Roberts K. Evaluation of the upper lip bite test in predicting difficult laryngoscopy. J Clin Anesth. 2010;22(3):174–8.
18. Mallampati SR, Gatt SP, Gugino LD, Desai SP, Waraksa B, Freiberger D, Liu

PL. A clinical sign to predict difficult tracheal intubation: a prospective study. Can Anaesth Soc J. 1985;32(4):429–34.
19. Tse JC, Rimm EB, Hussain A. Predicting difficult endotracheal intubation in surgical patients scheduled for general anesthesia: a prospective blind study. Anesth Analg. 1995;81(2):254–8.
20. Butler PJ, Dhara SS. Prediction of difficult laryngoscopy: an assessment of the thyromental distance and Mallampati predictive tests. Anaesth Intensive Care. 1992;20(2):139–42.
21. Hester CE, Dietrich SA, White SW, Secrest JA, Lindgren KR, Smith T. A comparison of preoperative airway assessment techniques: the modified Mallampati and the upper lip bite test. AANA J. 2007;75(3):177–82.
22. Khan ZH, Mohammadi M, Rasouli MR, Farrokhnia F, Khan RH. The diagnostic value of the upper lip bite test combined with sternomental distance, thyromental distance, and interincisor distance for prediction of easy laryngoscopy and intubation: a prospective study. Anesth Analg. 2009; 109(3):822–4.
23. Salimi A, Farzanegan B, Rastegarpour A, Kolahi AA. Comparison of the upper lip bite test with measurement of thyromental distance for prediction of difficult intubations. Acta Anaesthesiol Taiwanica. 2008;46(2):61–5.
24. Faramarzi E, Soleimanpour H, Khan ZH, Mahmoodpoor A, Sanaie S. Upper lip bite test for prediction of difficult airway: a systematic review. Pak J Med Sci. 2018;34(4):1019–23.
25. Sahin SH, Yilmaz A, Gunday I, Kargi M, Sut N, Taskinalp O, Ulucam E. Using temporomandibular joint mobility to predict difficult tracheal intubation. J Anesth. 2011;25(3):457–61.
26. Lundstrom LH, Vester-Andersen M, Moller AM, Charuluxananan S, L'Hermite J, Wetterslev J. Poor prognostic value of the modified Mallampati score: a meta-analysis involving 177 088 patients. Br J Anaesth. 2011;107(5):659–67.
27. Huh J, Shin HY, Kim SH, Yoon TK, Kim DK. Diagnostic predictor of difficult laryngoscopy: the hyomental distance ratio. Anesth Analg. 2009;108(2):544–8.
28. Safavi M, Honarmand A, Zare N. A comparison of the ratio of patient's height to thyromental distance with the modified Mallampati and the upper lip bite test in predicting difficult laryngoscopy. Saudi J Anaesth. 2011;5(3):258–63.
29. Liu Y, Lowe AA, Zeng X, Fu M, Fleetham JA. Cephalometric comparisons between Chinese and Caucasian patients with obstructive sleep apnea. Am J Orthod Dentofac Orthop. 2000;117(4):479–85.
30. Porter JP, Lee JI. Facial analysis: maintaining ethnic balance. Facial Plast Surg Clin North Am. 2002;10(4):343–9.
31. Solmaz I, Raberin M. Is the ethnic factor an orthodontic therapeutic instructor? Orthod Fr. 2011;82(4):347–58.
32. Chang HP, Liu PH, Tseng YC, Yang YH, Pan CY, Chou ST. Morphometric analysis of the cranial base in Asians. Odontology. 2014;102(1):81–8.
33. Frerk CM. Predicting difficult intubation. Anaesthesia. 1991;46(12):1005–8.
34. Wajekar AS, Chellam S, Toal PV. Prediction of ease of laryngoscopy and intubation-role of upper lip bite test, modified mallampati classification, and thyromental distance in various combination. J Family Med Prim Care. 2015; 4(1):101–5.

25

Role of inferior vena cava collapsibility index in the prediction of hypotension associated with general anesthesia

Marcell Szabó[1,2*], Anna Bozó[1], Katalin Darvas[2], Alexandra Horváth[1] and Zsolt Dániel Iványi[2]

Abstract

Background: Intraoperative hypotension increases 30-day mortality and the risks of myocardial injury and acute renal failure. Patients with inadequate volume reserve before the induction of anesthesia are highly exposed. The identification of latent hypovolemia is therefore crucial. Ultrasonographic measurement of the inferior vena cava collapsibility index (IVCCI) is able to detect volume responsiveness in circulatory shock. No current evidence is available regarding whether preoperative measurement of the IVCCI could identify patients at high risk for hypotension associated with general anesthesia.

Methods: A total of 102 patients undergoing elective general surgery under general anesthesia with standardized propofol induction were recruited for this prospective observational study. The IVCCI was measured under spontaneous breathing. A collapsing (IVCCI≧50%) (CI+) and a noncollapsing (CI-) group were formed. Immediate postinduction changes in systolic and mean blood pressure were compared. The performance of the IVCCI as a diagnostic tool for predicting hypotension (systolic pressure < 90 mmHg or a ≥ 30% drop from the baseline) was evaluated by ROC curve analysis.

Results: A total of 83 patients were available for analysis, with 20 in the CI+ and 63 in the CI- group, we excluded 19 previously eligible patients due to inadequate visualization of the IVC (7 cases), lack of adherence to the protocol (8 cases), missing data (2 cases) or change in anesthesiologic management (2 cases). The mean decrease in systolic pressure in the CI+ group was 53.8 ± 15.3 compared to 35.8 ± 18.1 mmHg in CI- patients ($P = 0.0001$). The relative mean arterial pressure change medians were 34.1% (IQR 23.2–43.0%) and 24.2% (IQR 17.2–30.2%), respectively ($P = 0.0029$). The ROC curve analysis for IVCCI showed an AUC of 64.8% (95% CI 52.1–77.5%). The selected 50% level of the IVCCI had a sensitivity of only 45.5% (95% CI 28.1–63.7%), but the specificity was high at 90.0% (78.2–96.7%). The positive predictive value was 75.0% (95% CI 50.9–91.3%), and the negative predictive value was 71.4% (95% CI 58.7–82.1%).

Conclusion: In spontaneously breathing preoperative noncardiac surgical patients, preoperatively detected IVCCI≧50% can predict postinduction hypotension with high specificity but low sensitivity. Despite moderate performance, IVCCI is an easy, noninvasive and attractive option to identify patients at risk and should be explored further.

Keywords: Anesthesia, Hypotension, Propofol, Vena cava, Inferior, Echocardiography

* Correspondence: szabo.marcell@med.semmelweis-univ.hu
[1]1st Department of Surgery, Semmelweis University, Üllői út 78, Budapest 1082, Hungary
[2]Department of Anesthesiology and Intensive Therapy, Semmelweis University, Üllői út 78B, Budapest 1082, Hungary

Introduction

Maintaining hemodynamic stability is essential for reducing the rate of postoperative complications. Although intraoperative hypotension has no universal definition, it has a serious impact on myocardial injury, acute kidney injury, septic complications [1], the risk of 30-day mortality [2], as well as the risk of one-year mortality in selected patient populations [3] after noncardiac surgery. Prevention of an undesired hypotensive event has a key role in providing patient safety. To date, available prediction models used for estimation of the risk of hypotension are mostly based on nonmodifiable factors (e.g., age, comorbidities) [4, 5]. There is a need to identify easily available variables that can help clinicians recognize patients with a modifiable risk level, such as those with impaired preload.

Hypovolemia is probably the most common factor provoking postinduction hypotension, despite worldwide improvement in preoperative optimization and changing practices promoting the avoidance of unnecessary fasting and mechanical bowel preparation, optimized fluid therapy remains the cornerstone of treatment with excellent effectiveness [5]. The identification of latent hypovolemic patients affords clinicians a chance to implement proper fluid replacement before inducing general anesthesia. Without a universal definition, we consider latent hypovolemia a clinical condition corresponding to a decrease in circulating blood volume without obvious hemodynamic changes and/or organ dysfunction, which increases the risk of the development of hypoperfusion in response to external impacts such as anesthesia and surgery.

Several invasive devices (e.g., pulmonary arterial catheter, PiCCO®, Vigileo®, etc.) are available for evaluating preload among other elements of hemodynamic status, but their universal use is not a reasonable option due to financial constraints, relatively high complication rates, known limitations and unnecessary invasiveness compared to most surgical procedures [6].

The use of noninvasive ultrasound examination by anesthesiologists is a widespread and useful aid in the safe application of anesthesia. In a recent meta-analysis, Ferreira et al. reported an approximately 31% change in anesthesia management when ultrasound was used. Thirty-five percent of the performed ultrasonographies were transthoracic echocardiographies [7]. A standard transthoracic echocardiography revealing all relevant cardiologic details takes a significant amount of time, even when performed by adequately trained cardiologists; however, focused goal-directed scans are much faster while maintaining important clinical relevance [8]. The proper training of anesthesiologists is an issue because all types of sonographies are operator-dependent exams. However, a French center reported that parameters of high anesthesiological importance such as global left ventricular function, ventricular diameters, pericardial effusion or the diameter of the inferior vena cava were adequately evaluated by trainees who had taken part in a 12 h learning program [9]. Concerning volemic status, the variability of the diameter of the inferior vena cava (IVC), which follows the respiratory cycle, is considered to be a valuable predictor of volume responsiveness in cases of circulatory failure in ventilated [10–13] and spontaneously breathing patients [14, 15] even in the presence of nonfatal cardiac arrhythmias [16]. In these studies, clinically evident volume responsiveness was defined as an at least 10% increase in cardiac output in response to bolus fluid administration.

In the present study, we aimed to characterize the collapsibility index of the IVC as a potential screening tool to identify patients who were candidate for hypotensive events related to general anesthesia in an otherwise hemodynamically stable population.

Materials and methods

Patients

This prospective, observational study was conducted between 26/07/2016 and 30/10/2018 in the 1st Department of Surgery, Semmelweis University, Budapest, Hungary. Ethics approval for this study was provided by Semmelweis University Regional and Institutional Committee of Science and Research Ethics, Budapest, Hungary (Registration number: 144/2016, date of approval: 25/07/2016). Informed consent was obtained from each subject. Patients aged ≥18 years who were scheduled for elective general surgery under general anesthesia on predetermined weekdays were included if they met the eligibility criteria and all necessary data were available. The inclusion and exclusion criteria are shown in Table 1. As a conceptual summary, we included elective, premedicated patients and excluded those who were already hypotensive or severely

Table 1 Inclusion and exclusion criteria

Inclusion criteria	Exclusion criteria
Age ≥ 18 years	ASA physical status > 3
Elective surgery	Dyspnea
General anesthesia	Systolic blood pressure ≥ 180 mmHg
	Systolic blood pressure < 90 mmHg
	Decompensated heart failure
	Elevated pulmonary arterial pressure > 40 mmHg
	Significant valvular disease
	Significant carotid stenosis
	Documented negative fluid balance > 1.000 ml on preceding day
	Pheochromocytoma
	SOFA score > 1
	Agitation (RASS > 1)
	IVC non visualized
	Epidural catheter in use

ASA American Society of Anesthesiology, *IVC* inferior vena cava, *RASS* Richmond Agitation Sedation Scale, *SOFA* Sepsis-related Organ Failure Assessment hypertensive, those considered to be at high risk or those having a clinical condition that would prevent the adequate evaluation of either the IVC (e.g., significant tricuspid regurgitation) or blood pressure changes (e.g., pheochromocytoma).

Study design

Eligible patients were screened using ultrasonography. The inferior vena cava was identified, and characteristics were recorded in the dorsal recumbent position under light sedation (RASS 0- -1) and spontaneous breathing. The collapsibility index (IVCCI) was calculated, and two groups were formed according to the measured IVCCI: the collapsing group characterized by IVCCI≥50% (CI+) and the noncollapsing group (CI-) (in whom the IVCCI was< 50%). This level was arbitrarily set with regard to the results in previously published literature, verifying that IVCCI values between 40 and 50% measured in spontaneously breathing patients are predictive for volume responsiveness in different clinical settings [14–16].

Vital signs were recorded, and protocolled anesthesia induction was performed. Two minutes after drug administration but before intubating the trachea, the vital signs were measured again. The hemodynamic response was characterized in each group with the change in systolic blood pressure as the end point. Anesthesia-related hypotensive events were recorded if the systolic blood pressure dropped below 90 mmHg or a ≥ 30% drop in initial systolic pressure was observed.

Ultrasonographic measurements

Patients in the surgical ward were evaluated before transportation to the operating room. Ultrasonographic scans were performed by one of four adequately trained independent anesthesiologists who had undergone institutional training for ultrasound use in anesthesia and who had at least 2 years of experience in the field. One of two ultrasound machines was used (Sonosite Titan - FUJIFILM SonoSite, Inc. Bothell, Washington, United States and Hitachi Aloka Noblus, Hitachi Healthcare, Tokyo, Japan). Both machines were equipped with a curvilinear transducer (5 MHz). The inferior vena cava was visualized in B-mode from a longitudinal paramedian subxyphoid view; when a good echographic window was not available, an intercostal, transhepatic lateral view was used. The last section of the vein, which was proximal to the hepatic vein inflow and 0.5–3 cm from the right atrium, was selected for the M-mode, and measurements were performed as recommended in the consensus document of the American and European Cardiologic Societies [17]. The maximal expiratory diameter of the vein was recorded (dIVC expiration) under normal breathing of the lightly sedated patient, and the collapsibility index (IVCCI) was calculated using the following formula: (dIVC expiration − dIVC inspiration) / dIVC expiration × 100 = IVCCI. The IVC diameter at expiration and inspiration had to be measured during the same respiratory cycle. Figure 1 represents a typical highly collapsing IVC.

Anesthesiologic practice

Routine premedication using alprazolam was given 1 hour before surgery. Regular cardiovascular medication of the patients was maintained on their established routine, except for diuretics and angiotensin-converting inhibitors, which were withdrawn. All patients were monitored continuously using ECG, pulse oximetry and capnography starting from the beginning of manual ventilation. Noninvasive blood pressure monitoring by oscillometry and invasive arterial blood pressure monitoring were used at the discretion of the anesthesiologist according to the details of the planned surgery and the risk level of the patient. Noninvasive measurements were obtained at 5 min intervals, and an additional measurement was obligatory 2 min after induction drug administration. This step preceded the intubation of the trachea. If invasive monitoring was used, an arterial cannula was inserted before induction, and postinduction vital signs were registered at the same time points as above. To induce general anesthesia, our institutional standard practice of using fentanyl (1–2 μg/kg), propofol (1,5–2 mg/kg) and nondepolarizing muscle relaxants (rocuronium or cis-atracurium) according to age, weight, chronic organ function and the needs of the surgery was not changed for study purposes.

Statistical analysis

Sample size

To calculate the sample size, the change in systolic blood pressure after induction drug administration was the variable of interest. A minimum difference of 15 mmHg was considered clinically important, and that in combination with a standard deviation of 25 mmHg coming from our pilot data of 103 patients not involved in the study were used for the calculations. A type one error of 0.05 and a required power of 0.80 were set. Assuming unequal study groups with a 1 to 3 ratio of patients having collapsing (CI+) and noncollapsing (CI-) IVC, we used corrected sample sizes [18]. A minimum of 81 patients were required based on the conditions detailed above. To maintain adequate power in cases of a lack of adherence to the protocol or methodological failure, an additional 25% was screened, and a total of 102 patients were enrolled.

Data analysis

Data were pooled for analysis in Microsoft Excel 2013 (Additional file 1); for the statistical analysis, we used

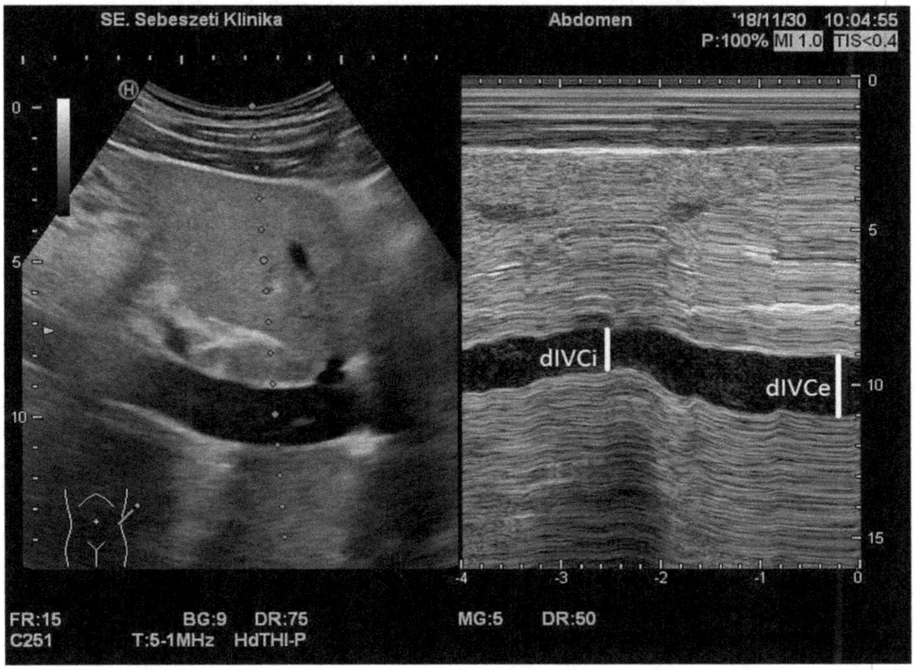

Fig. 1 Typical ultrasound image of the inferior vena cava near the heart. M-mode image represents high respiratory collapsibility. (dIVCe = IVC diameter in expiration, dIVCi = IVC diameter in inspiration)

StatsDirect Statistical Software (Version 3.1.20, Stats Direct Ltd., Grantchester, Cambridge, UK). Continuous variables are presented as the means±standard deviation if they were normally distributed as tested by the Shapiro-Wilk W test. Nonnormally distributed data are shown as the medians and interquartile ranges. Student's two-sample t-test and the Mann-Whitney U test were used for comparisons. Categorical variables are shown as percentages and absolute numbers of cases. The χ^2 and Fisher exact test were used for contingency table analysis as appropriate. Two-sided p-values are shown, and the limit of statistical significance was set to $p < 0.05$.

The 50% value of IVCCI as a diagnostic cutoff value was evaluated by calculating the sensitivity, specificity, and positive and negative predictive values. Previously cited literature [14] data highlight the potential cutoff level for IVCCI of 40%; this value was also tested. The receiver operating characteristics curve was plotted, and the area under the curve was calculated by Wilcoxon's method, and the standard error was calculated according to the method by DeLong. In these calculations, a composite definition of hypotension was used. Postinduction systolic pressure less than 90 mmHg and/or a more than 30% decrease from the baseline systolic pressure was needed to treat data as positive for hypotension.

Results

Population demographics and characteristics

A total of 102 patients were recruited. We had to exclude 19 previously eligible patients due to inadequately visualized IVC (7 cases), a lack of adherence to the protocol (8 cases), a lack of data (2 cases) or a change in anesthesiological management (2 cases). Finally, 83 patients who matched all inclusion criteria were enrolled. Twenty patients were evaluated in the CI+ group and 63 in the CI+ group. The list of surgical operations performed is provided in Table 2. Baseline characteristics in terms of anthropometry, physiologic status, comorbidities and important prescreening treatments are summarized in Table 3. All variables except age were similar in the two groups without any significant intergroup differences. The median age in the CI+ group was 8 years older than that in the CI- group.

Hemodynamic data

The mean postinduction decrease in systolic pressure in the CI+ group was 53.8 ± 15.3 mmHg, which was significantly higher than the 35.8 ± 18.1 mmHg observed among CI- patients ($P = 0.0001$). The same phenomenon was present in the case of a relative decrease in systolic pressures: CI+ patients had a mean of 36.4 ± 9.1%, while this was 24.7 ± 11.3% in the CI- group ($P < 0.0001$). The results are shown in Fig. 2a (absolute decrease) and 2b

Table 2 Surgical procedures in the CI+ and CI- groups

Surgery types	Collapsible (CI+) group (*N* = 20)	Noncollapsible (CI-) group (*N* = 63)	*P* value
Minor procedures	30.0%	34.9%	0.6851
minor laparoscopies, N	2	8	
hernia repairs, N	1	7	
breast and plastic surgeries, N	1	3	
minor perianal procedures, N	0	2	
endocrine surgeries, N	1	2	
Major procedures	70.0%	65.1%	
upper gastrointestinal, N	2	5	
hepatic resections, N	2	4	
pancreatic-biliary surgeries, N	3	10	
colorectal	7	20	
other intestinal	1	2	

(decrease relative to the preinduction level). Similarly, the relative MAP change medians were 34.1% (IQR 23.2–43.0%) and 24.2% (17.2–30.2%) ($P = 0.0029$) (data not graphed). Meanwhile, no difference was detectable in heart rate decrease, as CI+ patients presented a median of only 4 bpm (0 bpm–9.5 bpm), and 1 bpm (− 3 bpm–7 bpm) was observed among CI- patients ($P = 0.1901$).

Performance characteristics of IVC collapsibility

The ROC curve analysis of the ability of the IVCCI to predict hypotension after the induction of general anesthesia resulted in an AUC of 64.8% (95% CI 52.1–77.5%), demonstrating a poor to fair diagnostic accuracy (Fig. 3). As we previously and arbitrarily set our cutoff value of IVCCI to 50% to distinguish between the CI+ and CI- groups, this particular value was evaluated. The sensitivity was only 45.5% (95% CI 28.1–63.7%), but the specificity was as high as 90.0% (95% CI 78.2–96.7%), giving a positive likelihood ratio of 4.5 (95% CI 1.8–11.3). The positive predictive value was 75.0% (95% CI 50.9–91.3%), and the negative predictive value was 71.4% (95% CI 58.7–82.1%). The IVCCI cutoff of 40% was less promising. The sensitivity became 51.5% (95% CI 33.5–69.2%), and the specificity was 72.0% (95% CI 57.5–83.8%), with positive and negative predictive values of 54.8% (95% CI 36.0–72.7%) and 69.2% (95% CI 54.9 to 81.3%), respectively. In this case, the positive likelihood ratio was only 1.84 (95% CI 1.06–3.20). Setting the cutoff value to 50% was supported by the ROC curve's Youden index, indicating this value is the optimal cutoff value.

Discussion

Our prospective observational study compared the hemodynamic consequences of the induction of general anesthesia by propofol in patient groups defined on the basis of having collapsing (IVCCI ≥50%) or noncollapsing (IVCCI< 50%) IVC, and we evaluated the diagnostic value of a high IVCCI value in the prediction of postinduction hypotension. We detected important differences between the two groups, verifying that a high IVCCI value was associated with a more profound change in systolic blood pressure and mean arterial pressure. This remarkable phenomenon is consistent with the general concept that the IVCCI is able to detect volemic changes. The IVCCI had high specificity and low sensitivity in experiments by Mueller et al. when a cutoff level of > 40% was used to predict volume responsiveness [14]. However, this performance as a diagnostic tool is,

Table 3 Baseline population characteristics

Variable	Collapsible (CI+) group (*N* = 20)	Noncollapsible (CI-) group (*N* = 63)	*P* value
Age, years, median (IQR)	69 (60.5–77)	61 (51–82)	0.0066
Male sex, N (%)	7 (35.0%)	29 (46.0%)	0.3858
BMI, kg/m^2	24.15 ± 3.04	26.48 ± 4.94	0.0505
ASA 3, N (%)	9 (45.0%)	16 (25.4%)	0.0959
COPD, N (%)	2 (10.0%)	7 (11.1%)	0.9999
Hypertension, N (%)	14 (70.0%)	36 (57.1%)	0.3060
Peripheral arterial disease, N (%)	3 (15.0%)	4 (6.4%)	0.3510
Diabetes, any type, N (%)	4 (20.0%)	12 (19.1%)	0.9999
Preoperative fluid intake, ml (IQR)	700 (500–1400)	600 (100–1200)	0.1438
Baseline systolic pressure, mmHg	147 ± 16	143 ± 17	0.3218
IVC diameter in expiration, mm	17 ± 3	18 ± 4	0.2031
Propofol dose for induction, mg/kg	1.77 ± 0.15	1.81 ± 0.16	0.3756

ASA American Society of Anesthesiology, *BMI* body mass index, *COPD* chronic obstructive pulmonary disease, *IQR* interquartile range, *IVC* inferior vena cava

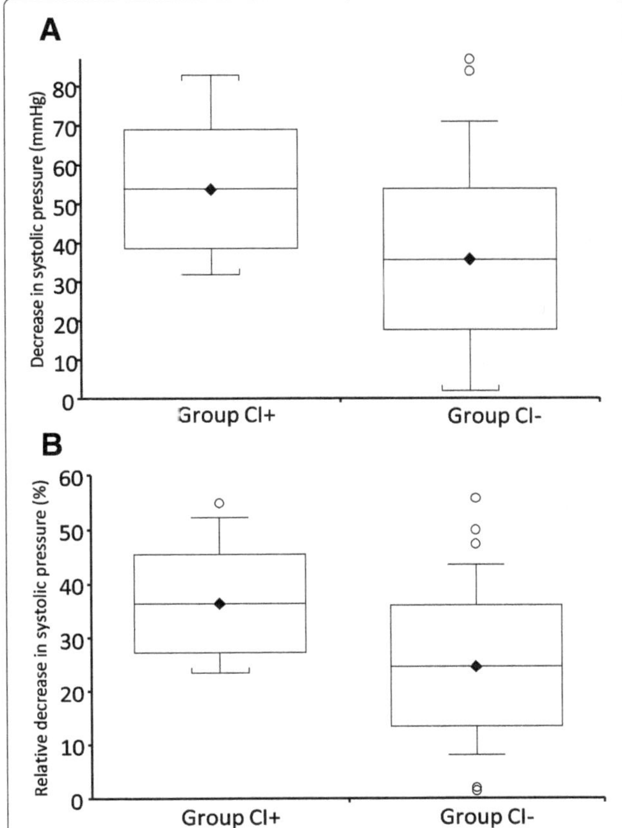

Fig. 2 Decrease in systolic pressure after the induction of anesthesia measured in the study groups. **a** absolute decrease in mmHg (mean, standard deviation and range). **b** relative decrease (percentage) from the baseline (mean, standard deviation and range). For group definitions, see the text

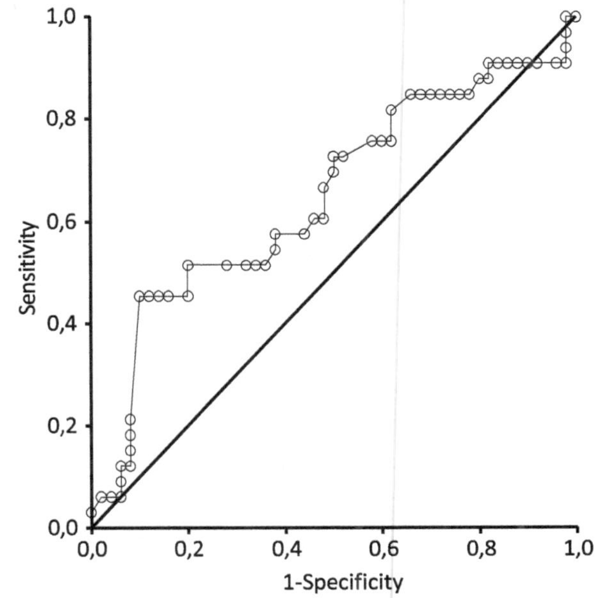

Fig. 3 Receiver operating characteristics (ROC) curve of IVC collapsibility for the prediction of hypotension

on the one hand, similar to that observed in our experiments in the case of the value of 50%, but on the other hand, the physiologic meaning is different: we consider values indicating high collapsibility measured in normotensive or even hypertensive patients as a sign of latent volume depletion when general anesthesia and the consequent deactivation of the sympathetic compensatory mechanisms might have profound effects.

Of note, most previous data are from intensive care settings in which IVC diameter and the IVCCI were used to identify volume-responsive patients in circulatory shock [10–16]. Our approach has several new aspects. First, although it is not entirely unique, we performed IVC measurements in a general anesthesiologic setting. Such studies are still controversial in spinal anesthesia, in which sympathetic denervation could also reveal inadequate fluid reserve. Mačiulienė et al. failed to detect a prognostic role of the IVCCI [19], while another recent trial reported an IVCCI-based fluid replacement strategy as a useful tool to reduce the incidence of hypotension [20].

Second, contrary to the results of the abovementioned articles, the IVCCI was evaluated in an otherwise hemodynamically stable patient population. Despite our systematic screening of the relevant literature, we were not aware of a similar study at the preparation of our study protocol. However, Zhang et al. reported the use of the IVCCI for the prediction of hypotension attributable to general anesthesia [21]. Some important differences must be emphasized here. An important proportion of their patients came from a cardiac surgical population, which probably contributed to the choice of etomidate as an intravenous anesthetic. The more prominent hypotension frequency (42/90) in that study compared to ours (33/83) despite the relatively safe agent is important and most likely attributable, at least in part, to the high proportion of cardiac surgical patients. Our choice of propofol comes from its widespread use for everyday purposes and consequently high variability of the affected population. This choice is Janus-faced, as propofol has a well-known potential to provoke hypotension itself by several mechanisms, the most important of which is vasodilation [22, 23], making the agent an independent risk factor for hypotension [24], but the protocolized anesthetic strategy, provided to all the enrolled patients, excludes the induction agent as an independent risk factor.

Our observational trial has limitations. First, we had to exclude 19 patients despite a slightly better visualization rate compared to that in the previously cited study with a similar approach [21], but adherence to the protocol was lower than optimal. The final population was still large enough to not jeopardize our statistical power. Second, spontaneous breathing is difficult to standardize, and we hypothesized that premedicated patients without obvious signs of agitation (RASS≤1) and respiratory efforts constitute an adequate setting for IVC measurements. Our protocol tends to follow physiologic airway pressure changes but therefore differs from that of some cited studies, which chose forced deep inspiration [15] or sniffing [14, 16]. Additionally, our study, by its observational nature, is not entirely free from intergroup differences: patients in the CI+ group were slightly older than those in the CI- group (median 69 vs 61 years.). Despite the statistical significance, both groups represent a population otherwise highly susceptible (older than 50 years) to hypotension [24]. As an older population is generally more susceptible to profound volume disturbances, we consider this finding a pathophysiologic consequence and not a biasing factor. This feature also characterized the hypotensive population in the study by Zhang et al. [21], and the randomization process allowed Ceruti et al. to characterize their IVCCI-based fluid replacement strategy without this confounder [20].

When we focus on IVCCI's diagnostic performance, our AUC of 64.8% together with the sensitivity and specificity levels should be evaluated in the context of the models currently available for the prediction of hypotension associated with general anesthesia. A recent multicenter observational study identified age, degree of high blood pressure prior to surgery and type II diabetes as risk factors [5]. As these results, which were similar to former findings [24], are hard to use to stratify individual patients' risk in everyday practice, a simplified scoring system was also developed by Cheung et al. [4]. In their 'HEART Score' model in which preexisting hypotension or bradycardia, elderly age, preoperative renin-angiotensin blockade, revised cardiac risk index (≥3 points), and type of surgery (major surgery) were valuable risk factors, the ROC analysis showed moderate usefulness (AUC 75%). As our protocol ruled out unstable patients, and ACE inhibitors were withdrawn, we consider that IVCCI measurement can reveal additional patients at risk who were potentially not identified by the abovementioned factors. It is important to emphasize that, in contrast to previous models, our observations point to a potentially modifiable variable.

Conclusion

As a clinical interpretation of our results in spontaneously breathing preoperative noncardiac surgical patients, preoperative IVCCI measurement is feasible and can predict postinduction hypotension with high specificity but low sensitivity. Despite its moderate performance, IVCCI is an easy, noninvasive and attractive option to identify patients at risk of postinduction hypotension and should be explored further. The potential involvement of the IVCCI in multifactorial models can be a field of future studies.

Abbreviations

ASA: American Society of Anesthesiology; CI: Collapsibility Index; IQR: Interquartile range; IVC: Inferior vena cava; IVCCI: Inferior vena cava collapsibility index; MAP: Mean arterial pressure; RASS: Richmond Agitation Sedation Scale; ROC: Receiver Operating Characteristics; SOFA: Sepsis-related Organ Failure Assessment

Acknowledgments

Not applicable.

Authors' contributions

MS: proof of concept, design, ultrasound measurements, data collection and analysis, manuscript preparation. AB: ultrasound measurements, data collection, data entry. KD: data collection, manuscript oversight. AH: ultrasound measurements, data collection. ZDI: design, manuscript oversight. All authors read and approved the final manuscript.

References

1. Haynes AB, Regenbogen SE, Weiser TG, Lipsitz SR, Dziekan G, Berry WR, et al. Surgical outcome measurement for a global patient population: validation of the surgical Apgar score in 8 countries. Surgery. 2011;149:519–24.
2. Gu WJ, Hou BL, Kwong JSW, Tian X, Qian Y, Hao J, et al. Association between intraoperative hypotension and 30-day mortality, major adverse cardiac events, and acute kidney injury after non-cardiac surgery: a meta-analysis of cohort studies. Int J Cardiol. 2018;258:68–73.
3. Bijker JB, van Klei WA, Vergouwe Y, Eleveld DJ, van Wolfswinkel L, Moons KG, et al. Intraoperative hypotension and 1-year mortality after noncardiac surgery. Anesthesiology. 2009;111:1217–26.
4. Cheung CC, Martyn A, Campbell N, Frost S, Gilbert K, Michota F, et al. Predictors of intraoperative hypotension and bradycardia. Am J Med. 2015; 128:532–8.
5. Jor O, Maca J, Koutna J, Gemrotova M, Vymazal T, Litschmannova M, et al. Hypotension after induction of general anesthesia: occurrence, risk factors, and therapy. A prospective multicentre observational study. J Anesth. 2018; 32:673–80.
6. Vincent JL, Pelosi P, Pearse R, Payen D, Perel A, Hoeft A, et al. Perioperative cardiovascular monitoring of high-risk patients: a consensus of 12. Crit Care. 2015;19:224.
7. Ferreira Albuquerque Costa NT, Gomar Sancho C. Perioperative ultrasound applied to diagnosis and decision making in anesthesia. Minerva Anestesiol. 2018;84:94–107.
8. Cowie B. Focused cardiovascular ultrasound performed by anesthesiologists in the perioperative period: feasible and alters patient management. J Cardiothorac Vasc Anesth. 2009;23:450–6.
9. Vignon P, Mucke F, Bellec F, Marin B, Croceb J, Brouqui T, et al. Basic critical care echocardiography: validation of a curriculum dedicated to noncardiologist residents. Crit Care Med. 2011;39:636–42.
10. Barbier C, Loubieres Y, Schmit C, Hayon J, Ricome J, Jardin FO, et al. Respiratory changes in inferior vena cava diameter are helpful in predicting fluid responsiveness in ventilated septic patients. Intensive Care Med. 2004;30: 1740–6.
11. Feissel M, Michard F, Faller JP, Teboul JL. The respiratory variation in inferior vena cava diameter as a guide to fluid therapy. Intensive Care Med. 2004;30: 1834–7.
12. Vignon P, Repesse X, Begot E, Leger J, Jacob C, Bouferrache K, et al. Comparison of echocardiographic indices used to predict fluid responsiveness in ventilated patients. Am J Respir Crit Care Med. 2017;195: 1022–32.
13. Huang HJ, Shen QK, Liu YF, Xu H, Fang YX. Value of variation index of inferior vena cava diameter in predicting fluid responsiveness in patients with circulatory shock receiving mechanical ventilation: a systematic review and meta-analysis. Crit Care. 2018;22:204–10.
14. Muller L, Bobbia X, Toumi M, Louart G, Molinari N, Ragonnet B, et al.

Respiratory variations of inferior vena cava diameter to predict fluid responsiveness in spontaneously breathing patients with acute circulatory failure: need for a cautious use. Crit Care. 2012;16:R188.

15. Preau S, Bortolotti P, Colling D, Dewavrin F, Colas V, Voisin B, et al. Diagnostic accuracy of the inferior vena cava collapsibility to predict fluid responsiveness in spontaneously breathing patients with Sepsis and acute circulatory failure. Crit Care Med. 2017;45:e290–7.
16. Bortolotti P, Colling D, Colas V, Voisin B, Dewavrin F, Poissy J, et al. Respiratory changes of the inferior vena cava diameter predict fluid responsiveness in spontaneously breathing patients with cardiac arrhythmias. Ann Intensive Care. 2018;8:79.
17. Rudski LG, Lai WW, Afilalo J, Hua L, Handschumacher MD, Chandrasekaran K, et al. Guidelines for the echocardiographic assessment of the right heart in adults: a report from the American Society of Echocardiography endorsed by the European Association of Echocardiography, a registered branch of the European Society of Cardiology. J Am Soc Echocardiogr. 2010;23:685–713.
18. Whitley E, Ball J. Statistics review 4: sample size calculations. Crit Care. 2002; 6:335–41.
19. Maciuliene A, Gelmanas A, Jaremko I, Tamosiunas R, Smailys A, Macas A. Measurements of inferior vena cava diameter for prediction of hypotension and bradycardia during spinal anesthesia in spontaneously breathing patients during elective knee joint replacement surgery. Medicina (Kaunas). 2018;54:49.
20. Ceruti S, Anselmi L, Minotti B, Franceschini D, Aguirre J, Borgeat A. Prevention of arterial hypotension after spinal anaesthesia using vena cava ultrasound to guide fluid management. Br J Anaesth. 2018;120:101–8.
21. Zhang J, Critchley LA. Inferior vena cava ultrasonography before general anesthesia can predict hypotension after induction. Anesthesiology. 2016; 124:580–9.
22. Billard V, Moulla F, Bourgain JL, Megnigbeto A, Stanski DR. Hemodynamic response to induction and intubation. Propofol/fentanyl interaction. Anesthesiology 1994;81:1384–93.
23. Muzi M, Berens RA, Kampine JP, Ebert TJ. Venodilation contributes to propofol-mediated hypotension in humans. Anesth Analg. 1992;74:877–83.
24. Reich DL, Hossain S, Krol M, Baez B, Patel P, Bernstein A, Bodian CA. Predictors of hypotension after induction of general anesthesia. Anesth Analg. 2005;101:622–8.

Permissions

All chapters in this book were first published by BioMed Central; hereby published with permission under the Creative Commons Attribution License or equivalent. Every chapter published in this book has been scrutinized by our experts. Their significance has been extensively debated. The topics covered herein carry significant findings which will fuel the growth of the discipline. They may even be implemented as practical applications or may be referred to as a beginning point for another development.

The contributors of this book come from diverse backgrounds, making this book a truly international effort. This book will bring forth new frontiers with its revolutionizing research information and detailed analysis of the nascent developments around the world.

We would like to thank all the contributing authors for lending their expertise to make the book truly unique. They have played a crucial role in the development of this book. Without their invaluable contributions this book wouldn't have been possible. They have made vital efforts to compile up to date information on the varied aspects of this subject to make this book a valuable addition to the collection of many professionals and students.

This book was conceptualized with the vision of imparting up-to-date information and advanced data in this field. To ensure the same, a matchless editorial board was set up. Every individual on the board went through rigorous rounds of assessment to prove their worth. After which they invested a large part of their time researching and compiling the most relevant data for our readers.

The editorial board has been involved in producing this book since its inception. They have spent rigorous hours researching and exploring the diverse topics which have resulted in the successful publishing of this book. They have passed on their knowledge of decades through this book. To expedite this challenging task, the publisher supported the team at every step. A small team of assistant editors was also appointed to further simplify the editing procedure and attain best results for the readers.

Apart from the editorial board, the designing team has also invested a significant amount of their time in understanding the subject and creating the most relevant covers. They scrutinized every image to scout for the most suitable representation of the subject and create an appropriate cover for the book.

The publishing team has been an ardent support to the editorial, designing and production team. Their endless efforts to recruit the best for this project, has resulted in the accomplishment of this book. They are a veteran in the field of academics and their pool of knowledge is as vast as their experience in printing. Their expertise and guidance has proved useful at every step. Their uncompromising quality standards have made this book an exceptional effort. Their encouragement from time to time has been an inspiration for everyone.

The publisher and the editorial board hope that this book will prove to be a valuable piece of knowledge for researchers, students, practitioners and scholars across the globe.

List of Contributors

Wouter Droog, Sanne E. Hoeks, D-Yin Lin, Robert Jan Stolker and Eilish M. Galvin
Department of Anaesthesia, Erasmus University Medical Centre Rotterdam, 3000, CA, Rotterdam, The Netherlands

G. Peter van Aggelen
Department of Anaesthesia, Franciscus Gasthuis & Vlietland, 3004, BA, Rotterdam, The Netherlands

J. Henk Coert
Department of Plastic Surgery, University Medical Centre Utrecht, 3508, GA, Utrecht, The Netherlands

Ting Ting Oh
Department of Women's Anaesthesia, KK Women's and Children's Hospital, Singapore, Singapore

Mohammad Ikhsan and Kok Kiong Tan
Department of Electrical and Comupter Engineering, Faculty of Engineering, National University of Singapore, Singapore, Singapore

Sultana Rehena
Center for Quantitative Medicine, Duke-NUS Medical School, 8 College Road, Singapore, Singapore

Nian-Lin Reena Han
Division of Clinical Support Services, KK Women's amd Children's Hospital, Singapore, Singapore

Alex Tiong Heng Sia and Ban Leong Sng
Department of Women's Anaesthesia, KK Women's and Children's Hospital, Singapore, Singapore Anesthesiology and Peroperative Sciences Academic Clinical Program, Duke-NUS Medical School, 8 College Road, Singapore, Singapore Department of Women's Anaesthesia, KK Women's and Children's Hospital, 100 Bukit Timah Road, Singapore, Singapore

Toru Matsuoka, Masakazu Kotoda and Takashi Matsukawa
Department of Anesthesiology, Faculty of Medicine, University of Yamanashi, Chuo, Yamanashi, Japan

Tadahiko Ishiyama, Noriyuki Shintani and Kazuha Mitsui
Surgical Center, University of Yamanashi Hospital, University of Yamanashi, 1110 Shimokato, Chuo, Yamanashi 409-3898, Japan

Wendong Lin and Jiehao Sun
Department of Anesthesiology, The First Affiliated Hospital of Wenzhou Medical University, Wenzhou 325000, China

Shuying Fu
Department of Anesthesiology, The Second Affiliated Hospital and Yuying Children's Hospital of Wenzhou Medical University, Wenzhou 325000, China

Seok-Jin Lee, Tae-Yun Sung and Choon-Kyu Cho
Department of Anaesthesiology and Pain Medicine, Konyang University Hospital, Myunggok Medical Research Center, Konyang University College of Medicine, 158, Gwangeodong-ro, Seo-gu, Daejeon 35365, South Korea

Chen Gao and Liqiang Yu
Department of Nephrology, The Hangzhou Fuyang Hospital of Traditional Chinese Medicine, Zhejiang, Hangzhou, China

Chunyan Weng and Jingli Xu
The First Clinical Medical of Zhejiang Chinese Medicine University, Zhejiang, Hangzhou, China

Chenghai He
Department of Internal Medicine, The Affiliated Hospital of Hangzhou Normal University, 126 Wenzhou Road, Zhejiang, Hangzhou, China

Jun Xiong and Yongxing Sun
Department of Anesthesiology, Sanbo Brain Hospital, Capital Medical University, No. 50 Yikesong, Xiangshan, Haidian District, Beijing 100093, China

Huijun Wang, Yin Bao and Yuliang Guo
Department of Anesthesiology, Tongren Hospital, Capital Medical University, No. 1 Dongjiao Minxiang, Dongcheng District, Beijing 100730, China

Nan Wang and Mingyu Wang
Department of Anesthesiology, Cancer Hospital of China Medical University, Liaoning Cancer Hospital & Institute, Dalian Medical University Clinical Oncology College, Shenyang 110042, Liaoning, China

Alireza Mirkheshti, Alireza Shakeri, Elham Memary and Ardeshir Tajbakhsh
Department of Anesthesiology, Shahid Beheshti University of Medical Sciences, Tehran 1985717443, Iran

Mansoureh Baniasadi and Jalal Zaringhalam
Department of Physiology, School of Medicine, Shahid Beheshti University of Medical Sciences, Tehran, Iran

Marzieh Mirzaei
Department of Gynecology, Tehran Azad University, Tehran, Iran

Elena Lak
Department of Gastroenterology, Shahid Beheshti University of Medical Sciences, Tehran, Iran

Fang Wang, Jianmin Zhang, Jie Yu, Muyang Tian and Xiaohuan Cui
Department of Anesthesiology, Beijing Children's Hospital, Capital Medical University, National Center for Children's Health, No. 56 Nanlishi Road, Beijing 100045, China

Anshi Wu
Department of Anesthesiology, Beijing Chaoyang Hospital, Capital Medical University, No. 8 Gongti South Road, Chaoyang District, Beijing 100020, China

Guanhua Zhu, Ling Zhang and Jiapeng Dan
Department of Anesthesiology, Jingzhou Central Hospital, Jingzhou, Hubei Province, China

Qiong Zhu
Department of Anesthesiology, The First Affiliated Hospital of Yangtze University, Hangkong Road 8, Jingzhou 434020, Hubei Province, China

Yang Liu, Wei Li, Hao Yuan and Cheng Yang
Department of Orthopedics, Chengdu Aerospace Hospital, Chengdu 610100, China

Mang Su
Department of Anesthesia, Chengdu Aerospace Hospital, Chengdu 610100, China

Lixin Sun, Qiujie Li, Qiang Wang, Fuguo Ma and Mingshan Wang
Department of Anesthesiology, Qingdao Municipal Hospital, Qingdao 266011, Shandong, China

Wei Han
Department of Respiratory Medicine, Qingdao Municipal Hospital, 1 Jiaozhou Road, Qingdao 266011, Shandong, China

Jillian C. Belrose and Ruediger R. Noppens
Department of Anesthesia & Perioperative Medicine, Western University, London Health Sciences Center, 339 Windermere Rd, London, ON N6A 5A5, Canada

Hon Sen Tan
Department of Women's Anaesthesia, KK Women's and Children's Hospital, 100 Bukit Timah Road, Singapore, Singapore

Shi Yang Li and Wei Yu Yao
Department of Anesthesiology and Perioperative Medicine, Quanzhou Macare Women's Hospital, Quanzhou, Fujian Province, China

Yong Jing Yuan
Department of Anesthesiology, Qinghai University Affiliated Hospital, Xining, Qinghar Province, China

Rehena Sultana
Center for Quantitative Medicine, Duke-NUS Medical School, 8 College Road, Singapore, Singapore

Nian-Lin R. Han
Division of Clinical Support Services, KK Women's and Children's Hospital, 100 Bukit Timah Road, Singapore, Singapore

Huai-Zhen Wang, Ling-Yu Wang, Hui-Hong Liang, Yan-Ting Fan, Xing-Rong Song and Ying-Jun She
Department of Anesthesiology and Perioperative Medicine, Guangzhou Women and Children's Medical Center, Guangzhou Medical University, 9# Jinsui Road, Guangzhou 510623, China

Patrick Schäfer, Rolf Rossaint, Mark Coburn and Ana Kowark
Department of Anaesthesiology, Medical Faculty RWTH Aachen University, Pauwelsstr. 30, 52074 Aachen, Germany

Astrid Fahlenkamp
Department of Anaesthesiology and Intensive Care Medicine, Campus Virchow-Klinikum, Charité–Universitätsmedizin Berlin, Berlin, Germany

Yeojung Kim, Ann Misun Youn, Hyun Rhim and Seok-Hwan Hong
Department of Anesthesiology and Pain Medicine, Chungnam National University Hospital, 282 Munhwa-ro, Jung-gu, Daejeon 35015, Republic of Korea

Boohwi Hong, Sunyeul Lee, Yoon-Hee Kim, Seok-Hwa Yoon and Chaeseong Lim
Department of Anesthesiology and Pain Medicine, Chungnam National University Hospital, 282 Munhwa-ro, Jung-gu, Daejeon 35015, Republic of Korea
Department of Anesthesiology and Pain Medicine, Chungnam National University College of Medicine, 266 Munhwa-ro, Jung-gu, Daejeon 35015, Republic of Korea

Minhee Lee
MediRedox (Biomedical convergence Research Center), 266 Munhwa-ro, Jung-gu, Daejeon 35015, Republic of Korea

Jung Min Lee, Soo Kyung Lee, Kyung Mi Kim, You Jung Kim and Eun Young Park
Department of Anesthesiology and Pain Medicine, Hallym University Sacred Heart Hospital, College of Medicine, Hallym University, 22, Gwanpyeong-ro 170beon-gil, Dongan-gu, Gyeonggi-do, 14068 Anyang-si, Republic of Korea

Ruizhu Liu, Kai Li and Guoqing Zhao
Department of Anesthesiology, China-Japan Union Hospital of Jilin University, No. 126 Xiantai Road, Changchun 130000, Jilin Province, China

Haiyan Qin
Department of Plastic Surgery, China-Japan Union Hospital of Jilin University, Changchun 130000, Jilin Province, China

Meng Wang
Department of Cardiology, No. 965 Hospital of PLA, Jilin 132000, Jilin Province, China

Xu-hao Zhang, Yu-jie Li, Wen-quan He, Chun-yong Yang, Jian-teng Gu, Kai-zhi Lu and Bin Yi
Department of Anesthesia, Southwest Hospital, Army Medical University, Chongqing 400038, China

Xi Yang, Jing Ma, Ke Li, Lei Chen, Rui Dong, Yayuan Lu, Zongze Zhang and Mian Peng
Department of Anesthesiology, Zhongnan Hospital of Wuhan University, 169 Donghu Road, Wuhan, Hubei, China

Qinghong Zheng, Xiaohong Peng and Yaqin Zhang
Department of Anesthesia, Wuhan Fourth Hospital; Puai Hospital, Tongji Medical College, Huazhong University of Science and Technology, 473 Hanzheng Street, Qiaokou District, Wuhan 430033, Hubei, China

Jong Chan Kim, Yumin Ki, Jihee Kim and So Woon Ahn
Department of Anesthesiology and Pain Medicine, CHA Bundang Medical Center, CHA University, 59 Yatap-ro, Bundang-gu, Seongnam-si, Gyeonggi-do 13496, South Korea

Anna Bozó and Alexandra Horváth
1st Department of Surgery, Semmelweis University, Üllői út 78, Budapest 1082, Hungary

Marcell Szabó
1st Department of Surgery, Semmelweis University, Üllői út 78, Budapest 1082, Hungary
Department of Anesthesiology and Intensive Therapy, Semmelweis University, Üllői út 78B, Budapest 1082, Hungary

Katalin Darvas and Zsolt Dániel Iványi
Department of Anesthesiology and Intensive Therapy, Semmelweis University, Üllői út 78B, Budapest 1082, Hungary

Index

www.ingramcontent.com/pod-product-compliance
Lightning Source LLC
LaVergne TN
LVHW060606210926
848485LV00005B/1379